Recent Advances of Chemistry & Molecular Biology in Cancer Research

International Symposium on Recent Advances of Chemistry & Molecular Biology in Cancer Research held in Beijing/China, July 23rd— 26th, 1991

Dai Qianhuan, Margaret-Ann Armour
Zheng Qingying(Eds.)

Recent Advances of Chemistry and Molecular Biology in Cancer Research

International Symposium on Recent Advances of Chemistry and Molecular Biology in Cancer Research held in Beijing/China, July 23rd—26th, 1991

Science Press
Beijing Hong Kong New York

Springer-Verlag
Berlin Heidelberg New York
London Paris Tokyo
Hong Kong Barcelona
Budapest

Responsible Editors: SHI Shu-De
HUA Wan-Jun

Published by Science Press
16 Donghuangchenggen North Street
Beijing 100717, China

* Distribution rights throughout the world, excluding
China, are granted to Springer-Verlag, Berlin Heidelberg
Tiergartenstraße 17, D-69121 Heidelberg, Germany

Printed by C & C Joint Printing Co. (H. K.) Ltd.
Binding: K. Triltsch, Würzburg

ISBN 7-03-003627-1/0.451 Science Press, Beijing
ISBN 3-540-57384-4 Springer-Verlag Berlin Heidelberg New York
ISBN 0-387-57384-4 Springer-Verlag New York Berlin Herdelberg

Dedicated to my Respected Teacher
Academician, Prof. XING Qi-Yi
on Occasion of his Eightieth Birthday

DAI Qianhuan
Nov. 11, 1991

Preface

In May of 1989, Professor I. G. Csizmadia, President of the World Association of Theoretical Organic Chemists (WATOC) entrusted me, on behalf of the Association, with the task of organizing an international symposium on the recent advances of chemistry and molecular biology in the cancer research. So a presidium, an international scientific board, a national organizing committee and a local secretariat were established and there was a strong support from both the domestic and the international communities. I would like to mention in particular the support of Prof. R. Daudel, President of European Academy, Dr. Per-Olov Löwdin, Professor Emeritus of Uppsala University in Sweden, Professors B. and A. Pullman, both pioneers in quantum chemical research on chemical carcinogens, my respected teacher, Academician, Professor Xing Qiyi, to whom this volume is dedicated, and three renowned theoretical chemists in this country, Professors Tang Aoqing, Tang Youqi and Xu Guangxian. I am also extremely grateful to the sponsors of the symposium. Without their support the symposium could not have taken place.

After two years of preparation, the symposium took place at the Xiangshan Hotel in Beijing from July 23 to 26, 1991. With the thirty foreign scholars from fourteen different countries the attendance at the symposium was over one hundred. The co-chairmen of the symposium were Professor Liu Hsing-Jang of Canada, Professor John Cassady of the United States, Professor Koichi Shudo of Japan, and me.

Until recently, much of the research on cancer was conducted in the medical and toxicological fields. Thus, compounds which can mitigate pain caused by the disease were sought after and clinically tested. Considerable effort has also been dedicated to identifying chemicals which may incite cancer. However, the fundamental theories which could explain the experimental results have only recently begun to be developed. WATOC supports the exchange of results in this growing field of research. As can be seen from the papers given at the symposium and reproduced in this volume, a wide range of work at the cutting edge of the fundamental theoretical research on cancer is represented.

It was the view of the participants at the completion of the symposium that the meeting had been very successful in promoting the exchange of recent advances in fundamental research on cancer and they suggested that a similar symposium should again be held in the future. Professor Schleyer, the new President of WATOC who spoke highly of the success of the CMBC Symposium, told me that he would like to encourage a second international conference in this field in Beijing.

This volume was prepared in collaboration with my coeditors, Dr. Margaret-Ann Armour and Professor Zheng Qingying.

However, I would like to express my heartfelt thanks to all the members in CMBC Secretariat, for their cooperation in preparing the manuscript. Of course, the three editors warmly thank all the participants for their valuable contributions to the success of the CMBC symposium.

DAI Qianhuan

Contents

Welcoming and Congratulatory Speeches at the Opening Ceremony

Welcoming Speech, by Dr. ZOU Zuye ············(3)
Welcoming Speech, by Dr. ZHANG Lianzhong ············(5)
Congratulatory Speech, by Academician, Prof. LU Jiaxi ············(6)
Congratulatory Speech, by Prof. L. V. Szentpaly ············(7)
Congratulatory Speech, by Prof. WANG Yiming ············(8)
Opening Address, by Prof. DAI Qianhuan ············(9)
Closing Remarks by Profs. H. J. Liu, J. M. Cassady, K. Shudo ············(11)

Plenary Lectures at the Opening Ceremony

Recent Advances in the Discovery of Potential Cancer Chemopreventive Agents
············*John M. Cassady, Xiping Wang, Yong Long Liu et al.* (15)
Conformational Adjustments Associated With the Binding of Drugs to DNA ···
············*Michael Waring* (21)
Di-region Theory, Mechanism of Carcinogenesis Uncovered by the Theoretical Treatment of a Quantitative Structure-carcinogenic Activity Relationship ······
············*DAI Qianhuan* (29)
Studies on the Total Synthesis of Phyllanthocin ············
············*Hsing-Jang Liu, Virginia Wiszniewshi, Naim H. Al-Said et al.* (49)

Plenary Lectures

Antioxidant and Prooxidant Activity of Vitamin E in Micelles ············
············*LIU Youcheng, LIU Zhongli, HAN Zhengxu et al.* (59)
Synthesis and Structure-Activity Relationship of Potential Inhibitors of Benzo[a]-pyrene Carcinogenesis ············
············*David K. Ho, John M. Cassady, Young H. Chae et al.* (65)
ESR Studies on the Active Oxygen Radicals Produced in the Leukocytes of Malignant Lymphoma Patients and Healthy People ············
············*XIN Wenjuan, ZHAO Baolu, LI Xiaojie et al.* (71)

Flexible and Rigid Chain-linked Bis-pyrimidine and Bis-purine Derivatives as Potential Intercalating Agents ……… *Cyril Párkányi, Hui Liang Yuan, Martha C. Marin-Montes et al.* (77)

On Control Strategy of Environmental Carcinogens and the Catalytic Elimination of Carcinogenic Polycyclic Aromatic Hydrocarbons in Combustion Exhaust ……… *ZHENG Qingying, WANG Shoulan, SHI Xuejun et al.* (85)

Storage and Active Forms of N-*myc* Oncoprotein in Mammalian Embryos and Their Role in the Tumorigenesis and Embryogenesis ……… *Hiroyuki Shimatake, Chizuru Nakagawa, Tahahiko Yokoyama et al.* (91)

Synergism Between Environmental Ester Carcinogens ……… *R. Schoental* (97)

Study on Cyclonucleotides ……… *ZHANG Lihe* (105)

The Cross-linking Ability Between DNA Double Strands as a New Method for the Identification of Carcinogens… *PEI Shu, ZHU Xujing, XIANG Mang et al.* (111)

Nucleic Acid Biosynthesis and Repair Errors Induced by Mispair Formation as a Pathway of Mutations and Carcinogenesis ……… *V. I. Poltev, N. V. Shulyupina, V. I. Bruskov* (121)

Structure-Activity Studies of Some Methyl and Phenyl Derivatives of the Food Mutagen 2-Amino-3-methylimidazo[4, 5-*f*]quinoxaline (IQx) in the Ames Test ……… *Spiros Grivas, Rose Vikse, Anne Knapstad et al.* (127)

Unwound States of DNA in Gene Control……… *Frida Shimron, Gad Yagil* (133)

Transgenic Mice Aberrantly Expressing Human Ornithine Decarboxylase, a Growth-related Enzyme ……… *J. Jänne, L. Alhonen, M. Halmekytö et al.* (141)

Section A The Biochemistry and Molecular Biology of Cancer

Pleiotypic Changes in Expression of the N-*myc* Gene in Neuroblastoma Cell Lines Treated With Anti-cancer Drugs ……… *Hikoji Shindo, Chizuru Nakagawa, Hiromichi Hemmi et al.* (149)

Modes of Binding and Internalization of Monoclonal Antibodies Against Human Gastric Cancer ……… *CHEN Xitao, CAI Xuejun, HU Jialu et al.* (155)

A Method to Determine the Affinity Constant of an Antibody and Antigen Density on Cell Surfaces ……… *GUO Xuegang, CHEN Xitao, HU Jialu et al.* (161)

Effect of 6-Thioguanine and Interferons on c-*myc* Protooncogene Expression in HL-60 Cells ……… *TAN Yuying, SUN Xinghua, TAN Huiying et al.* (167)

The Purification and Characterization of a Carbohydrate Recognized by Concanavalin A in Gastric Cancer Tissue and Its Significance in the Diagnosis of Patients With Malignancies ……*ZHANG Jiren, ZHANG Xueyong* (177)

Quantum Biological Studies of DNA Methylation and PAH Carcinogenic Activity ………… *WANG Ying, LIU Ciquan, HUANG Jingfei* (183)

Changes of Immunological Properties of Serum Copper-Zinc Superoxide Dismutase in Cancer Patients and Their Clinical Application ………… *SHEN Wenmei, TIAN Yaping, JIANG Chaoguang et al.* (189)

Studies on Antibody-IgY Against Stomach Cancer ………… *LIU L. R., WANG H. P., YONG T. L. et al.* (195)

Observations on Manganese-containing Superoxide Dismutase Activity in Human Lung Cancer ………… *JIANG Chaoguang, HU Zhongyang, JIN Yuquan et al.* (201)

Section B The Molecular Mechanism of Carcinogenesis by Chemical, Virus or Physical Factors

Antitumor Activity of Diazoketones in Terms of Physical and Quantum Chemistry ………… *L. I. Kirkovsky* (207)

pH-dependent Protease-inhibitory Activity of v-Ha-*ras* p21 Toward Cathepsins B and L, and Papain ………… *Takaki Hiwasa* (215)

Why Are Arene Imines More Metagenic Than Arene Oxides? ………… *László von Szentpály, Peter Schwerdtfeger* (219)

Isomerism of Active Species and Molecular Biology ………… *Zdenék Slanina* (225)

Anti-mutagenic Effects of Kiwi Fruit Drink on Benzo(a)pyrene and Benzene ………… *XU Hou'en, CHEN Jidi, ZHOU Zongcan et al.* (231)

Urinary 1-Hydroxypyrene as an Index for Human Exposure to Ambient PAH ………… *ZHAO Zhenhua, QUAN Wenyi, TIAN Dehai* (235)

The Examination of Intermolecular Weak Interaction Between Bases of DNA by Using Fast Atom Bombardment Mass Spectrometry (FAB-MS) and Surface-enhanced Raman Scattering (SERS) ………… *LONG Yaoting, MO Yujun, CAO Enhua* (241)

The Cytogenetic, Morphological and Clinical Study of M2/*t* (8 : 21) Acute Nonlymphocytic Leukemia (ANLL) ………… *CHENG Fanjun, YANG Aide, FEI Hongbao* (249)

Transcription and Methylation of Epidermal Growth Factor Receptor Genes and Ribosomal RNA Genes in Melanoma Cells During Differentiation Induced by Differentiating Agents ………… *YAN Yongshan* (255)

Sections C and D The Reaction-Metabolic Fate and Control of Chemical Carcinogens; Promoter, Inhibitor of Carcinogenesis Structure-Carcinogenic Activity Relationship, Other Structure-Activity Relationship Related to Cancer Research

Bionic Catalysis of Polycyclic Aromatic Hydrocarbons With Metalloporphyrins ……………………………………*ZHAI Fudong, WANG Xiaoyi, MA Binglun et al.* (263)
Molecular Surface Areas of Polycyclic Aromatic Hydrocarbons and Di-Region Theory ……………………………………*WANG Liansheng, WANG Xiaojiang* (271)
Superoxide Radical in Human Esophageal, Gastric Cancer and Chronic Gastritis ……………………………………*WENG Qiliang, ZHANG Yulin, LIU Zhen et al.* (277)
Effect of Rhodamine B on Transplanted Mouse Tumor ……………………………………*HE Fengying, WANG Liufang, YANG Zhengyin et al.* (281)
A High-Yield New Synthesis Method of Benzo[k]fluoranthene ……………………………………*WANG Lihui, WANG Zhiqiang, LI Yunxiang et al.* (285)
Studies on the Interaction of an Adriamycin-Calf Thymus DNA Complex With Nickel (II) Ions……………………*YANG Pin, YANG Zuoyin, YANG Binsheng* (295)
QSAR Study on the Activity of Some Biological Fluorescent Agents Against ECa109 ……………………*LI Bingrui, WANG Liufang, PENG Zhouren et al.* (301)

Sections E and F Chemical Factors in the Environment and Etiology of Cancer, Chemical Protection Against Cancer Antitumor Agents, Structure-Activity Relationship in Cancer Chemotherapy

Disposal Methods for Some Known or Suspect Chemical Carcinogens ……………………………………*Margaret-Ann Armour* (309)
Carcinogenicity of Dinitrobenzo[a]pyrenes and Dinitrofluoranthenes in F344 Rats ……………………*Kazumi Horikawa, Nobuyuki Sera, Koichi Murakami et al.* (319)
Quantum Chemical Study of Antitumor Agents——Lycobetaine and Its Derivatives ……………………………………*GAN Ling, CHEN Kaixian, WU Ji'an et al.* (327)
Synthesis and Antitumor Activity of 4-Methyl-6-carbazoyl-pyridazinone-3 ……………………*WANG Liufang, CHEN Xingguo, PENG Zhouren et al.* (335)
Inhibition of Benzo[a]pyrene Binding to DNA by Ellagic Acid ……………………………………*K. L. Khanduja and S. Majid* (341)
Antitumor Activities of 5′-Iodo-indirubin ……………………………………*DU Deji, ZENG Qingtian, SI Xiaofeng et al.* (345)

Binding Between Beta-elemene and Nucleic Acids ······ *LI Deshan, QIN Liya, CUI Xiuyun et al.* (351)

The Effect of Chemotherapy on the Activity of NK Cells and T Cells in Peripheral Blood of Cancer Patients ······ *ZHOU Lizhong, WEN Fugang, LU Jinfang et al.* (357)

Design and Synthesis of Antineoplastic Agents Based on a Natural Blueprint ······ *Hsing-Jang Liu, Milan Ralitsch, Shu Yuan Yu* (361)

Conformational Analysis of the Antineoplastic Pentapeptide Dolastatin 10 and Its Analogue Without Nonstandard Amino Acids ······ *M. Toscano, T. Marino, E. Zasa et al.* (365)

The Anti-breast Cancer Effect of iRNA ······ *HUANG Huazhang, LI Weilian, ZHANG Yuqin et al.* (371)

Presence of a Urokinase Peak in the Urine of Mice Just Before Cancer Metastasis ······ *HUANG Huazhang, LI Guangyu, ZHANG Yuqin* (377)

Supplements

Studies on Fractal Dimensions for Cancer Growth Paths ······ *ZHAO Huaming, LI Houqiang* (387)

Effect of a Chinese Traditional Prescription "White Tiger Soup" to the Patient With High Fever After Chemotherapy ······ *HAO Qinling, ZHANG Jinghua* (393)

The Action of Chemotherapy in the Combined Therapy for Carcinoma of the Nasopharynx
—— A Report of 49 Cases ······ *SHENG Hongzheng, ZHENG Guangwen* (395)

On Essentials of the Acupuncture Channel ······ *JIN Chengzhe* (403)

A Regression Analysis of Influence of Atmospheric Pollution on Cancer Incidence ······ *HAN Zhinong, BAI Yunfeng, HUANG Zhuhan* (405)

Welcoming and Congratulatory Speeches at the Opening Ceremony

Welcoming Speech by Dr. Zou Zuye, Chairman, Beijing Commission for Science and Technology

On behalf of Dr. Lu Yucheng, Vice Mayor of Beijing Municipality Administration

First of all, please allow me, on behalf of the Municipal Government of Beijing and Mr. Lu Yucheng, Vice Mayor, to express our warm congratulations to this International Symposium on Recent Advances in Chemistry and Molecular Biology of Cancer Research, and to extend our warm welcome to all of you, the outstanding scientists and experts from more than twenty countries.

This is an important meeting, for we have noticed with concern that the global ecological environment has been gradually damaged by the civilization, man has created through thousands of years of labour. Air, food, water, and even clothes may be potential sources of danger to the residents of the globe. Cancer has posed a constantly serious threat to the health of mankind; and to relieve that threat, we will have to devote every effort, in a joint struggle together with the scientists and experts of all countries. I am glad to see that this meeting, which is both well attended and broadly representative has set a good example of cooperation.

The varied and interesting program of the meeting has struck me as being significant in that it reflects in a comprehensive manner the recent advances both in the chemistry and molecular biology of the carcinogenesis mechanism. The contributions of the meeting should mark a milestone in the rapidly expanding experimental and theoretical "universe" of this field. To some, they will be introductory; to others, a summary; and to all, critical comments on the future of research.

I also noted that most cancers today appear to be induced by chemical elements originating from the environment that we live in, and with the increasing number of news reports regarding hazardous components of the environment, the average citizens in the world, especially in highly advanced industrial countries, consider themselves immersed in an uncontrollable sea of carcinogens. For this reason I perceive that this meeting is just one of many that will take place over the years. Additionally, as you are probably more aware than I, public concern over cancer is widespread. The field of oncology is divided into three major areas: etiology, biology, and therapy. However, our knowledge is expanding. New problems are being identified.

Again I express my thanks for your coming to Beijing. “Beijing has undergone great changes and become more beautiful than ever before.” There are many historic spots worth seeing and I sincerely hope that you will all have a good time here. We stand ready to provide any assistance to make your stay in Beijing a pleasant one.

In conclusion, I wish the meeting brilliant success.

Welcoming Speech by Zhang Lianzhong

Deputy Director, International Cooperation Bureau, National
Natural Science Foundation of China

I feel greatly honoured to have the opportunity of being present at the opening ceremony of International Symposium on Recent Advances of Chemistry and Molecular Biology in Cancer Research. First of all, I would like, on behalf of the National Natural Science Foundation of China (NSFC), to express my sincere congratulations on the opening of this grand gathering, to extend our hearty welcome to the foreign guests present here who have come to China and to wish them a pleasant stay in this country.

NSFC is an organization which aims to support basic and applied basic research in the natural sciences in China. Cancer research is one of the topics to which the Foundation attaches great importance. We greatly appreciate the joint efforts made by Chinese and foreign scientists in research in this field. The International Cooperation Bureau of NSFC has been trying its best to promote academic exchanges between scientists at home and abroad in all the fields we support. Holding international conferences in China is one of the exchange activities. In 1990, we supported 72 conferences of this kind and we will support even more conferences which will be held in China this year.

We hope that a more intimate relationship of cooperation between Chinese and foreign scientists, such as carrying out joint research, can be developed through the contacts made at conferences.

Finally, I would like to wish the symposium great success and all the participants good health.

Thank you.

Congratulatory Speech by Academician Prof. Lu Jiaxi,

Ex-president, Chinese Academy of Sciences

Ladies and Gentlemen,

On this pleasant occasion of the opening ceremony of the International Symposium on Recent Advances in Chemistry and Molecular Biology of Cancer Research, I would like to extend to you all colleagues from various parts of China as well as friends from other parts of the world, on behalf of the Chinese Academy of Sciences and on my personal behalf as a scientist, my heartiest welcome and warmest greetings. Cancer research is an interesting field, and is winning attention from the viewpoints of chemistry and molecular biology. Some months ago, I accepted an invitation to give a plenary lecture on quasi-aromaticity of certain $[Mo_3S_4]^{4+}$ clusters, which might have some bearing on this new field. But unfortunately I had to be hospitalized on account of some recent troubles with my gastro-intestinal tract. I am here this morning to wish this Symposium great success and hope you all have a good time exchanging new ideas in this beautiful part of Beijing.

Congratulatory Speech by Prof. L. V. Szentpaly

On behalf of World Association of Theoretical Organic Chemists (WATOC)

It is a pleasure to extend to you cordial greetings on behalf of the World Associa ion of Theoretical Organic Chemists and its President Prof. Paul von Rague Schleyer. One of the aims of WATOC is to bring together scientists working in different fields for a hopefully inspiring exchange of views. Typically the congresses organized or sponsored by WATOC consist of an optimal mix of theoretical and experimental presentations. This scheme developed during the presidency of Prof. Imre Csizmadia, who has strongly promoted the present CMBC congress. Prof. Csizmadia is particularly sorry that he is unable to attend, and I know how much he enjoyed Chinese hospitality at the Beijing Polytechnic University during his earlier visits, a hospitality, which all of us are experiencing now, during our stay in China.

As a result of the worthy efforts of the local CMBC organization committee headed by Profs Dai and Zheng, we, the attendees, have finally assembled for deliberations on the state of the art of cancer research in the beautiful surroundings of the Xiangshan Hotel in the Fragrant Hills.

However, the congress is not an end in itself. The importance of scientific investigation on cancer is obvious. and has been stressed repeatedly. Cancer is known as a very complex phenomenon, and consequently, there are a number of different approaches and models. Let us hope that this meeting will deepen the mutual understanding and give rise to further discussions and more action on this important subject.

Since this congress has brought together a large number of researchers from different parts of China and the world, and also scientists with very different backgrounds, I hope every speaker will make a special effort to give his presentation in a lucid manner, which is understandable and also inspiring to all the listeners.

I welcome you all once again and pass the microphone to the next speaker.

Congratulatory Speech by Wang Yiming

Professor, Vice-President, Beijing Polytechnic University

It is a great pleasure to be here even if time limitations preclude my participation in all of these very interesting events.

On behlf of this university and our President, Professor Wang Hu, I would like to add my welcoming remarks to those of the former distinguished speakers and I would like to express my warm congratulations to all of you now, at the opening of this international symposium.

I take this opportunity to voice my appreciation of the various sponsors of this symposium, the World Association of Theoretical Organic Chemists, the National Natural Science Foundation of China, the Chinese Chemical Society, the Beijing Commission for Science and Technology as well as the Beijing Commission of Municipal Service for their moral or financial supports. Without their help, it would have been difficult to have this symposium convened in such a beautiful place, The Fragrant Hill Hotel designed by the famous architect, Dr. Peter P. Pei.

The presence of so many international scholars from Japan, from Europe, from America, and from universities and institutes throughout this country, ensures the success of our symposium.

I am sure that much will be contributed to the basic science of cancer research. I hope that you will enjoy these four days of concentrated work and wish you all the best of luck and success.

Opening Address

DAI Qianhuan
Chief, Ctr. Chem. & Bioengineering of Cancer, Beijing Polytechnic University, Chinese National Representative of the World Association of Theoretical Organic Chemists

I am greatly honored to have been entrusted by the World Association of Theoretical Organic Chemists (WATOC), with chairing this international symposium. We have done our best in making preparations and I am sure that our work in the coming days will greatly advance the knowledge of theoretical chemistry and molecular biology in cancer research. The enthusiastic response accorded to the symposium reflects the high priority given by the international community to basic scientific research on cancer, which along with Aids has been increasingly threatening human life.

The President, and the honorary President of WATOC, Professor P. von R. Schleyer, Erlangen-Nürnberg Universität, Academician, Professor R. Dandel, European Academy, and Professor I. G. Csizmadia, University of Toronto, had asked Professor J. Ladik, a scientific board member of WATOC and the President of the International Society of Theoretical Chemical Physics, to congratulate, on behalf of them, the opening of this symposium. Unfortunately, Professor Ladik is now hospitalized with ankle trouble. So, Professor Schleyer and Professor Csizmadia have asked me to make the congratulatory speech instead. Throughout the past two years, I have greatly benefited from the moral and financial support of the various organizations listed by Professor Wang. I would like to thank all of you for coming to Beijing and I would like to thank specially the following distinguished scholars: Academician, Professor XING Qiyi; Academician, Professor HUANG Liang, Academician, Professor JIANG Lijin; and Academician, Professor XU Guangxian, the Ex-Chairman of the Chinese Chemical Society for their presence at the symposium. Representing the medical section are: Professor GU Fangzhou, the President of the Chinese Medical Society; Professor CHEN Miaolan, Vice-President of the Chinese Medical Science Academy; Professor WU Dechang, President of the Chinese Academy of Military Medical Sciences and Professor HAN Rui, Chairman of the Chinese Pharmaceutical Committee. Their presence clearly indicates the great concern of the Chinese medical community.

I am happy to note that this year marks the eightieth anniversary of the birthday of my respected teacher, Professor XING Qiyi, and I shall feel greaty honoured to dedicate the proceedings of the symposium to him. I am also very pleased to announce that the proceedings of this symposium will be co-published by Science Press, Beijing, China and Springer-Verlag, Heidelberg, Germany.

Dr. ZHU Lilan, Vice-Chairman of the Chinese Committee of Science and Technology, Professor CHANG Chunhao, Chairman of the National Natural Science Foundation of China, Academic an, Professor TANG Aoqing and Academician, Professor TANG Youqi, who are unable to participate in this ceremony, have asked me to pass on their greetings to all of you.

Professor CHEN Shengwu, the Ex-Vice-Chairman of the Chinese Science and Technology Association and Dr. LU Yucheng, Vice-Mayor of Beijing municipality, who are also absent from the meeting, have given us much encouragement in the preparation of this symposium.

It goes without saying that we are most grateful for the participation of our foreign colleagues here at this meeting and for the special efforts they have made in helping to bring about complete success of the meeting. On behalf of WATOC, I now invite Professor Cassady, Ohio State University, Professor Hsing-jang Liu, University of Alberta, and Professor K. Shudo, University of Tokyo, to be the vice-presidents of this symposium. After this ceremony, Prof. Cassady, Dr. Waring, Cambridge University, Prof. Liu and myself will give the key note lectures.

I declare that the International Symposium "Recent Advances of the Chemistry and Molecular Biology in Cancer Research" is now open.

Closing Remark by

H. J. Liu
Professor, Department of Chemistry, University of Alberta, Canada
J. M. Cassady
Professor, College of Pharmacy, Ohio State University, Columbus, USA
K. Shudo
Professor, Faculty of Pharmaceutical Sciences, University of Tokyo, Japan

On behalf of the International Scientific Advisory Committee and the foreign participants, we wish to congratulate Professor Dai Qianhuan and the local organizing committee for the arrangement of a highly successful Symposium on Recent Advances of the Chemistry and Molecular Biology in Cancer Research held in Beijing from July 23— 26, 1991. Participating in the meeting were 25 foreign visitors from more than 15 countries and so a very appropriate forum was provided for the presentation and discussion of a wide variety of current research on cancer. Because of the inestimable value of this exchange of ideas, we propose that a similar meeting be held again in two years' time.

Plenary Lectures at the Opening Ceremony

Recent Advances in the Discovery of Potential Cancer Chemopreventive Agents*

John M. Cassady, Xiping Wang, Yong Long Liu, David K. Ho

(Division of Medicinal Chemistry and Pharmacognosy, College of Pharmacy, The Ohio State University, Columbus, Ohio 43210, U.S.A.)

William M. Baird, Young H. Chae and Vanessa M. Cook

(Department of Medicinal Chemistry and Pharmacognosy, School of Pharmacy and Pharmacal Sciences, Purdue Univeristy, West Lafayette, Indiana 47907, U.S.A.)

Abstract The use of a benzo[a]pyrene metabolism based bioassay has directed the isolation from plants of a number of potential cancer chemopreventive agents. They include biochanin A from *Trifolium pratense,* flavone from *Feijoa sellowiana,* a series of flavones and flavanones from *Eriodictyon californicum*, and coumarins from *Heracleum lanatum.*

I. Introduction

Dietary factors are now recognized as one of the major determinants in the incidence of human cancer[1—3]. These dietary influences on cancer incidence in humans involve the complex interaction of a number of factors; however, a number of dietary components have been clearly related to a decreased incidence of tumors in humans. Consumption of cruciferous vegetables is linked to a decreased incidence of colorectal cancer in humans[2]. Wattenberg and his co-workers have succeeded in isolating two major classes of chemopreventive agents from cruciferous vegetables, a series of indoles including indole 3-acetonitrile, 3, 3′-diindolylmethane, and indole-3-carbinol[4, 5] and a series of aromatic isothiocyanates such as benzyl or phenethyl isothiocyanate[4, 6]. Onion and garlic oils have also demonstrated anticarcinogenic activity[7, 8]. Allylsulfide compounds from garlic and onions have been shown to inhibit tumorigenesis[9, 10].

The biochemical effects of the above compounds and other naturally occurring inhibitors of carcinogenesis such as certain terpenoids[11—13] and coumarins[14] are complex and may result from various biochemical alterations in the target organs. Some other compounds with potential to be chemopreventive agents include reserpine[15], protoanemonin[16], calcium glucarate[17, 18], curcumin[19], glabrene[20], hydroxychavicol[21], 9-hydroxyellipticine[22], and certain fatty acids[23]. The various types of inhibitors of carcinogenesis and mutagenesis and their mechanisms have been reviewed by others[4, 24, 25].

---

* Project supported by the National Cancer Institute Grant CA38151 (JMC and WHB).

Wattenberg[4] described three categories of inhibitors: (a) agents that prevent the formation of carcinogens, (b) "blocking" agents that prevent carcinogens from binding to critical targets, (c) "suppressive agents" that prevent the development of tumors after exposure to a carcinogen. Many chemicals act by more than one of these mechanisms. The blocking agents that may act by several mechanisms to inhibit various classes of chemical carcinogens offer excellent potential for finding widely useful inhibitors of carcinogenesis.

The blocking agents themselves can be divided into several subcategories[4]. One type inhibits the metabolic activation of carcinogens to their ultimate carcinogenic forms. Another increases the activity of the detoxification system, and a third scavenges the reactive forms of carcinogens[26]. This diversity of action has resulted in the development of a number of types of assays for the detection of the blocking agent group of chemopreventive agents. One of the best characterized assays involves examining the effect of potential chemopreventive agents on the detoxifying enzyme glutathione transferase[4]. This assay has been used by Wattenberg and his co-workers to isolate active compounds from a number of classes of plants including cruciferous vegetables, green coffee beans, onions, and garlic[4, 10, 11]. Another assay which has been widely used for the detection of potential chemopreventive agents is the mutation assay in *Salmonella typhimurium*[27]. This assay takes advantage of the fact that many classes of chemical carcinogens are also mutagens and may be rapidly detected by a reversion assay in *S. typhimurium*[25, 27]. A third major approach has been the use of assays that measure either the metabolism of the carcinogen itself or the interaction of carcinogens with DNA. Carcinogen DNA interactions are known to correlate with carcinogenic activity for a number of classes of chemical carcinogens. Such assays can be carried out either in tissue culture[28] using mammalian cells or in animals[29, 30]. A major requirement for such assays is the ability to carry them out in a short time period to permit efficient activity-directed fractionation of plants. This has resulted in the majority of activity-directed fractionation studies to date being carried out with either the Ames mutation assay or the carcinogen metabolism assays.

II. Benzo[a]pyrene Metabolism Bioassay

The assay which we have developed for use in isolating potential chemopreventive agents from plants is based upon the effect of these plant extracts on metabolism of the carcinogen benzo[a]pyrene (B[a]P) in hamster embryo cells in tissue culture[28, 31]. B[a]P is a common environmental contaminant that is metabolized in cells by a number of enzyme systems[32]. It is activated to an ultimate carcinogenic form through two oxidations by the mixed function oxidase (cytochrome P_{450}) system and an intermediate conversion of the initial arene oxide to a dihydrodiol by epoxide hydrase[32]. It is subject to multiple pathways of oxidation as well as conjugation with glucuronic acid, sulfate, and glutathione. The interrelationship of all of these activities determines the relative proportion of hydrocarbon detoxified compared with that activated to ultimate carcinogenic diol-epoxides. These reactive metabolites may be measured by analyzing the binding of B[a]P to DNA[33]. Hamster embryo cells were chosen for these studies because they are k own to have very high metabolizing and metabolic activation capacity for B[a]P. The assay involves plating hamster embryo cells in culture vessels and then adding the test compound and tritiated B[a]P[28]. After an incubation of approximately 18— 24 h, the culture medium is removed and aliquots are extracted with a mixture of $CHCl_3$, MeOH, and H_2O. The $CHCl_3$ phase contains the primary hydrocarbon oxidation products as well as unmetabolized B[a]P. Multiple oxidation products as well as conjugates remain in the aqueous phase. The amount of radioactivity in each phase is determined by liquid scintillation counting, and the ratio provides a rapid measure of the relative effect of the test compound on the metabolism of B[a]P[28]. A change of 20% or more in the water soluble metabolites is considered active in the assay. The advantage in such studies is that further analysis may be carried out through the use of HPLC or ion-pair chromatography to determine which specific pathways of hydrocarbon metabolism are altered by the test compound[28].

III. Isolation and Identification of Chemopreventive Natural Products

1. *Feijoa Sellowiana* (*O. Berg.*) *O. Berg.* (*Myrtaceae*)

The fruit of pineapple guava, *Feijoa sellowiana,* was fractionated based on activity exhibited in the preliminary screening process. This waxy, dark green fruit has a delightful flavor and grows in Brazil, Uruguay, Paraguay, Argentina, New Zealand and California. The large scale recollection (65.9 kg fresh fruit) was blended and percolated with 95% EtOH and further fractionated to give a 90% MeOH fraction. Subsequent chromatography yielded a pure compound, which was identified as flavone (3.23 g, 0.005% yield) by spectroscopic analysis. Flavone showed good B[a]P inhibitory activities of −69% at 20 μg/ml and −54% at 10 μg/ml.

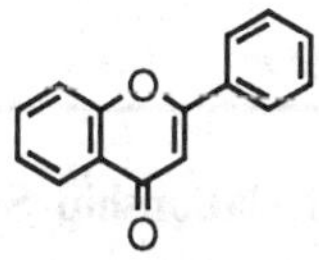

Flavone

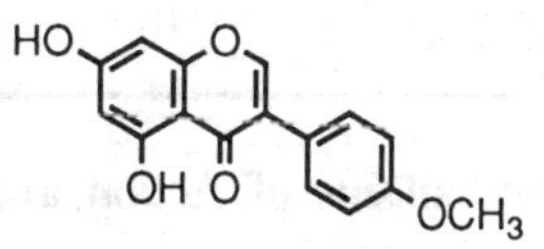

Biochanin A

2. *Eriodictyon californicum* (*Hook. & Arn.*) *Torr.* (*Hydrophyllaceae*)

The plant *Eriodictyon californicum,* a sticky shrub whose dried leaves are used medicinally, showed very good activity in the preliminary screening program. Bioactivity-directed fractionation of this plant resulted in the isolation of various flavones and flavanones (Table 1). Most of the structures of the active compounds have been determined by MS and NMR. In general, the flavones are more active than the corresponding flavanones. Prior research of our group has uncovered a series of active flavones and isoflavones[28] related to biochanin A.

Table 1

Compound	Substituents	Activity	Structure
Flavones:			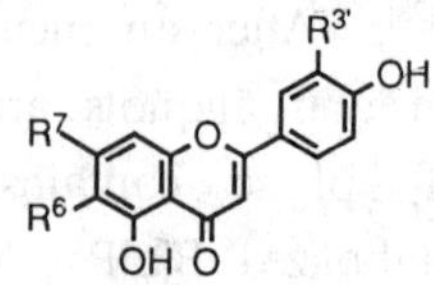
Chrysoeriol	$R^6=H$; $R^7=OH$; $R^{3'}=OMe$	−96% at 20 μg/ml	
Hispidulin	$R^6=OMe$; $R^7=OH$; $R^{3'}=H$	−92% at 20 μg/ml	
Cirsimaritin	$R^6=R^7=OMe$; $R^{3'}=H$	−88% at 20 μg/ml	
Flavanones:			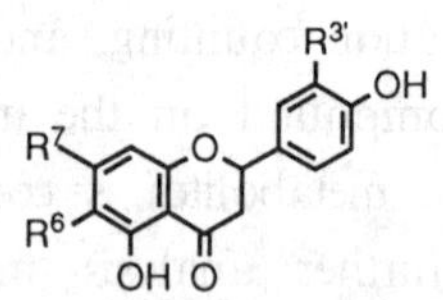
Eriodictyol	$R^6=H$; $R^7=R^{3'}=OH$	−57% at 20 μg/ml	
5, 7, 4′-Trihydroxy-6, 3′-dimethoxyflavanone	$R^6=R^{3'}=OMe$; $R^7=OH$	−46% at 20 μg/ml	
Homoeriodictyol	$R^6=H$; $R^7=OH$; $R^{3'}=OMe$	−36% at 20 μg/ml	
5, 4′-Dihydroxy-6, 7-dimethoxyflavanone	$R^6=R^7=OMe$; $R^{3'}=H$	−36% at 20 μg/ml	

3. *Heracleum lanatum Michx.* (*Apiaceae*)

The plant *Heracleum lanatum*, cow parsnip, has an edible root. It was fractionated due to outstanding bioactivity in the screen. Systematic fractionation of the fruit, leaf stalk, and root is underway. The initial results indicated that some of the B[a]P active compounds are of the furanocoumarin-type, which are known to be the common constituents of this plant (Table 2). According to the extraction scheme, it is conceivable that the most active compounds are yet to be isolated.

Table 2

Compound	Activity	Structure	Compound	Activity	Structure
Psoralen; R=H	−29% at 5 μg/ml	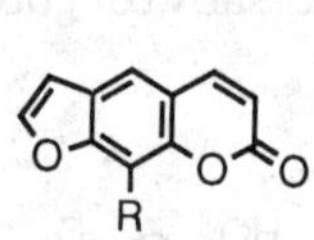	Pimpinellin	−36% at 10 μg/ml	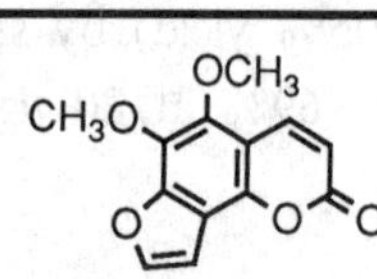
Imperatorin; R=O-Prenyl	−53% at 10 μg/ml				

IV. Mechanisms of Action and Structure-Activity Relationship Studies

The mechanisms by which biochanin A inhibited B[a]P activation were investigated in hamster embryo cell cultures. Biochanin A inhibited both the oxidation of B[a]P by cytochrome P_{450} and the glucuronidation of B[a]P-phenols. Biochanin A was an effective inhibitor of B[a]P-induced mutagenesis, however, the most effective doses caused some toxicity[34]. To determine if other flavonoids had similar ability to inhibit B[a]P activation at doses even further below those which induced any toxicity, we tested a series of structurally related isoflavones and flavones. Two flavones, acacetin and kaempferide, had high activity at nontoxic doses and merit testing for chemopreventive activity *in vivo*. The ability of biochanin A to inhibit the activation of B[a]P by cytochrome P_{450} led us to examine the effect of a series of structurally related flavonoids in B[a]P etabolism by liver homogenates or microsomes from rats induced with various types of P_{450} inducers. These studies demonstrate that the most effective compounds were effective inhibitors of P_{450} from rats induced with β-naphthoflavone (P_{4501A1} and/or P_{4501A2})[35].

V. Future Direction

The use of animal models to screen the efficacy of candidate chemopreventive compounds has recently been reviewed by Boone, Kelloff and Malone[13]. The NCI Chemoprevention Branch Screen consists of studies of tumor induction in skin (mouse-2 stage; DMBA, TPA), breast (rat; DMBA, MNU), lung (hamster; MNU), bladder (mouse; OH-BBN), and colon (rat and mouse; 1, 2-dimethylhydrazine). Chemoprevention studies with a series of compounds including isothiocyanates[15] such as phenethyl isothiocyanate[36] have made extensive use of the mouse lung tumor and the rat esophageal tumor models[37—39]. The most active compounds from our work such as biochanin A, acacetin and kaempferide will be further evaluated as dietary chemopreventive agents on lung tumor induction in strain A mice. Compounds with the greatest chemopreventive potency will then be submitted to the Chemoprevention Branch of NCI for additional *in vivo* tests and consideration for human chemoprevention trials. Numerous clinical trials are being carried out in humans in high risk groups with vitamins A, C and E, β-carotene, 4-HPR, calcium carbonate, difluoromethylornithine, piroxicam, dehydroepiandrosterone, *N*-acetylcysteine and selenite[13]. Isotretinoin (13-*cis*-retinoic acid) has already been demonstrated to reduce the incidence of second primary tumors in patients[40, 41] and other compounds show promise as inhibitors of oral leukoplakia. The long-range objectives of these studies are to identify chemopreventive agents which, at nontoxic concentrations, inhibit tumor initiation and progression in man.

References

1 Doll, R. and Peto, R., *J. Natl. Cancer Inst.*, **66**(1981), 1191.

2 *Diet, Nutrition and Cancer*, National Academy Press, Washington, 1982.

3 Reddy, B. S. and Cohen, L. A., eds., *Diet, Nutrition and Cancer: A Critical Evaluation*, CRC Press, Boca Raton, Florida, 1986.

4 Wattenberg, L. W., *Cancer Res.*, **45**(1985), 1.

5 Wattenberg, L. W. and Loub, W. D., *Cancer Res.*, **38**(1978), 1410.

6 Wattenberg, L. W., *J. Natl. Cancer Inst.*, **58**(1977), 395.

7 Belman, G. S., *Carcinogenesis*, **4**(1983), 1063.

8 Wargowich, M. J., *Carcinogenesis*, **8**(1987), 487.

9 Sparnins, V. L., Mott, A. W., Barany, G. *et al.*, *Nutr. Cancer,* **8**(1986), 211.
10 Sparnins, V. L., Barany, G. and Wattenberg, L. W., *Carcinogenesis,* **9**(1988), 131.
11 Wattenberg, L. W., *Cancer Res.*, **41**(1981), 2991.
12 Elson, C. E., Maltzman, T. H., Boston, J. L. *et al.*, *Carcinogenesis,* **9**(1988), 331.
13 Boone, C. W., Kelloff, G. J. and Malone, W. E., *Cancer Res.*, **50**(1990), 2.
14 Sparnins, V. L., Chuan, J. and Wattenberg, L. W., *Cancer Res.*, **42**(1982), 1205.
15 Lupulescu, A., *J. Natl. Cancer Inst.*, **71**(1983), 1077.
16 Minakata, H., Komura, H., Nakanishi, K. *et al.*, *Mutat. Res.*, **116**(1983), 317.
17 Walaszek, Z., Hanausek-Walaszek, M. and Webb, T. E., *Carcinogenesis,* **5**(1984), 766.
18 Walaszek, Z., Hanausek-Walaszek, M., Minton, J. P. *et al.*, *Carcinogenesis,* **7**(1986), 1463.
19 Nagalbhushan, M., Amonkar, A. J. and Bhide, S. V., *Food Chem. Toxicol.*, **25**(1987), 545.
20 Mitscher, L. A., Drake, S., Gollapudi, S. R. *et al.*, in *Antimutagenesis and Anticarcinogenesis Mechanisms* (eds. Shankel, D. M. *et al.*), Plenum Press, 1986, p. 156.
21 Amonkar, A. J., Nagabhushan, M., D'Souza, A. V. *et al.*, *Food Chem. Toxicol.*, **24**(1986), 1321.
22 Lesca, P. and Mansuy, D., *Chem. Biol. Interact,* **30**(1980), 181.
23 Au, Y. L., Grimm, N. K. and Pariza, M. W., *J. Agric. Food Chem.*, **37**(1989), 75.
24 Fiala, E. S., Reddy, B. S. and Weisburger, J. H., *Annu. Rev. Nutr.*, **5**(1985), 295.
25 Ames, B. N., *Science,* **221**(1983), 1256.
26 Wattenberg, L. W., *Cancer Res.*, **43**(1983), 2448s.
27 Ames, B. N., McCann, J. and Yamasaki, E., *Mutat. Res.*, **31**(1975), 347.
28 Cassady, J. M., Zennie, T. M., Chae, Y. H. *et al.*, *Cancer Res.*, **48**(1988), 6257.
29 Das, M., Mukhtar, H., Bik, D. P. and Bickers, D. R., *Cancer Res.*, **47**(1987), 760.
30 Das, M., Khan, W. A., Asokan, P. *et al.*, *Cancer Res.*, **47**(1987), 767.
31 Cassady, J. M., Baird, W. M. and Chang, C. -J., *J. Nat. Prod.*, **53**(1990), 23.
32 Osborne, M. R. and Crosby, N. T., eds., *Benzopyrenes,* Cambridge University Press, Cambridge, England, 1987.
33 Baird, W. M. and Pruess-Schwartz, D., in *Polycyclic Aromatic Hydrocarbon Carcinogenesis: Structure-Activity Relationships* (eds. Yang, S. K. and Silverman, B. D.), CRC Press, Boca Raton, Florida, Vol. II, P. 141.
34 Chae, Y. -H., Coffing, S. L., Cook, V. M. *et al.*, *Carcinogenesis,* **12**(1991), 2001.
35 Chae, Y. -H., Marcus, C. B., Ho, D. K. *et al.*, *Cancer Letters,* **60**(1991), 15.
36 Morse, M. A., Reinhardt, J. C., Amin, S. G. *et al.*, *Cancer Lett.*, **49**(1990), 225.
37 Mandal, S. and Stoner, G. D., *Carcinogenesis,* **11**(1990), 55.
38 Daniel, E. M. and Stoner, G. D., *Cancer Lett.*, **56**(1991), 117.
39 Stoner, G. D., Morissey, D. T., Heur, Y-H. *et al.*, *Cancer Res.*, **51**(1991), 2063.
40 Hong, W. K., Lippman, S. M., Itri, L. M. *et al.*, *New Eng. J. Med.*, **323**(1990), 795.
41 Meyskens, Jr., F. L., *New Eng. J. Med.*, **323**(1990), 825.

Conformational Adjustments Associated With the Binding of Drugs to DNA

Michael Waring

(Department of Pharmacology, University of Cambridge, Tennis Court Road, Cambridge, CB2 1QJ, England)

Many anti-cancer drugs owe their biological activity to interaction with DNA in such a manner as to distort its structure and function (Waring, 1981; Gale *et al.*, 1981). Thirty years ago the first explicit description of a drug-induced structural distortion of DNA was advanced by Lerman (1961) in his intercalation hypothesis for the binding of acridine frameshift mutagens to DNA. Since then the early notion of DNA as a rigid, ten-base-pairs-per-turn right-handed B-form helix has been systematically demolished. Not only can the binding of ligands alter the regularity and even the handedness of the helix, but they can perturb its structural characteristics in many more subtle respects.

Firstly, the gross conformational arrangement of the sugar-phosphate backbones can be modified by drug binding. A well-known example is the substantial helical unwinding provoked by the binding of intercalating drugs which serves as a most useful criterion for diagnosing intercalation itself (Waring, 1970; Gale *et al.*, 1981). Another example is the perturbation of the width of the minor groove caused by antibiotics such as netropsin and distamycin (Kopka *et al.*, 1985; Coll *et al.*, 1987, 1989). Typically these ligands cause a marked narrowing of the groove at the AT-rich regions where they bind, but it has recently been shown that by forcing two drug molecules to bind effectively at the same site (or overlapping sites) the groove can be widened (Pelton & Wemmer, 1990). Thus the gross helical conformation of DNA is far from rigid, and is susceptible to deformation by drug binding in a variety of ways.

Secondly, the disposition of the base pairs with respect to the helix axis can be altered. During the last few years crystallographic studies have revealed that the base pairs enjoy many degrees of freedom: they can move in various planes and about various axes to tip, tilt, roll, shear, slide, propeller twist and buckle (Dickerson *et al.*, 1989). When crystallographic data are available it is clear that drug binding commonly changes one or more of these parameters. For example, an intercalating drug which comes to lie with the long axis of its aromatic chromophore stacked more or less parallel to the principal axis of the base pairs (i. e. the line joining the glycosidic base-sugar bonds of the nucleosides) tends to flatten out the base pairs at the binding site, so that any pre-existing propeller twist or buckle is diminished. Conversely, when drugs such as the important anti-cancer anthracycline antibiotics (daunorubicin and congeners) bind by a "spearing" mode with their long axis more nearly perpendicular to the principal axes of the base pairs, the stacking is relatively poor and substantial buckling or propeller twisting occurs (Frederick *et al.*, 1990).

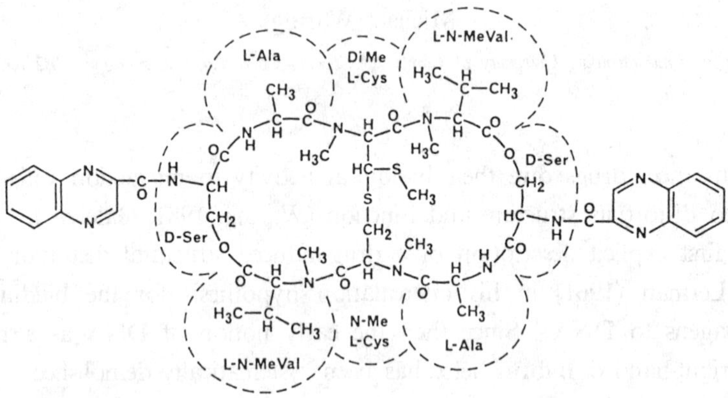

Echinomycin

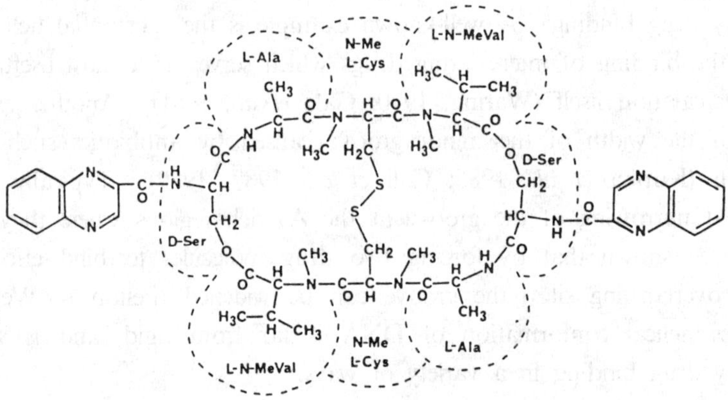

Triostin A

Fig. 1 Structures of the quinoxaline antibiotics echinomycin and triostin A. The binding of these substances to DNA, and molecular aspects of their mode of action, have been reviewed by Waring (1979 and 1990) and Waring & Fox (1983).

However, until 1985 one cardinal feature of DNA structure seemed to remain inviolate, that is the Watson-Crick association of the A-T and G-C base pairs. Then a series of reports from the laboratory of Alex Rich changed that: it was found that complexes of the bis-intercalating antibiotics echinomycin and triostin (Fig. 1) with short oligonucleotide

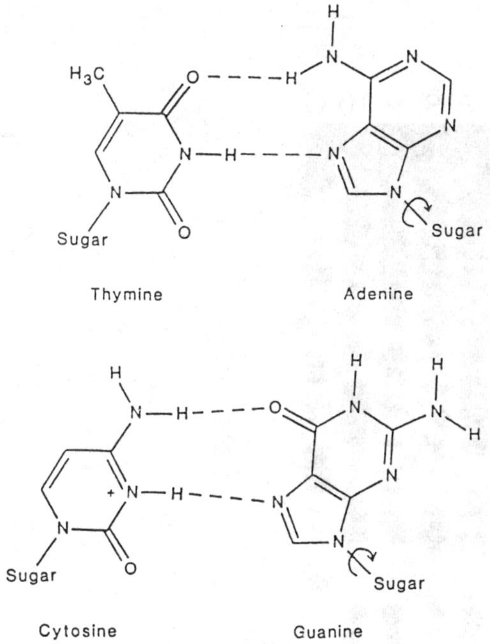

Fig. 2 Purine-pyrimidine base pairing according to the Hoogsteen scheme. The placement of the pyrimidines is much the same as in the Watson-Crick scheme, but the purines are turned over. Note that the C:G Hoogsteen base pairing requires protonation of the cytosine at N3.

double helices contained Hoogsteen base pairs (Fig. 2) flanking the antibiotic binding sites (Ughetto *et al.*, 1985; Quigley *et al.*, 1986). These initial findings, from crystallography, were subsequently confirmed by NMR studies (Gao & Patel, 1989; Gilbert & Feigon, 1991).

Do these antibiotics cause base pairs flanking their binding sites in long, macromolecular DNA to swi ch from Watson-Crick to Hoogsteen pairing? It is important to seek an answer to this question if only to guide the efforts of medicinal chemists attempting to design sequence-specific ligands to effect selective suppression (or activation) of gene function. Their task is likely to be made considerably more difficult if their models have to contend with altered base pairing in addition to the conformational variations noted above.

Several groups used diethylpyrocarbonate (DEPC) to probe for echinomycin-induced changes in base pairing but with inconclusive results (Mendel & Dervan, 1987; Portugal *et al.*, 1988; Jeppesen & Nielsen, 1988). It appears that DEPC is not a satisfactory reagent for detecting the formation of Hoogsteen pairs under such conditions. An attempt to adduce evidence of the formation of protonated cytosine-guanine Hoogsteen pairs in the presence of echinomycin at low pH also failed (McLean & Waring, 1988), as did efforts to secure an unequivocal result using a variety of other more-or-less-specific chemical probes. It was only by synthesizing DNA having its deoxyadenosine residues substituted by 7-deaza-deoxyadenosine (deoxytubercidin) residues (Fig. 3) that a direct test for Hoogsteen A-T pairing was devised because the tubercidin residues lack the purine N-7 atom essential as a hydrogen bond acceptor in Hoogsteen pairs such substituted DNA should be incapable of forming Hoogsteen A-T pairs. It was found to bind echinomycin at the same sites, provoking the same degree of reactivity towards at least one chemical probe, osmium tetroxide, as did normal

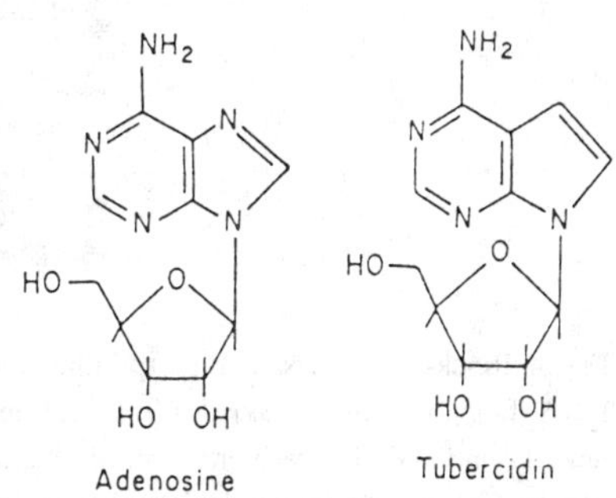

Fig. 3 Chemical structures of adenosine and tubercidin.

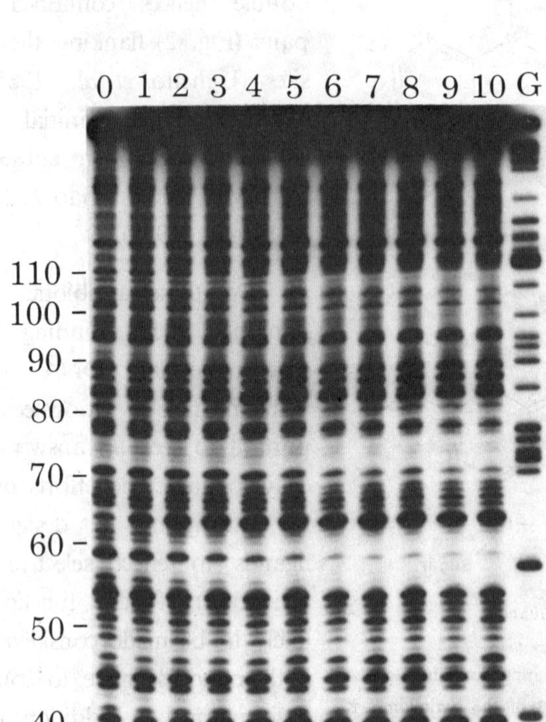

Fig. 4 Results of a DNase I footprinting titration experiment performed on the Watson strand of the 160 bp *tyr* T DNA fragment from *Escherichia coli*. All reactions were performed at 37°C. The concintration of echinomyc n in μmol/L included in each reaction is indicated by the number above each lane. The Lane marked with 'G' is a Maxam-Gilbert DMS/piperidine track specific for guanosine. Bond numbers are indicated along the left side of the autoradiogram. Each binding site is centred on a CpG step in the sequence. Experimental details, and full sequence of the DNA, are given in Low *et al.* (1984) and McLean & Warin (1988). Unpublished experiment of E Sayers.

DNA (McLean, Seela & Waring, 1989). Thus an ability to form Hoogsteen A-T pairs is not an essential requirement for bis-intercalative binding of echinomycin to DNA.

But the adoption of Hoogsteen base pairs adjacent to echinomycin or triostin binding sites in oligonucleotides is believed to be favoured by the formation of additional van der Waals contacts between antibiotic and nucleic acid, primarily as a result of the shortened

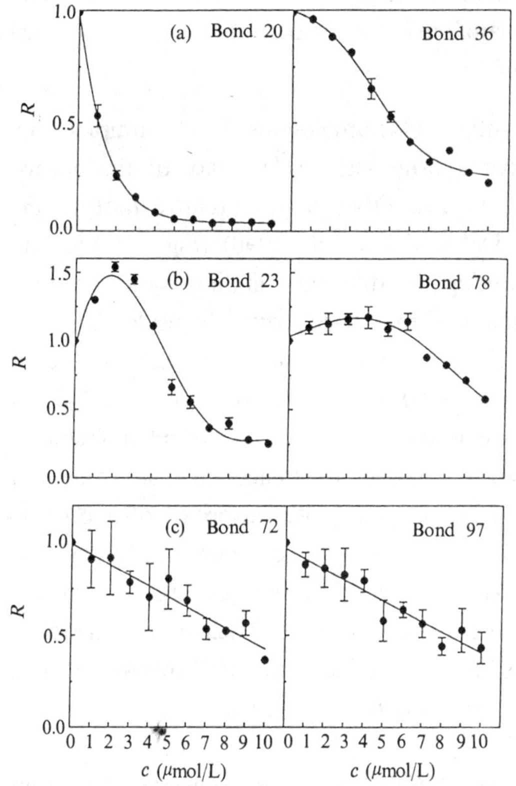

Fig 5 Footprinting plots for selected bonds in *tyr* T DNA which typify the various kinds of echinomycin-induced behaviour: a) bonds which correspond to straightforward footprints of varying sensitivity to the antibiotic; b) bonds where enhanced cleavage occurs before the intensity is suppressed; c) bonds where no clear end-point is reached. All plots display data collected at 37°C. The quantity R is the relative band intensity, and c is the concentration of echinomycin. In all the cases, the points shown are the mean R values of three scanning trials, and the error bars indicate the standard error of the mean. The curves shown were fitted by either a linear or nonlinear least-squares algorithm as appropriate. Unpublished results of E Sayers.

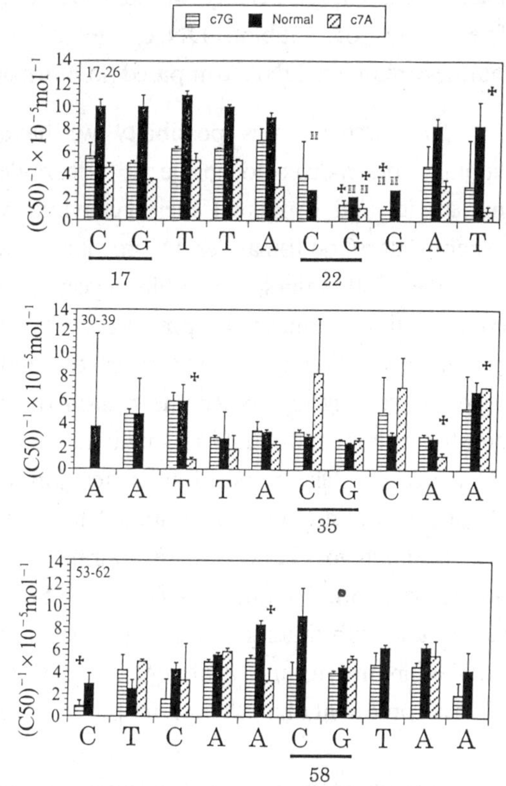

Fig. 6 Analysis of regions on the Watson strand showing echinomycin-induced protection from DNAase I cleavage at 37°C in normal DNA compared to DNA substituted with 7-deaza-guanosine (c7G) or 7-deaza-adenosine (c7A). All the CpG steps (which are the common feature of the antibiotic binding sites) are underlined, with the corresponding bond number indicated below. All bonds displayed behaviour of the type (a) illustrated in Fig. 5 except those marked II which fell into class (b) and those marked + which were of type (c). Hence bars plotted for the latter two categories are less reliable and can only be regarded as estimates. Note that the ordinates correspond to reciprocal values of C50. Unpublished results of E Sayers.

inter-glycosidic bond distance which in turn is attributable to the rotation of the purine bases to the *syn* conformation necessary for Hoogsteen pairing. Even without forming Hoogsteen pairs the purines could rotate to the *syn* conformation if that were a sufficiently important change to facilitate binding of echinomycin, though the loss of Watson-Crick hydrogen bonding would presumably incur an energy penalty (especially with 7-deaza purines which could, at best, form only a single H-bond to the pyrimidine base). The energy penalty would have to be made good by a subtraction from the total free energy of antibiotic-DNA interaction, manifested by weaker binding to 7-deaza purine-containing DNA compared to normal DNA.

To investigate this possibility we have synthesized homologous DNA samples containing 7-deaza-deoxyadenosine or 7-deaza-deoxyguanosine residues in place of the normal nucleosides and compared their behaviour with normal DNA in quantitative footprinting experiments (Goodisman & Dabrowiak, 1985; Dabrowiak *et al.*, 1990) (Fig. 4). We find that the C50 values for echinomycin footprinting at different binding sites, i. e. the concentrations required to produce 50% of the maximal effect, differ considerably—presumably reflecting differences in the intrinsic association constant at each individual binding site (Fig. 5). When the measured values of C50 are compared among the 7-deaza substituted or control DNAs small differences are found, but rarely exceeding a factor of 2. Moreover, there is no clear correlation between apparent differences in C50 values for 7-deaza substituted DNAs compared to control DNA at prime sites suspected of a propensity to undergo changed base pairing, such as A or T residues immediately flanking strong antibiotic binding sites (Fig. 6). So far as the present analysis goes we see little evidence that substituting 7-deaza purines for normal bases leads to weakened interaction with echinomycin, and therefore little reason to believe that the antibiotic provokes an *anti* → *syn* conformational change in purine nucleotides flanking its binding sites.

Original research from the author's laboratory reported here was supported by grants from the Cancer Research Campaign, the Medical Research Council, and the Royal Society. For his willing and expert technical assistance I am deeply grateful to Dean Gentle.

References

Coll, M., Frederick, C. A., Wang, A. H. J. *et al.*, *Proc. Natl. Acad. Sci. USA*, **84**(1987), 8385—8389.

Coll, M., Aymami, J., van der Marel, G. A. *et al.*, *Biochemistry*, **28**(1989), 310—320.

Dabrowiak, J. C., Goodisman, J. and Kissinger, K., *Biochemistry*, **29**(1990), 6139—6145.

Dickerson, R. E. *et al.*, *EMBO J.*, **8**(1989), 1—4.

Frederick, C. A., Williams, L. D., Ughetto, G. *et al.*, *Biochemistry*, **29**(1990), 2538—2549.

Gale, E. F., Cundliffe, E., Reynolds, P. E. *et al.*, *The Molecular Basis of Antibiotic Action*, 2nd ed., Wiley, Chichester, 1981.

Gao, X. and Patel, D. J., *Q. Rev. Biophys*, **22**(1989), 93—138.

Gilbert, D. E. and Feigon, J., *Biochemistry,* **30**(1991), 2483—2494.

Goodisman, J. and Dabrowiak, J. C., *J. Biomolec. Struct. Dynamics,* **2**(1985), 967—979.

Jeppesen, C. and Nielsen, P. E., *FEBS Lett.,* **231**(1988), 172—176.

Kopka, M. L., Yoon, C., Goodsell, D. *et al., Proc. Natl. Acad. Sci. USA,* **82**(1985), 1376—1380.

Lerman, L. S., *J. Mol. Biol.,* **3**(1961), 18—30.

Low, C. M. L., Drew, H. R. and Waring, M. J., *Nucleic Acids Res.,* **12**(1984), 4865—4879.

McLean, M. J. and Waring, M. J., *J. Molecular Recognition,* **1**(1988), 138—151.

McLean, M. J., Seela, F. and Waring, M. J., *Proc. Natl. Acad. Sci. USA,* **86**(1989), 9687—9691.

Mendel, D. and Dervan, P. B., *Proc. Natl. Acad. Sci. USA,* **84**(1987), 910—914.

Pelton, J. G. and Wemmer, D. E., *J. Am. Chem. Soc.,* **112**(1990), 1393—1399.

Portugal, J., Fox, K. R., McLean, M. J. *et al., Nucleic Acids Res.,* **16**(1988), 3655—3670.

Quigley, G. J., Ughetto, G., van der Marel, G. A. *et al., Science* (Wash. DC), **232**(1986), 1255—1258.

Ughetto, G., Wang, A. H. J., Quigley, G. J. *et al., Nucleic Acids Res.,* **13**(1985), 2305—2323.

Waring, M. J., in *Antibiotics* (ed. Hahn, F. E.), Vol. 5/part 2: *Mechanism of Action of Antieukaryotic and Antiviral Compounds,* Springer-Verlag, Heidelberg, 1979, pp. 173—194.

Waring, M. J., in *Molecular Basis of Specificity in Nucleic Acid-drug Interactions* (eds. Pullman, B. & Jortner, J.), Kluwer, Dordrecht (23*rd Jerusalem Symposium on Quantum Chemistry and Biochemistry*), 1990, pp. 225—245.

Waring, M. J., *Ann. Rev. Biochem.,* **50**(1981), 159—192.

Waring, M. J., *J. Mol. Biol.,* **54**(1970), 247—279.

Waring, M. J. and Fox, K. R., in *Molecular Aspects of Anti-cancer Drug Action* (eds. Neidle, S. and Waring, M. J.), Macmillan, London, 1983, pp. 127—156.

Di-region Theory, Mechanism of Carcinogenesis Uncovered by the Theoretical Treatment of a Quantitative Structure-carcinogenic Activity Relationship

DAI Qianhuan

(*Centre of Chemistry & Bioengineering of Cancer, Beijing Polytechnic University, Beijing 100022, China*)

Abstract This paper reviews recent advances in this author's di-region theory, a new conception of the mechanism of carcinogenesis proposed in 1979. The hypothesis of tumorigenesis being turned on by transcription genes was put forward for the first time in di-region theory. The theory has been supported by experimental evidence 8 years after this work was published. The di-region theory can explain reasonably the puzzling QSCAR of various series of carcinogens as an understandable structure-chemical reactivity relationship. Two cis-platin congeners with higher therapeutical indices than cis-platin or carboplatin, have been developed after being designed using the principles of di-region theory.

It is 12 years since the publication of the di-region theory, a new understanding of the mechanism of carcinogenesis or oncogenesis[1]. Di-region theory resulted from quantum chemical treatment of the experimental data from studies of the relationship between quantitative structure and carcinogenic activity (QSCAR) in 1979 in this laboratory. In recent years, much kind encouragement has been given to this theory from the domestic and international communities because of its success in advancing the mechanism of tumorigenesis, in explaining the QSCAR of various series of compounds, as well as in the application to the design of anticancer agents with high selectivity. The aim of this paper is to review the basic results and the development of di-region theory.

I. Discovery of the Mechanism of Carcinogenesis Through QSCAR

The goal of quantitative structure-biological activity relationship research (QSAR or QSBAR), is to relate the biological activity to the relationship between structure and chemical reactivity or to the relationship between structure and physical properties or to a combination of both. Once this aim has been achieved, we must get a deep insight into the mechanism of related biological phenomena. The QSCAR research has long been the focus of the attention of QSBAR research, because of its importance in environmental or occupational cancer. The pioneers of this challenging problem have always worked on the QSCAR of the parent benzenoid polycyclic aromatic hydrocarbons (PAH) by considering it as the possible key to QSCAR research. The highlights of the early historical development were the Toroid (anchor) region conception proposed by C. Schmidt, and the meso region conception put forward by R. Daudel, both in the forties. R. Daudel modified systematically the hypothesis of the mechanism of arcinogeneses[2]. He proposed that it was turned on by tautomerism of the protein which was induced by chemicals, radiation or virus. This proposal obviously had an important influence on the development of the later "oncogene" hypothesis in the medical field for oncogenesis. During the fifties, B. and A. Pullman[3] put forward the famous K-region theory, which laid the foundation of modern quantum biology. However, the nucleophilic character of chemical carcinogenesis proposed by K-region theory has been shown to be inconsistent with later metabolic experiments. The bay-region or fjord-region theory proposed by D. M. Jerina *et al.* between 1976— 1978, in practice, is the summerization of metabolic experiments using PAH. These experiments showed that the carbonium ion formed on the bay region might play an important role in the alkylation of DNA[4]. Unfortunately, neither the sophisticated K-region theory based upon quantum mechanics nor the bay region theory developed in terms of metabolic experiments could explain the QSCAR of PAH. In order to find the correlation between certain quantum chemical parameters and the carcinogenicities of PAH, much work had been done before the eighties, but the efforts seemed to be futile. Various advanced quantum chemical calculations including the *ab initio* method have been used in the theoretical treatment of some typical carcinogenic PAH, such as benz[a]pyrene, but they did not reveal useful information related to the carcinogenesis of PAH at the end of the seventies, the QSCAR of PAH and other series of compounds were still a problem waiting to be resolved. The historical aspects of QSCAR research can be learned by referring to the references[5, 6], and it is unnecessary to go into further detail.

Since the beginning of the seventies, this author has engaged in theoretical research on the QSCAR of PAH. Now, some of the strategies of our research indicating the starting points and emphasizing the differences from earlier authors will be summarized in the following paragraphs, together with a discussion of di-region theory.

Biological phenomena are very complex and in order to guarantee the reliability of the theoretical treatment, it is necessary to collect experimental data for as large a set of compounds as possible. To be statistically significant, the minimum number of samples in the set should be at least 50. Therefore, the present author tried to collect as many as possible the parent benzenoid PAH with dependable carcinogenicity data. By deleting those PAHs for which reliable animal test results were not available, 49 PAHs were used as the basis for the theoretical treatment of their QSCAR research. It is not appropriate to arbitrarily neglect some compounds which appear to be abnormal. Some variation of QSCAR in a surprising manner might give us more information. For example, benz[a]pyrene is a potent carcinogen (++++), but its slightly different isomer, benz[e]-

pyrene is a non-carcinogen; and benzo[a, h]anthracene is carcinogenic (+ +), but its analogue with an additional ring, dibenzo[a, j]naphthacene is non-carcinogenic(−). In practice, those are the inevitable outcome of the molecular mechanism of carcinogenesis, which had already been reasonably explained by di-region theory[1].

The level of biological activity shows characteristic uncertainty. Experimental determinations often use different species, different age groups and different conditions in various laboratories, and it is implied that the obtained data can be extrapolated seemingly to all animals as well as to human beings. In terms of the statistics, extrapolation of the data resulting from limited numbers of animals and from special cases to the general condition, must result in uncertainty, and we can determine this sort of quantity only as a range but not as an exact value. The Ibell index has attempted to approximately divide the carcinogenicity into a hundred-grade system, however, by using this index, the carcinogenic tests in different laboratories using the same compound show outstanding variation. In contrast the Badger index divides the carcinogenicity into 5 degrees, i.e. non (−), slight (+), certain (+ +), marked (+ + +) and potent (+ + + +), and it has been shown to result in agreement between the data obtained by different authors. Therefore, a simple method of quantum chemical calculation might get the analogous result as the advanced one. This would also be easier to do for the large amount calculation required in QSCAR research. However, at the same time as the development of the di-region theory, an artificial intelligence package calculation for the automatic calculation of a whole class of compounds called as wholesale molecular orbital calculation was developed in 1980. This is more convenient for advanced calculations than considering one compound at a time[7].

Because of the complex and puzzling character of carcinogenesis, the theoretical treatment should depend even more on experiment results purely than chemical problems. Although the carcinogenicity must be the manifestation of the physical or chemical properties of the molecule in a complex biological system, simple quantum chemical parameters which are connected directly with the physical or chemical properties are not able to correlate the QSCAR of PAH. So, the task of the theoretical treatment of the QSCAR of PAH is to summarize the experimental facts related to the metabolic fate of PAH. It has been shown by metabolic experiments *in vivo* or *in vitro* that almost all carcinogens are metabolized to an electrophilic intermediate species, and that bio-alkylation occurs on DNA through those species. Thus, chemical carcinogens, after metabolic activation, show the ability to cause mutagenesis through electrophilic alkylation on DNA. J. A. and E. C. Miller have summarized the characteristics of the metabolic activation of carcinogens through an electrophilic species[8], and it was them who named the monofunctional electrophilic intermediate the "ultimate" carcinogen and the original compound the precarcinogen[8]. The work conducted by Sims[9] and many others has shown that the

7, 8-dihydro-9, 10-epoxide of benz[a]pyrene might be the "ultimate" carcinogen, since it formed a covalent adduct with DNA in a culture containing benz[a]pyrene. D. M. Jerina from the results of metabolic experiments with se eral PAH proposed the bgy-re ion theory[4], which emphasizes the importance of the carbonium ion at the bay-region, the 4, 5-positions in phenanthrene like structures. The stability or the reactivity of the carbonium ion is easily estimated by the carbocation delocalization energy (ΔE_{deloc}) calculated using the perturbational molecular orbital theory (PMO). The bay-region theory implies that the higher the value of the bay-region carbonium ion, the more potent the carcinogenic activity of the PAH would be . In a chemical reaction, it is more difficult to epoxidize the angular ring on the bay-region or the non-bay region of PAH, because the bond-localization energies on the angular ring are relatively higher. However, in biological systems, its epoxidation and further transformation are much easier. Obviously, the facility for epoxidation of the projected angular ring in PAH including the one on the bay-region might be closely related to the "lock-key" mechanism between the PAH substrate and the monooxygenase, as a result of the PAH molecule being adsorbed on the surface and inserting its projected ring into the cavity around the active center of enzyme. The bay-region carbocation and the metabolism and alkylation of angular ring are illustrated in Fig. 1.

The projected angular ring in PAH, particularly the one in the bay-region, could make an important contribution to the electrophilic alkylation of DNA. However, calculated values of the least square regressions between the highest delocalization energies on the angular rings of 36 PAH show almost no correlation with their carcinogenic activities, and the activities fluctuate violently on both sides of the regression line. Therefore, it was expected that another electrophilic alkylation center important during the metabolism of PAH remained to be found.

After systematic calculations on the theoretical prediction of the metabolic fate of all 49 PAHs, it was discovered[1] that the K-regions, the 9, 10-positions of phenanthrene-like

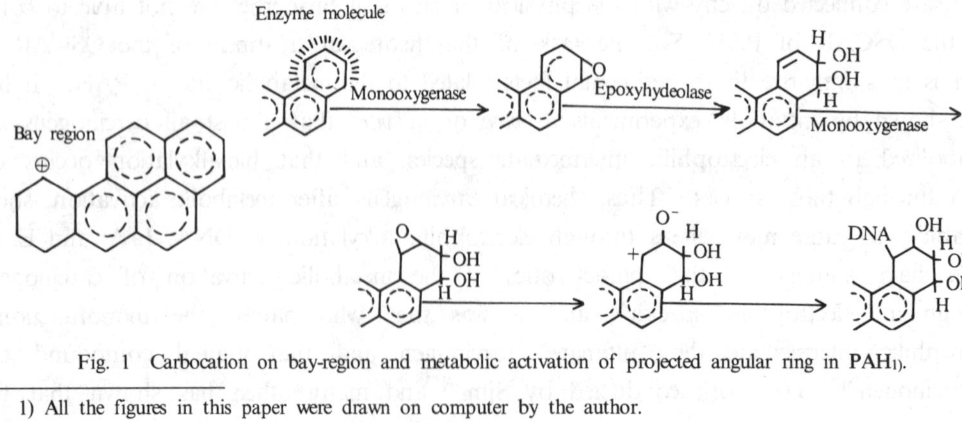

Fig. 1 Carbocation on bay-region and metabolic activation of projected angular ring in PAH1).

1) All the figures in this paper were drawn on computer by the author.

structures, which had been thought of as the crucial regions for the carcinogenesis of PAH by B. and A. Pullman in their famous K-region theory, can be divided into two distinct categories. For example, the ion in position 11 of BaP has a very high ΔE_{deloc}, 0.833β, while for the one in position 12, it is only 0.597β. Therefore, the 11, 12-epoxide of BaP must be a very strong electrophilic alkylating agent through the formation of the carbocation at the 11-position. This K-region of the 11, 12-positions is called the active K-region and should be a bio-alkylation species not yet recognised. On the other hand, the K-region of the 4, 5-positions has an identical ΔE_{deloc} for both atoms, and is called an equivalent or inert K-region, thus the 4, 5-epoxide reacts with water to form BaP-4, 5-dihydrodiol, but it has not been found to form a covalent adduct by reaction with DNA. So, there are two types of the most important alkylating species present during the metabolism of PAH, i.e. the carbocation on the bay-region or the angular ring, and the carbocation formed in the active K-region. It has been found that the epoxide on 5, 6-positions of 7, 12-dimethyl-benz[a]anthracene can link with DNA in culture[10]. The epoxide would also be very reactive if both ΔE_{deloc} are over 0.75β in spite of the equivalency of both the K-region atoms. The definitions and different reactions of these two types of K-region are illustrated in Fig. 2.

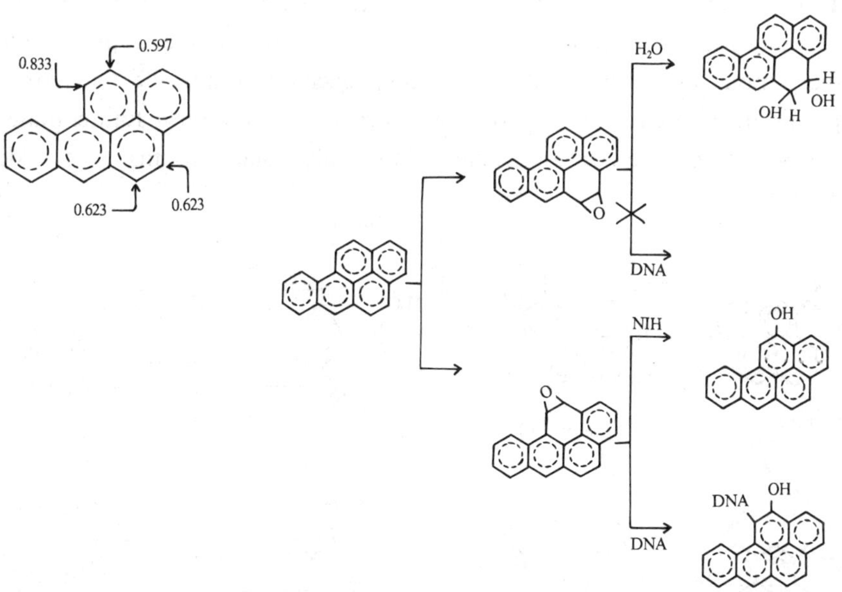

Fig. 2 Definitions and different reactions of active and inert K-regions

After the careful analysis of the data on these 49 PAHs from numerous calculation, it has been found[1] that during the metabolic course, all of the carcinogenic PAHs produce two electrophilic alkylating centers, and all the non-carcinogenic PAHs produce at most only one reactive center, which would imply that chemical carcinogenesis must require the cross-linking in DNA to occur through bifunctional alkylation. For xample, the potent carcinogen, BaP, would produce two very active centers at the 10- and 11-positions, while the 4, 5-positions in the non-carcinogen, BeP, are an inert K-region (both $\Delta E_{deloc}=0.586\beta$). Therefore, BeP can have only one reactive center on the 9- or 12-position. Furthermore, the most favorable distance between these two reactive centers for the carcinogenic potential of PAH is just about 2.80— 3.00 Å. In fact, the distances between the two predicted reactive centers in the four most potent carcinogens among the 49 PAHs are all close to 2.80 Å. However, if the distance between both predicted reactive centers in the PAH is very different from 2.80— 3.00 Å, then the corresponding PAH will have no carcinogenic activity at all, even if the ΔE_{deloc} of both centers are very high. This characteristic distance of 2.80 — 3.00 Å just matches the distance between the hydrogen-bonded twin negative centers of the complementary base pairs of DNA, which implies that carcinogenesis requires covalent cross-linking between DNA complementary base pairs. This specific distance requirement for PAH carcinogenesis and its match with the twin nucleophilic centers in DNA complementary base pairs is illustrated in Fig. 3. Therefore, this author concluded in 1979 that the key step for carcinogenesis would be cross-linking between the DNA complementary base pairs, which might induce a complementary frameshift along the DNA double helix, and finally trigger the cell to become cancer cell. In order to reasonably explain these conclusions, the author wrote in 1979[1], "Another serious alternative is that this complementary frameshift mutation occurs in a gene producing transcriptase, thus coding information for reverse transcriptase. The erroneous DNA from the complementary frameshift mutation may be hidden in the

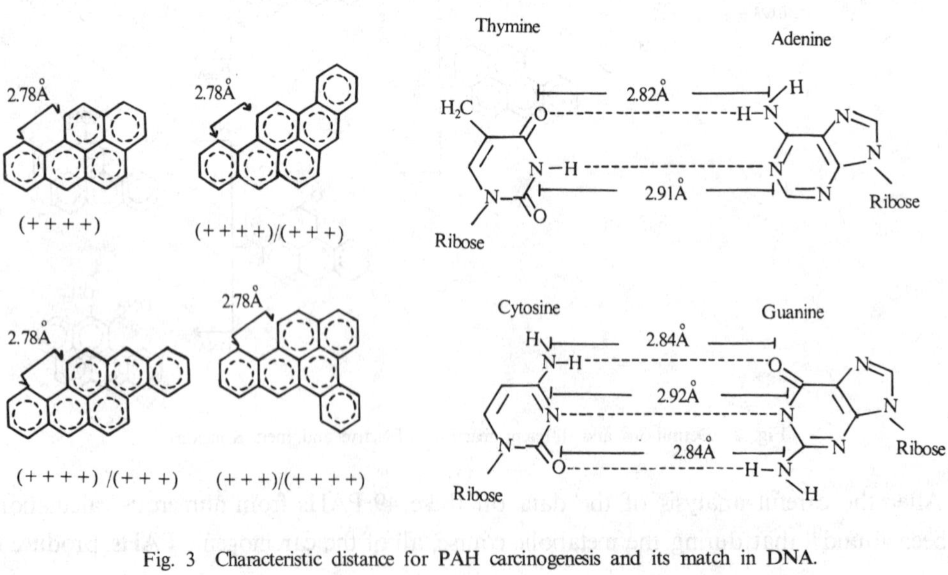

Fig. 3 Characteristic distance for PAH carcinogenesis and its match in DNA.

chromosome as a system and replicated by itself, and analogously the reverse transcriptase system may integrate its erroneous RNA information into the normal DNA by reverse transcriptase. For these cells, the reverse transcription mechanism would, therefore, cause damage to the repair mechanism causing an antagonistic imbalance. After a certain incubation period and through inducement by other factors, the malignant tumor may appear". It was known at that time that transcriptase and reverse transcriptase from different sources had structures with a certain analogy with each other. Both are zinc bonded complex proteins, and furthermore, the reverse transcriptase has been found in most of the studied leukemia cells[11].

The above ideas about carcinogenesis, which were uncovered by theoretical treatment of the QSCAR of PAH, have been named the di-region theory. In the author's paper first describing this theory and in his successive works[5, 6], the general significance of the di-region theory for the chemical, physical as well as viral carcinogenesis or oncogenesis, has been emphasized. However, in 1979, this new concept of oncogenesis was in sharp contrast to the "oncogene" hypothesis, put forward in 1969 by Huebner and Todaro[12]. Their hypothesis proposed that a sort of anomalous, harmful progenitor gene named an "oncogene" originated from the ancestor of all living organisms, the virus, and can potentially exist in the genes of all the higher animal cells. Thus, cancer will appear once the "oncogene" has been turned on by the action of a chemical, viral or physical factor. As a result of this hypothesis, much research has been carried out on the homologous cellular genes of the retroviral oncogene, known as "proto-oncogene". To date, about 17 such cellular "proto-oncogenes" or cellular "oncogenes" have been identified[13]. In 1987, 8 years after the establishment of the di-region theory, the work of Tjian's group showed by experiment that the cellular progenitor, c-*jun*, of the retroviral oncogene, v-jun, is closely related to the gene for the transcription factor AP-1[14]. Hence, the so-called "oncogene" is simply related to the transcription gene. In an invited paper published in the same issue of Science (USA), entitled "Oncogenes and Transcriptional Control" by H. Varmus valued Tjian's work highly, since it provided evidence of the identity between "oncogenes" and transcription control genes[15]. It is a pity that both Tjian's work and Varmus' perspective missed citating this author's works, since the di-region theory was known in America[16, 17]. However, now, in scientific cycles, it is well-known that Huebner's hypothesis has been negated, and the recognition that oncogenesis or carcinogenesis is induced by transcription control genes is considered to have been a breakthrough. In 1989, the Nobel Prize for Medicine and Physiology was given to J. M. Bishop and H. Varmus for their experimental contribution to research on the "proto-oncogene". One of the reasons that the award was made is that their result was a tool, which led at last to the later essential change in the mechanism of oncogenesis or carcinogenesis[18]. In practice, this author is more an experimental organic chemist, but he admires the principle advocated by the World Association of Theoretical Organic Chemists (WATOC), which encourages the combination between quantum mechanical calculations and experimental organic chemistry. It might be expected that the conscientious theoretical treatment of the experimental facts would uncover some natural mysteries which would not be understood only by pure experiment or pure theory.

II. Results of Di-region Theory as Examples for Non-em irical QSBAR

Quantitative structure-biological activity relationship (QSBAR) research is still in the empirical phase. The basic method is to establish a "lead" compound, then change the substituents by using the Hammett linear free energy equation. The general equation is as follows:

$$\log C = K_1\rho_1\sigma_1 + K_2\rho_2\sigma_2 + \cdots + K_i\rho_i\sigma_i + \cdots + K_n,$$

where C is a measure of the special biological activity; ρ_i describes the specific effect, i.e. electronic, conjugated, field, stereo and other effect; σ_i is a constant characteristic of the variable substitute on the parent structure. Based on numerous experiments, and using regression analysis, certain correlations can be found between the biological activities and the parameters. By taking into account the importance of the permeability of the cell membrane using the oil-water partition coefficient, P, an index, has been developed by Hansch and his method is called the Hansch analysis. The linear model of this analysis is

$$\log l/C = K_0\pi + K_1\rho_1\sigma_1 + \cdots + K_i\rho_i\sigma_i + \cdots + K_n,$$

where C represents the molar concentration of the number of a congeneric series necessary to produce a defined biological response. Sometimes, quadratic functions may be used. Recently, much study has been done on QSBAR using the above-mentioned measures and some successful results have been achieved[19]. However, these measures are pure empirical, the simulations, in general, are decided by the experimental constants and the variation of the molecular structure is often limited only to the change of the substituent while the parent structure is kept constant. Therefore, this measure can only follow a known mechanism, or do without any mechanistic knowledge. To date, it seems that these calculations have failed to reveal any unknown molecular mechanism which account for related biological phenomena.

However, the quantitative structure-carcinogenic activity relationship (QSCAR) research required by environmental or sanitary problems forces us to tackle a series of compounds with distinct structure variations, even within one class of compounds. For example, in the QSCAR of PAH, we cannot find the "lead" compound, and it often drives us to our wits' end. So, the QSCAR should be regarded as a special case of the QSBAR, and could be classified as a non-empirical QSBAR, since its successful treatment must involve the molecular mechanism of the related biological phenomenon.

The requirements of QSCAR as an example of a non-empirical QSBAR, i.e. the statistical character of the sample number, the uncertainty of the biological quantity and the experimental determination of the theoretical treatment, have been discussed above.

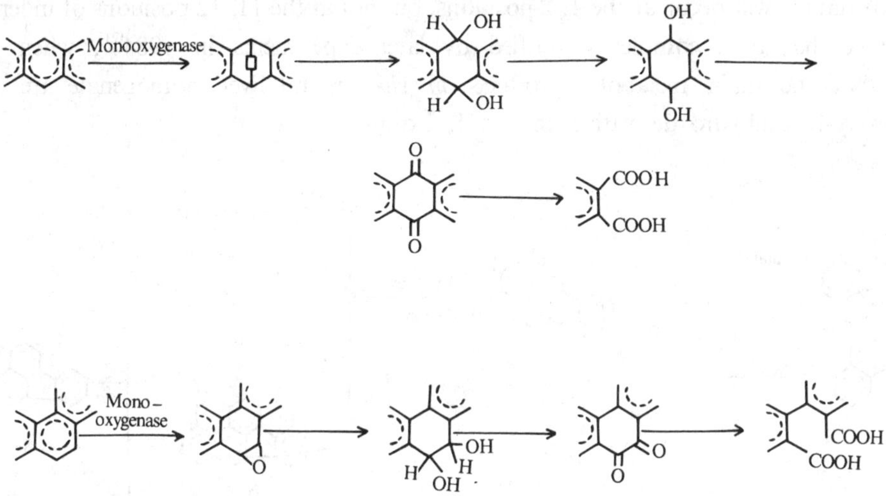

Fig. 4 Detoxication of PAH through the L-region and inert K-region.

For the QSCAR of PAH, the metabolic fate of PAH has two basic aspects, i.e. metabolic activation and metabolic detoxication. In the quantitative treatment, it is necessary to consider both aspects of this comprehensive metabolic process. Details of the activation have been discussed above. Similarly, the detoxication mechanisms for PAH can also be elucidated by quantum chemical calculations. One of the detoxication regions is simple the L-region, the 9, 10-positions in anthracene like structures, proposed by the Pullmans. These result in easy detoxication by formation of the quinone and then the di-carboxylic acid because the localization energies (ΔE_{loc}) of both positions are the lowest among all the positions. Another region useful in the detoxication of PAH would be the inert K-region passing through the dihydrodiol. Both processes have been discovered already by experiments and are summarized in Fig. 4. By simulating Gibbs' relationship through the extrathermodynamic hypothesis, and in consideration of the contribution of the cross-linking, a quantitative equation can be derived:

$$\log K = 4.751 \Delta E_1 \cdot \Delta E_2^3 - 0.0512 \cdot n \cdot \Delta E_2^3.$$

ΔE_1 is the delocalization energy of the most active carbocation, i.e. the ion with the highest energy, ΔE_2 is the second most active ion with the second highest localization energy and n is the number of detoxication regions. With K value lower than 6, 6−15, 15−45, 45−75 and above 75, the corresponding carcinogenic grades are (−), (+), (++), (+++) and (++++). The calculation is in excellent agreement with the experimental results and the consistency ratio is as high as 98%.

The same equation can be extended to 11 nonalternant PAH showing the carcinogenic activity in tests with animals. By using the Hückel molecular orbital theory (HMO) to obtain

ΔE_1, ΔE_2, calculation and experiment are completely consistent. The prediction in 1982[20] that epoxidation will occur at the 1, 2-positions, but not at the 11, 12-positions of indeno[1, 2, 3-cd]pyrene, has been completely verified by later experiments in 1984[21], when it was shown that the main metabolic products *in vivo* in rat liver homogenate are the 1, 2-dihydroxy-1, 2-dihydro derivative and its 1, 2-quinone.

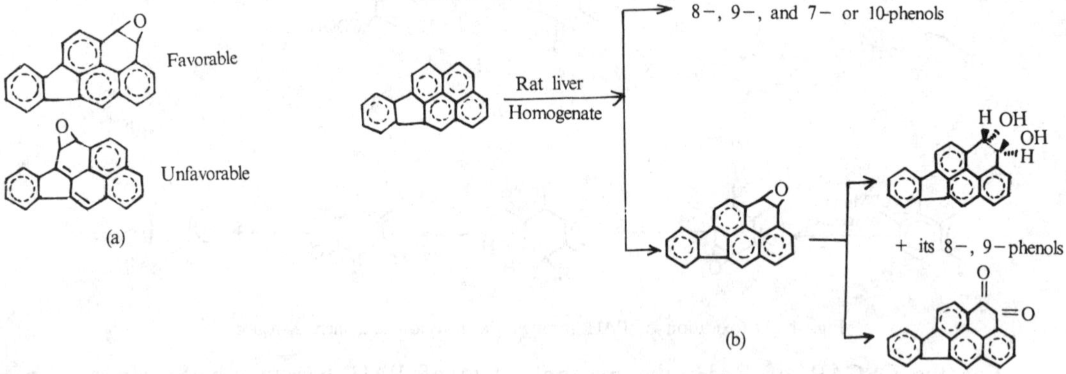

Fig. 5 Prediction of metabolism on indeno[1,2,3-cd]pyrene and its verification.

In addition to the molecular orbital calculation, an artificial intelligence method, i.e. pattern recognition, has been applied successfully to the theoretical treatment of the QSCAR of 153 N-nitroso compounds. Our work with the pattern recognition is somewhat different from that described previously. To start with the potential of pattern recognition to analyse abstract rules without any subjective bias should be fully utilized. Also, if we use the terms representing the regularity of biological metabolism as descriptors, the inherent rules which cannot be seen even by intelligent human eyes can be obtained. Furthermore, the traditional pattern recognition is only classification in two dimensions (i.e. yes or no), which is not in tune with the variety of biological possibilities achievable in the real world. Our work aims at harmonizing the theoretical method with five-degree real carcinogenic indexes, i.e. non(−), slight(+), certain(++), marked (+++) and potent carcinogenicity (++++). It is based on our previous work[22], which brings the strong capacity of pattern recognition for revealing inherent law into full play. This new strategy is called quantitative analysing pattern recognition (QAPR). The carcinogenic activity of 153 N-nitroso compounds (NNC) was correctly predicted 97.3% of the time. From the positive regression coefficients and variance ratios of the 10 descriptors with unequivocal biochemical meaning, it can be concluded that the bifunctional alkylation occurs between the α- and β-positions and between the α- and γ-positions if the γ-position is also ω-position. It is very interesting to note that the distance between both α- and β-positions and between α- and γ-positions closely approach 2.80—3.00 Å as illustrated in Fig. 6, which reflects the facility of cross-linking between complementary base pairs.

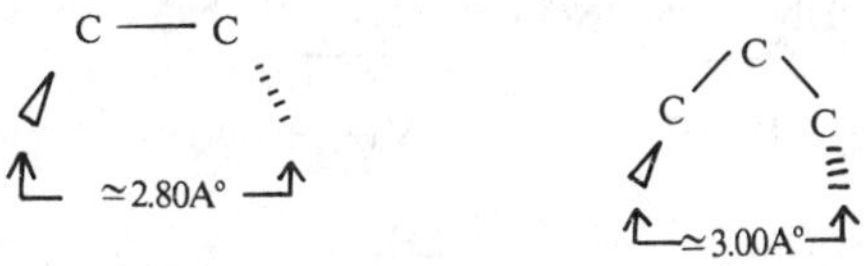

Fig. 6 Favorable distances between α- and β- or between α- and γ-positions.

Obviously, the activation and detoxication of NNC in terms of metabolic experiments and QAPR can be summarized as in Fig. 7. The specific bifunctional alkylation of the NNC metabolic species predicted by di-region theory relates the elusive QSCAR of NNC, to reasonable chemical behavior.

It has been invariably considered that the QSCAR of cyclic NNC is ver hard to explain[23]. Once the importance of the β and γ carbocations has been recognized, however, all the problems can be readily solved. In Fig. 8, the β carbonium ion on NNC I is stabilized by the +M effect of the oxygen atom, so the activity is higher than that of the parent II, but the stability of the β ion in III will be decreased because of oxidation of the sulfur atom. However, once the β Carbinol is formed in IV, V, the hydrogen atom

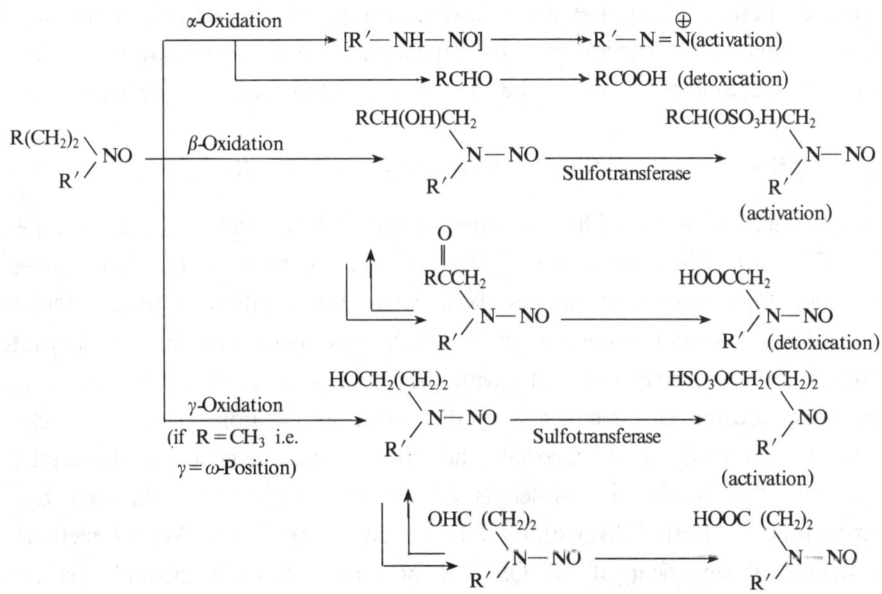

Fig. 7 The major routes of NNC for activation and detoxication.

will shift immediately to split the ring and form the aldehyde and amine according to fundamental organic chemistry rules. In the lower row (VI IX), the β methyl is a ω group, so the oxidation of the γ position would be the major tendency, then the active ester would get the neighboring group assistance from the nitrogens; the lowering of activity in IX would relate to steric hindrance of the blocking group to hydroxylation[24].

Additionally, the QSCAR of alkyl PAH including the methyl, polymethyl PAH and

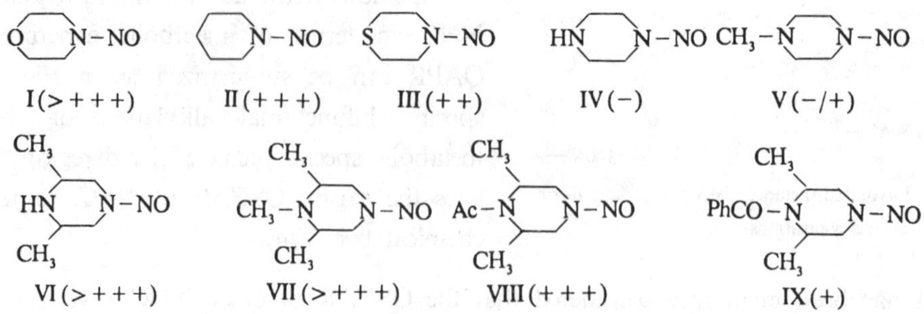

Fig. 8 The carcinogenicities of some cyclic N-nitroso compounds.

cholanthrene series (187 examples)[25], azo-dyes (20 examples)[26], amino-PAH (63)[28] have been expressed in reasonable structure-chemical reactivity relationships. It is surprising that by using the simple specific bifunctional alkylation conception defined in di-region theory, the quantitative relationships can be established in all of the above series. In the treatment of aromatic amines, taking the delocalization energy of the nitrenium ion as ΔE_1 and the highest energy of the carbonium ion formed through the epoxidation of the ring not substituted by the amino group as the ΔE_2, an equation may be developed as follows:

$$\log K = 1.687\Delta E_1 \cdot \Delta E_2^3 - 0.223 \cdot n \cdot \Delta E_2^{-3} - 0.222 \cdot (R-2.3)^2,$$

where R is the number of rings. The calculated carcinogenicity will be (−), (+), (++), and (+++), if $K<10$, $10<K<50$, $20<K<50$ and $K>50$, respectively. The agreement between calculation and experiment reaches 98% when this equation is used. Metabolic experiments involving 2-naphthylamine *in vitro* which were performed in this laboratory, give results which are completely consistent with the predictions of di-region theory, i.e. in terms of the bond localization energies and the atom localization energies, which can descriminate the formation trends of epoxides and phenols, the prediction of the content sequence of phenols, the 8->5->6->7-phenols of 2-naphthylamine, is evidenced by our metabolic experiment[29]. Both HMO and CNDO/2 based upon our WMO method are used in the theoretical treatment of the QSCAR of aza-PAH, both methods get almost equal results.

The success of di-region theory on the new knowledge of tumorigenesis and the QSCAR research might make the following deductions in terms of di-region theory. (1) For all the induced tumorigenesis by chemicals, viruses and the physical factors, such as the radiation and the foreign matter placement, the last trigger would be the cross-linking between the complementary base pair or the analogous action in DNA, the ultimate target might be the genes of transcriptase, through the complementary frameshift mutation, which transforms to the reverse transcription gene by remote chance, then the cell becomes cancer cell after long time incubation period[1]. (2) The mono-functional alkylation species formed after the metabolism of the carcinogen classified as the "ultimate" carcinogen might not be appropriate. The metabolites would be classified into three types, i.e. the non-active species, which includes all the species without the alkylation ability; the awaiting activation species, which includes all the mono-alkylation species, and the effect activation species, which includes bifunctional alkylation species combined already with DNA through one end or the corresponding free species[24]. (3) The cross-linking between DNA complementary base pairs on certain site of transcription control genes might be the key step for the carcinogenesis, so it would be expected that free radical reaction or the concerted reaction will induce the carcinogenesis too if the reaction can induce the cross-linking between DNA complementary base pairs[6]. (4) In terms of the characteristic distance required for the carcinogenesis, it would be considered that the alkylation on hydrogen-bonded negative atoms, such as O^6 in guanine, O^2 in cytosine, N^6 in adenine, O^4 in thymine, might be more important than on the other atoms outside the groove of DNA[24]. (5) A question about what the role of histone in eukaryote cell in biologic phenomena is, is still under discussion. It would be certainly that the histone is mainly a defence rampart to DNA, because the key step of carcinogenesis is only related to the cross-linking between the complementary base pair[30]. It was known that the tested carcinogens can induce the cross-linking between DNA and histone *in vitro* after their metabolism, which inhibit the carcinogenic damage on the genes. Although different types of complex multigene families for histone production are known in different species, the amino acid sequences of both its H3 and H4 proteins, rich with strong basic arginine, are nearly identical from one organism to the next. Whether the conservation of histone structure has any meaning for the defence mechanism is waiting to be investigated.

III. Application of Di-region Theory to the Design of Anticancer Agent

Futhermore, all the existing anticancer agents always show high toxicity to and marked carcinogenic effect on test animal. The selectivity is still a challenging task for the anticancer agent design. The so-called metastasis after the cancer chemotheraphy would be coming to a large degree from the oncogenesis of potentially injured cells. So far the screening and synthesis of anticancer agent has been almost a gemble even if we can seek the new natural products one by one in the same species in which an effective drug has been found, or synthesized seemingly at random by following the leading agent, but we could have no idea of their therapeutical effect beforehand because of the lack of understanding of the mechanism.

Just after the establishment of the di-region theory, author wondered if there were any possibility to design a new anticancer agent with high selectivity based upon this new understanding of the mechanism of carcinogenesis[30—32]. In the cellular experiments through culturing the carcinogens, the cross-linking between DNA double strands induced by carcinogens can be found in bacteria, fungus and cancer cell culture, but in mammal cell culture instead of the cross-linking product between DNA double strands, only the cross-linking between DNA and histone can be detected. It is evidenced widely *in vitro* that the cancer cell can be killed effectively by the bi-functional alkylation agents, but the mammal cells have much higher defence abilities and some damage can be repaired after certain time. Therefore, both the defence and repair abilities of the cancer cell are much lower than that of the mammal cells[33].

In light of di-region theory, it would be envisaged that an ideal anticancer agent can induce only the interstrand cross-linking between the non-complementary base pairs or between the bases within some strands, but cannot induce the interstrand cross-linking between complementary base pairs, because it would induce a carcinogenic effect. Theoretically, the former two sorts of cross-linking offer the tumor cell killing effect, which may be named as mitigative cross-linking and more easy to be repaired by normal cell, the latter named as critical cross-linking can offer the potentially carcinogenic effect in normal cells and is more difficult to be repaired, even this sort of cross-linking can kill tumor cell at the same time too. This classification of cross-linking into mitigative and critical ones is only for the convenience of description. It had been considered that for a cancer cell killing effect, the critical cross-linking contributes more, however, it was evidenced by recent experiment that the mitigative cross-linking shows a very strong cancer cell killing effect. Therefore, the design of new anticancer agent with high selectivity would strengthen the mitigative cross-linking, but inhibit the critical one.

In the late 1978 the Food and Drug Administration approved the use of cis-diamine dichloroplatinum, cis-DDP or cis-platin for the treatment of malignant disease in the United States, which soon became the leading drug for the treatment of cancer, especially of reproductive, urinary system and head-neck malignant tumors. Since 1980, this laboratory has made a systematic endeavor to synthesize new congeners of cis-platin based upon the above blueprint designed according to the di-region theory[31 – 33]. A problem had not been resolved at that time, namely, cis-platin shows excellent anticancer activity, but its trans isomer is inactive. It had been suggested that trans compounds are more reactive than cis compounds, the trans $Pt(NH_3)_2Cl_2$ aquating four times faster and ammonating some thirty times faster than the cis isomer, so this would mean that trans compound is likely to react faster and with a wider variety of body constituents than the cis isomer, and would not reside in the paritcular reactions with target molecules. However, both trans and cis platin are reacted in certain degree with DNA *in vivo* or *in vitro* and the above explanation might not be the main reason. From the beginning of our cis-platin congener research, a published idea of ours has constituted the guiding conception of our design on cis-platin congeners all the time, which would reasonably explain the strange difference between the cis and trans isomers.

cis-Platin is different from other bifunctional alkylation agents, *in vivo* or *in vitro* almost half of cross-linking occurs within the single strand, i.e. the intrastrand cross-linking, besides, another part of interstrand cross-linking occurs. At first, two ammonia ligands of cis-platin are attracted to the surface of histone through hydrogen bond interaction, and force the planar cis-platin molecule to overlap with the histone, then the two chlorine ligands have more chance to react within a single strand. However, consistent with experiments, in transplatin, one chlorine will react with DNA and another chlorine has to react with histone, so different from cis-platin the cross-linking product induced by trans-platin is formed mainly between DNA and histone, in which the combined histone molecule can be hydrolyzed by catalysis of proteinase. The reactions of cis-platin and trans-platin are illustrated in Fig. 9.

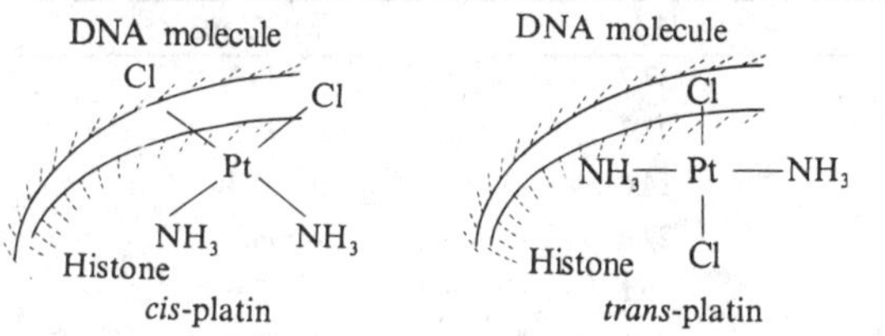

Fig. 9 Different reactions of cis-platin and trans-platin with DNA.

The distance between two chlorine atoms in cis-platin is 3.30 Å, which approaches the distance 2.80—3.00 Å, between the hydrogen bonded nucleophilic atoms, therefore, it might be expected that certain part of critical cross-linking should occur. In practice, cis-platin is not only a carcinogen[34] but a teratogen[35] also. It might be envisaged that if a rigid group with affinity to hydrogen bonds in histone, such as aromatic groups, introduces in both ammonia ligands, which will increase the content of intrastrand cross-linking and reduce the critical part in interstrand cross-linking, then the carcinogenic activity of the designed drug might be decreased.

From literature the therapeutic index of cis-dianilino dichloroplatinum, a synthesized compound in agreement with the above condition, is much lower than cis-platin itself perhaps due to the reducing electrophilic activities of chlorine atoms. Obviously, the aromatic rings conjugated with the leaving groups, two chlorine atoms, through the lone pairs on ammonia ligands and *d* orbitals on platinum atom, cause the decreasing of chlorine atom activities. Therefore, the activities of chlorine atoms should be kept if an aliphatic bridge inserts in the ligands between aromatic and amino groups. Since 1980, a systematic synthetic work related to the new cis-platin congeners and their efficacies has been done emphasizing the general structure on the left[32]. The Ar_1 and Ar_2, the aromatic group, Q_1 and Q_2, the aliphatic bridges, may be the same or different, or connecting with each other, X are chlorine, bromine, iodine, atoms or two oxygen atoms in a dibasic carboxylic acid, Z may be absent or the hydroxyl groups, R and R′ may be alkyl groups.

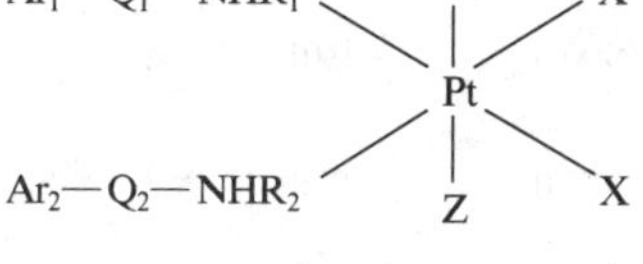

The tumor cell killing ratios (%) of the same congeners ($Ar_1=Ar_2, Q_1=Q_2=CH_2$, Z absent) by equivalent moles as the control cis-platin in DMSO are listed in Table 1. Among these 60 congeners, the animal test of some congeners are reported in Table 2.

Table 1 Tumor Cell Killing Ratio of New Cis-platin Congeners (%)

Sample	Mouse B16	Hela	MGC-803
DMSO	35.3	37.7	35.3
Cis-platin	70.6	77.2	75.9
Ar=C_6H_5—, X=I	91.0	14.6	55.4
Ar=C_6H_5—, X=Cl	100.0	27.6	74.9
Ar=o—Cl—C_6H_4—, X=I	70.0	66.1	62.6
Ar=o—Cl—C_6H_4—, X=Cl	91.0	74.6	88.6
Ar=m—Cl—C_6H_4—, X=I	50.0	76.9	83.8
Ar=m—Cl—C_6H_4—, X=Cl	91.0	62.9	43.0
Ar=p—Cl—C_6H_4—, X=I	53.0	24.8	57.8
Ar=p—Cl—C_6H_4—, X=Cl	100.0	42.8	86.4

Table 2 Animal Tests of New Cis-platin Congeners

(DBA/2, mice, S180 Sarcoma by i.p., Kill at 31th day)

Sample	Dosage (mg/kg)	Animal mumber (beginning/end)	Body weight (variation, g)	Average life-span (day)	Extended ratio, %	*P* value	Number of curative animals
Control		18/3	+5.8	>22.0			
Cis-platin	3.5*1	9/8	−2.3	>30.0	36.4	<0.01	8
Ar=p−Cl−C_6H_4− X=I	10*1	9/9	+2.0	>31.0	40.9	<0.01	9
Ar=p−Cl−C_6H_4− X=Cl	10*1	9/9	+1.2	>31.0	40.9	<0.01	9
CH_3 Ar=(+)Ph−CH X=I	17.5	9/9		>31.0	68.5	<0.01	9
Ar=(−)4−Ph-dioxane-1, 3-5-yl X=I	17.5	9/5		>27.1	47.3	<0.01	5
(DBA/2, Mice, L1210 by i.p.)							
Control		20/1	+4.0	>13.7			
Cis-platin	3.5*1	10/6	−0.5	>23.2	69.0	<0.01	6
Ar=C_6H_5 X=I	8*1	10/9	+0	>27.5	100.0	<0.01	9
Ar=p−Cl−C_6H_4− X=Cl	10*1	9/6	+0.2	>25.0	82.0	<0.01	6
Ar=p−Cl−C_6H_4− X=I	10*1	8/6	+0.3	>26.9	102.0	<00 1	6
Ar=o−Br−C_6H_4− X=I	10*1	10/7	+0	>27.7	102.2	<0.01	7

In recent years, almost 60 cis-platin congeners have been synthesized and tested with mice, most of them have certain efficacies in varying degrees and show relative lower toxicities. Now, two selected congeners, their LD_{50} both approach to 200 mg/kg (i.p.) as having lower toxicity than cis-platin (13 mg/kg, i.p.) and the new drug, carboplatin (140 mg/kg, i.p.) and their activities approach equal to or higher than those of the drugs, thus showing much higher therapeutical indices than currently used drugs. The preclinical tests of these two promising anticancer drugs are now in full swing[36].

Nevertheless, we do not know at this time whether the carcinogenic activities of those two congeners will be lower than those of cis-platin and carboplatin, even though the present results are encouraging. However, it would be possible to find a new drug with only very low carcinogenic activity, which might be an essential measure to control the cancer diseases.

IV. Concluding Remarks

Di-region theory has successfully expressed the puzzling QSCAR of most classes of carcinogen series and put them into an understandable structure-chemical reactivity relationship, it has even expressed the mysterious carcinogenic activities in approximate equations by using theoretical indices as the parameters. It was beyond the author's expectation that a simple theoretical treatment on experimental facts could get so surprising results, the author's good fortune was the accumulated wealth of metabolic investigation on chemical carcinogenesis. The author wonders whether the experience and principle of di-region theory might be extended non-empirically to other QSBAR and whether the non-empirical QSBAR can give a new deep insight into the molecular mechanism of other biologic phenomena.

Di-region theory went through a difficult time because it took the liberty of opposing such Huebner's "oncogene" hypothesis prevalent at that time. The author was not sure that transcription gene carcinogenesis or oncogenesis of di-region theory could be verified by experiment after such a short time and in such a manner. However, from the verification of di-region theory, it might be expected that a more concrete conclusion for carcinogenesis or oncogenesis induced by chemicals, viruses and physical factors, the crosslinking between DNA complementary base pairs, the complementary frameshift and the last step about the transformation of the transcriptase gene to reverse transcriptase gene would be verified in the not too distant future. The author considers with deep feelings that in the aspect of exploring natural mystery, the combination of theoretical and experimental methods would surpass the pure theoretical or experimental measure alone.

This project has been financially supported by the National Natural Science Foundation of China, Beijing Commission of Science and Technology. I indebted to Prof. Zheng

Qing-ying, Assoc. Prof. Zhong Rugang and a group of Masters of Science, Ms. Liu Ronghua, Mr. Fu Xing, Mr. Zhang Daping and Ms. Zhou Qialong, for their continuous work in this laboratory. The names of my colleagues, who were retired or went abroad, had participated in this works, are listed in the references.

References

1 Dai Qianhuan. *Scientia Sinica* (*Science in China*), **23**(1980), 453.

2 Daudel, R., *Rev. Sci.*, **84**(1946), 37.

3 Pullman, A. and Pullman, B., *Adv. Cancer Res.*, **3**(1955), 117.

4 Jerina, D. M. *et al.*, in *Origins of Human Cancer*, Book B(eds. Hiatt, H. *et al.*), Cold Spring Harbor Lab., 1977, p. 653.

5 Dai Qianhuan, in *Basic Mechanisms of Chemical Carcinogenesis: Chemical, Metabolic and Biological Aspects* (eds. Yao Zhen and Ji Ruyun), Shanghai, 1982, pp 41—49.

6 Dai Qianhuan, in *Polynuclear Aromatic Hydrocarbons: Mechanisms, Methods and Metabolism* (eds. Cooke, M. and Dennis, A.), Battelle Press, Columbus, 1984, pp. 1045—1073.

7 Dai Qianhuan, *Huanjing Kexue Congkan* (Series of Environmental Science), 1981, Combined issue of No. 6 & 7, 11; Dai Qianhuan and Shi Bingzhi, *Scientia Sinica* (Series B), **29**(1986), 1133—1146.

8 Miller, J. A. and Miller, E. C., in *Origin of Human Cancer*, Book B, 1977, pp. 605—627.

9 Sims, P. and Grover, P. L., *Adv. Cancer Res.*, **20**(1974), 166.

10 Jeffrey, A. M. *et al., Proc. Natl. Acad. Sci. USA,* **73**(1976), 2311.

11 Temin, H. M., *Science,* **192**(1976), 1075—1080.

12 Huebner, R. J. and Todaro, G. J., *Proc. Natl. Acad. Sci. USA,* **64**(1969), 1087.

13 Hathway, D. E., *Mechanism of Chemical Carcinogenesis,* Chapter 7, Butterworths, 1986, pp. 113—128.

14 Bohmann, D., Bos, T. J., Admon, A. *et al., Science,* USA, **238**(1987), 1386, 1392.

15 Varmus, H. E., *ibid.*, **238**(1987), 1337—1339.

16 Josephson, J., *ES & T,* **18**(1984), 3: 92A—95A (An outlook by using "A theory from China" as subtitle to recommend di-region theory) and c. f. Ref. [6].

17 The author had been invited to make lectures related to di-region theory in following American institutions: National Institute of Environmental Health (Oct. 1983, Research Triangle Park, NC), Duke University (Oct. 1985, Durham) University of North Carolina (Oct. 1985, Chapel Hill), The University of Michigan (Oct. 1985, Ann Arbor), FDA(Oct. 1985, Washington, DC), NIH (Oct. 1987, Baltimore) and so on.

18 Baum, R., *C & EN,* 1989, 10: 6—7.

19 Chapman, N. R. and Shorter, J. (eds.), *Advances in Linear Free Energy Relationships,* Plenum Press, New York, 1972.

20 Dai Qianhuan and Zhang Changyin, *Kexue Tongbao* (*Chinese Science Bulletin*), **27**(1982), 1347—1354.

21 Rice, J. C. *et al.*, in *Polynuclear Aromatic Hydrocarbons: Mechanisms, Methods and Metabolism* (eds. Cooks, M. and Dennis, A.), Battelle Press, Columbus, 1984, pp. 1097—1109.

22 Dai Qianhuan and Shi Chenxi, *Kexue Tongbao,* **30**(1985), 52—57.

23 Rao, T. K., Lijinsky, W. and Epler, J. L. (eds.), *Genotoxicology of N-Nitroso Compounds,* Plenum Press, New York, 1984.

24 Dai Qianhuan and Zhong Rugang, *Scientia Sinica,* **32**(1989), 7:776—790.

25 Dai Qianhuan and Zhang Dunxin, *Kexue Tongbao,* **25**(1980), 975; *Scientia Sinica,* **28**(1985), 160—187.

26 Zhang Dunxin, Li Hongshi and Dai Qianhuan, *Environmental Chemistry*, 1986, 2:1—8.

27 Dai Qianhuan, Zheng Qiangying and Wang Zhongyi, *Science in China,* **34**(1991), 5:547—559.

28 Zhong Rugang, Zhang Daping, WU Caicai and Dai Qianhuan, in preparation.

29 Li Tingshu, Dai Tianyou, Pei Shu and Dai Qianhuan, *J. Environ. Sci.*, (*China*), **3**(1990), 1:101—108.

30 Dai Qianhuan, Xu Peirong, Xiao Ping and Shi Bingzhi , *Journal of Beijing Polytechnic University* (*Beijing Gongye Daxue Xuebao*), 1985, 11:145—147.

31 Dai Qianhuan, Xu Peirong and Zheng Qingying, *Proceedings of Symposium on Noble Metal Anticancer Agents in China,* Kunming, 1987, pp. 15—17.

32 Dai Qianhuan, in *Proceedings of Xth World Congress of Pharmacology,* a Co-Chairman lecture on Cancer Chemotherapy Session.

33 Lippard, S. J. (ed.), Platinum, Gold and other metal chemotherapeutic agents, *ACS Symposium Series,* 1983.

34 Leopold, W. R., Miller, E. C. and Miller, J. A., *Cancer Res.,* **39**(1979), 913.

35 Lazar, R., Conran, P. C. and Danjanov, *Experimentia,* **35**(1979), 647.

36 British patent, 22069161 (Date of filing of 3rd June 1988, approved on 2nd, Oct. 1991; Inventor, Dai Qianhuan; Applicants, Beijing Polytechnic University and Xingnong Technique Development Company).

Studies on the Total Synthesis of Phyllanthocin

Hsing-Jang Liu, Virginia Wiszniewsky, Naim H. Al-Said and Milan Ralitsch

(Department of Chemistry, University of Alberta, Edmonton, Alberta, Canada T6G 2G2)

Abstract The work currently in progress in our laboratory, aimed at the total synthesis of phyllanthocin, the aglycone of the potent antineoplastic agent phyllanthoside, is described.

In the early 1960s, as part of a programme initiated by the National Cancer Institute (NCI) in the United States, Kupchan and coworkers became involved with the search for tumor inhibitors of plant origin. During the course of their investigations, Kupchan found that the crude ethanol extract obtained from the roots of the Central American tree *Pyllanthus acuminatus* Vahl (Euphorbiaceae) possessed anti-cancer properties. It exhibited potent antitumor activity against lymphocyte leukemia P-388 in mice. These significant pharmacological properties were traced to a bisabolane sesquiterpene glycoside, (+)-phyllanthoside (**1**)[1]. Methanolysis (Scheme 1) of phyllanthoside gave two crystalline compounds: a disaccharide (**2**) and the aglycone methyl ester phyllanthocin (**3**). The aglycone structure was elucidated by Kupchan and coworkers from a single-crystal X-ray diffraction study. The structure of the disaccharide phyllanthose (**2**) was likewise deduced by Pettit *et al.* several years later[2].

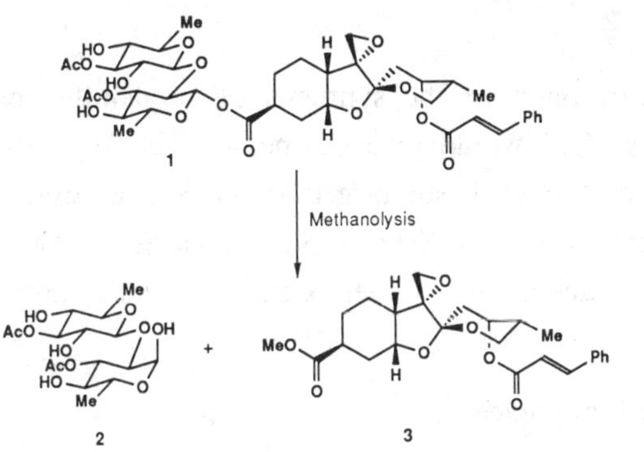

Scheme 1

Phyllanthoside has emerged as a particularly promising candidate for cancer chemotherapy, and pharmaceutical interest in this compound has escalated. The significant level of inhibition by phyllanthoside of the NCI murine B16 melanoma and the human mylloma cell line has led to extensive pre-clinical testing. More recently, NCI has advanced phyllanthoside to the level of clinical trials, where it will undergo human testing. This tremendous chemotherapeutic potential, in combination with its intriguing and challenging structure, renders phyllanthoside (**1**) and its aglycone (**3**) attractive synthetic targets and, over a rather short period of time, a number of elegant total syntheses of these

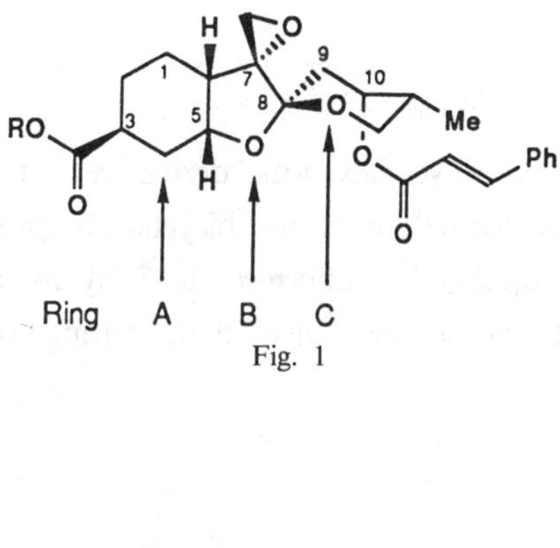

Fig. 1

compounds have been accomplished[3 — 8]. Common to all the syntheses reported is convergency: there is a basic dissection of the molecule into left and right sides. The approaches differ however with respect to which key carbon-carbon bond of the target molecule is constructed (C7—C8, C8—C9, or C9—C10), and the order in which the rings are formed (Fig. 1). In the McGuirk and Collum approach[3], for instance, the AB bicyclic butyrolactone ring system was built first, followed by attachment of a carbon chain to form the C8—C9 bond (Scheme 2), and which was eventually cyclized to form ring C.

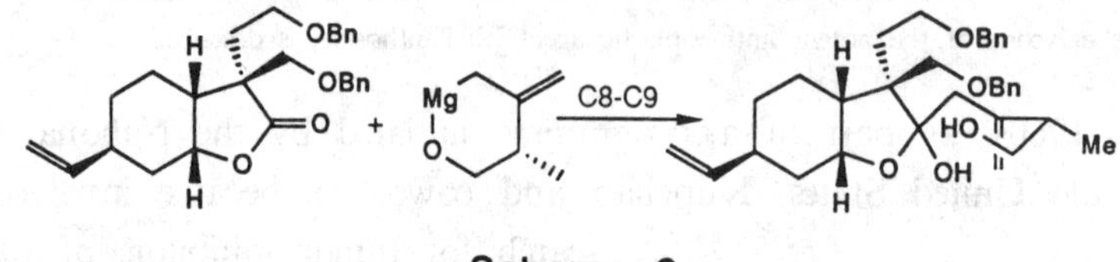

Scheme 2

We also chose to employ a convergent approach to the synthesis of phyllanthocin (**3**). First, dissection of the ester functionality at C10 would give ketone **4**. The key dissection at the C8 — C9 bond would yield two crucial sub-target molecules, a spiroepoxybutyrolactone **5** and the protected (P) keto alcohol **6** (Scheme 3). Towards the synthesis of the key intermediate **5**, two approaches are under current investigation. Preliminary results are described below.

I. Photochemical Approach

As shown in Scheme 4, the key operation in this approach is the photocycloaddition

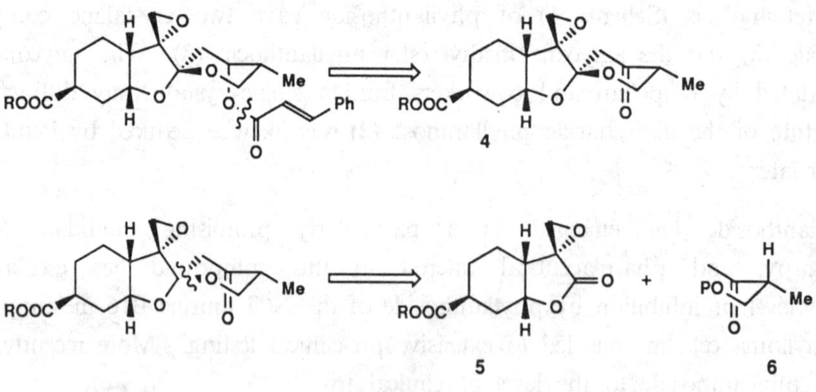

Scheme 3

of the cyclohexenone derivative 7 to vinyl acetate. The reaction is expected to facilitate the formation of the bicyclic compound **8** which could, in principle, be converted to the projected key intermediate **5** by an array of rather standard transformations, as outlined. It should be noted that, during the photochemical process, several chiral centers are simultaneously created. Although the bicyclo[4.2.0]octane system is known to be more stable when *cis*-fused, the C-7 chiral center is of no consequence to the synthesis as it will be destroyed subsequently, and the C-4 center is epimerizable, it is highly desirable to control the photocycloaddition in such a way that the desired stereoisomer **8** could be produced preferentially. This requires the addition of vinyl acetate from the sterically less hindered side (opposite to the substituent) of the counterpart **7**.

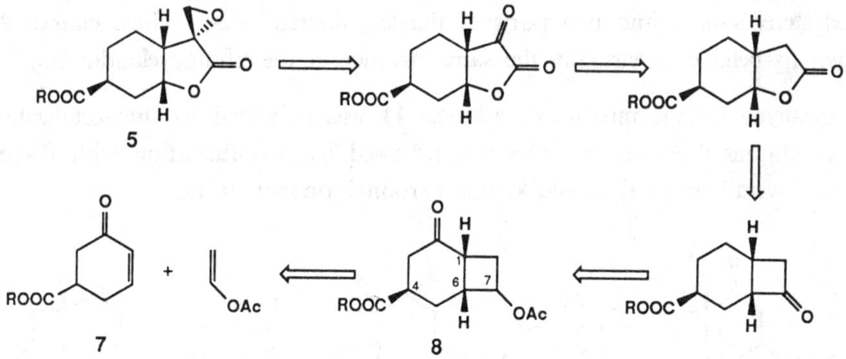

Scheme 4

In order to induce the stereoselectivity, two enones, **9** with a polar carboxyl group

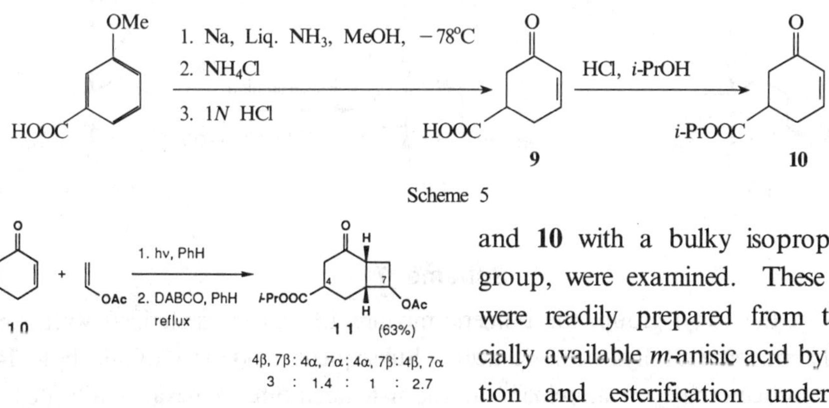

Scheme 5

and **10** with a bulky isopropoxycarbonyl group, were examined. These compounds were readily prepared from the commercially available *m*-anisic acid by Birch reduction and esterification under conditions which are summarized in Scheme 5.

Irradiation (450 W Hanovia medium pressure mercury lamp, quartz immersion well, and pyrex filter)[9] of a benzene solution of enone ester **10** and an excess of vinyl acetate for 12 h, followed by treatment of the resulting photoadducts with 1, 5-diazabicyclo[4.2.0]undec-5-ene[10] in refluxing benzene for 48 h, gave a mixture of all

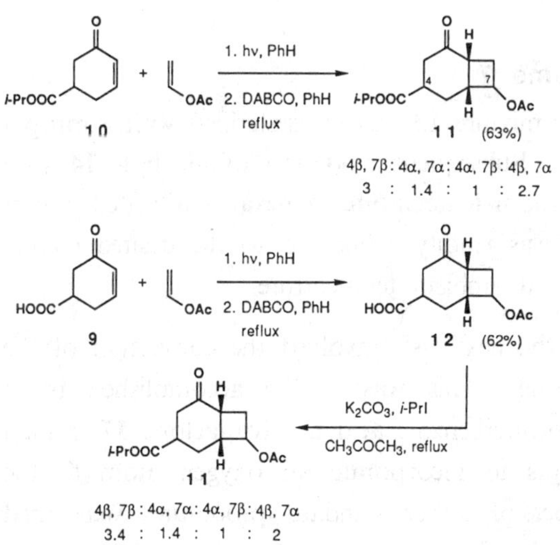

Scheme 6

four possible diastereoisomers of **11** (63% combined yield) resulting from head-to-tail addition (Scheme 6). A careful analysis of the mixture revealed the presence of *ca.* five parts of the desired 1β, 4β, 6β-stereoisomers and two parts of the less desired 1β, 4α, 6β-isomers. Similar irradiation of enone acid **9** and treatment of the resulting product mixture gave rise to a 62% yield of the head-to-tail adducts **12**, which were immediately esterified using potassium carbonate and isopropyl iodide in refluxing acetone. The mixture of esters **11** thus obtained was shown to contain again approximately five parts of the desired stereoisomers and two parts of the less desired ones. Thus, enones **9** and **10** were shown to behave in virtually the same manner in the photocycloaddition.

The diastereoisomeric mixture of adducts **11** was subjected to thioacetalization under standard conditions (Scheme 7). This was followed by desulfurization with Raney nickel, to effect the overall removal of the ketone carbonyl present in **11**.

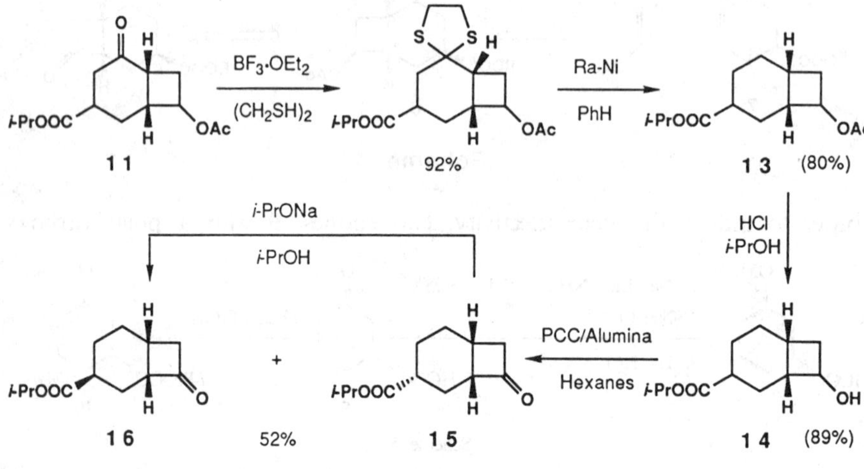

Scheme 7

To remove the acetyl group, the isomeric mixture **13** was transesterified with isopropyl alcohol in the presence of hydrochloric acid. Subsequent oxidation of alcohols **14** with pyridinium chlorochromate on alumina[11] at room temperature in hexanes afforded a pair of epimeric ketones **15** and **16**. The former was readily isomerized to the desired epimer **16** upon treatment with sodium isopropoxide at ambient temperature.

With the desired keto ester **16** in hand, the next task involved the conversion of the cyclobutanone ring into the required γ-lactone. This was readily accomplished by a Baeyer-Villiger oxidation reaction using *m*-chloroperbenzoic acid to give lactone **17** in high yield. Problems were encountered in attempts to incorporate an oxygen atom to the α-carbon of the lactone carbonyl. A number of rather standard procedures were tried unsuccessfully, as outlined in Scheme 8. Finally, this required synthetic operation was effected by first converting lactone **17** to the benzylidene derivative **18** *via* an aldol reaction

(Scheme 9). Subsequent ozonolysis gave rise to keto lactone **19**, an advanced intermediate towards the projected key segment required for our synthetic approach to phyllanthocin.

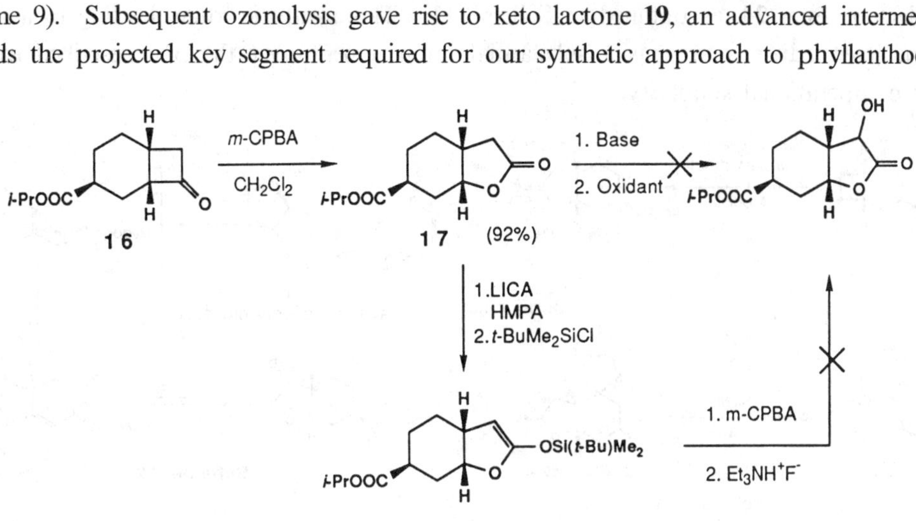

Scheme 8

While experimentation is underway to effect the conversion of the ketone carbonyl of **19** into an epoxy ring, we have also developed a considerably shorter synthetic sequence leading to an analog of the intermediate **17**. In this route, 1, 1-dimethoxyethene was applied in the initial photocycloaddition reaction. Its addition to enone ester **20** followed immediately by transketalization, gave the epimeric diketo esters **21** and **22** (1.4:1) in a combined yield of 70% (Scheme 10).

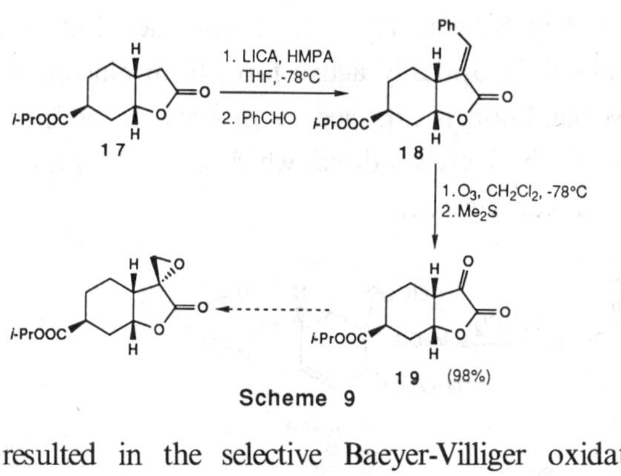

Scheme 9

Treatment of the major epimer **21** with *m*-chloroperbenzoic acid in the presence of disodium hydrogen phosphate as a buffer[12] resulted in the selective Baeyer-Villiger oxidation of the highly strained cyclobutanone moiety, giving rise to keto lactone **23**. The ketone carbonyl was subsequently reduced to the hydrocarbon level *via* a combination of thioacetal formation and desulfurization, to

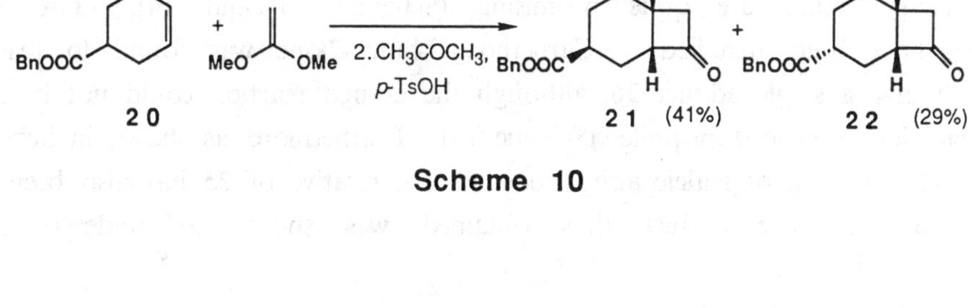

Scheme 10

give lactone ester **24**, as outlined in Scheme 11. This synthetic route, leading to a desired lactone intermediate, represents a substantial improvement over the one described early in terms of operational simplicity.

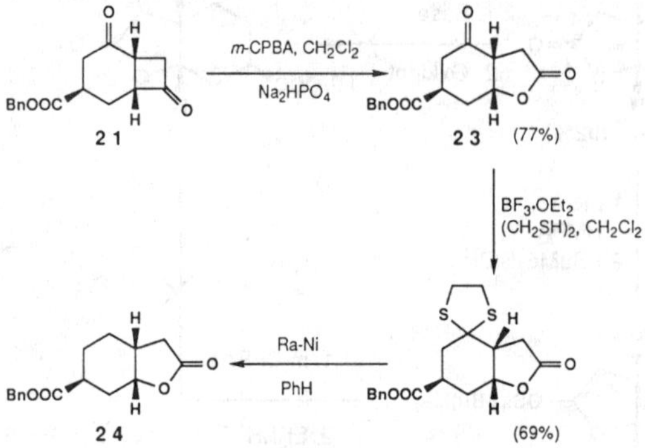

Scheme 11

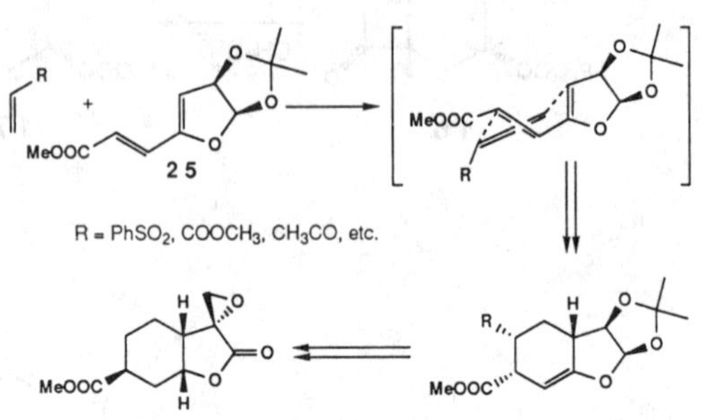

Scheme 12

Currently, we are studying the possible conversion of the minor epimer **22** into the desired lactone **24**, in order to enhance the overall efficiency of this improved photochemical approach.

II. Diels-Alder Approach

The core of the synthetic strategy illustrated in Scheme 12 is the Diels-Alder addition of diene **25**, a known compound readily available in optically active form from glucose in six steps[13], to a suitable dienophile. The cycloaddition is expected to proceed in the indicated regio- and stereo-selective manner to furnish the bicyclic adduct which could, in principle, be easily modified to provide the projected key segment.

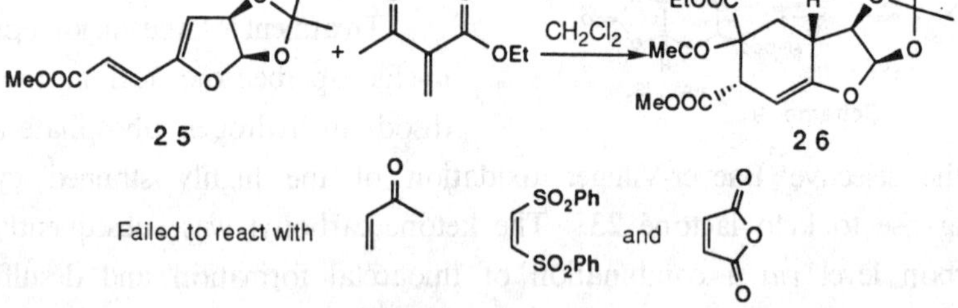

Scheme 13

Preliminary results are quite promising (Schemes 13 and 14). Two suitable dienophiles have been identified. 3-Carbethoxy-3-buten-2-one was found to react with diene **25** to give a single adduct **26**, although the desired reaction could not be induced using several less reactive dienophiles (Scheme 13). Furthermore, as shown in Scheme 14, the Diels-Alder reaction of maleic anhydride and a derivative of **25** has also been experimentally realized. The adduct thus obtained was shown to undergo catalytic hydrogenation readily to give the enantiomerically pure anhydride **27**.

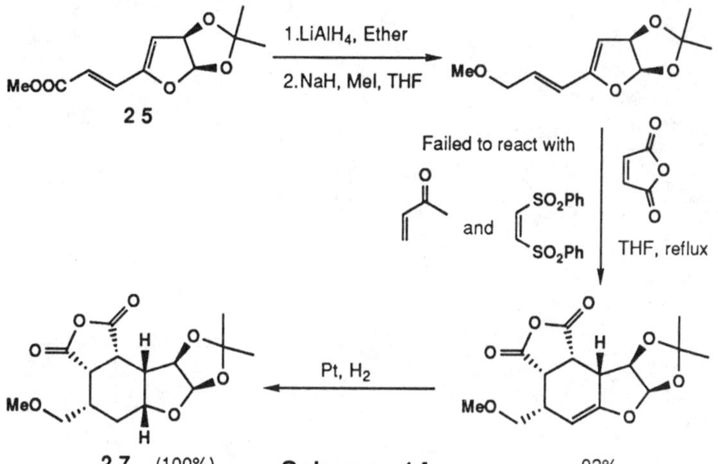

Scheme 14

Studies directed towards the total synthesis of phyllanthocin are being continued using the above approaches.

We are grateful to the Natural Sciences and Engineering Research Council of Canada for financial support and to the Alberta Heritage Foundation for Medical Research for a Studentship to M.R.

References and Notes

1 Kupchan, S. M., LaVoie, E. J., Branfman, A. R. *et al.*, *J. Am. Chem. Soc.*, **99**(1977), 3199.

2 Pettit, G. R., Cragg, G. M., Niven, M. L. *et al.*, *Can. J. Chem.*, **11**(1983), 2630.

3 McGuirck, P. R. and Collum, D. B., *J. Am. Chem. Soc.*, **104**(1982), 4496; *J. Org. Chem.*, **49**(1984), 843.

4 Williams, D. R. and Sit, S.－Y., *J. Am. Chem. Soc.*, **106**(1984), 2949.

5 Burke, S. D., Cobb, J. E. and Takeuchi, K., *J. Org. Chem.*, **50**(1985), 3420.

6 Smith, A. B., III and Fukui, M., *J. Am. Chem. Soc.*, **109**(1987), 1269; Smith, A. B., III and Rivero, R. A., *J. Am. Chem. Soc.*, **109**(1987), 1272; Smith, A. B., III, Hale, K. J. and Vaccaro, H. A., *Tetrahedron Lett.*, **28**(1987), 5591.

7 Martin, S. F., Dappen, M. S., Dupre, B. *et al.*, *J. Org. Chem.*, **52**(1987), 3708.

8 Trost, B. M. and Edsrom, E. D., *Angew. Chem. Intern. Ed. Engl.*, **29**(1990), 520; Trost, B. M. and Kondo, Y., *Tetrahedron Lett.*, **32**(1991), 1613.

9 For the apparatus used for the photocycloaddition reaction, see Valenta, Z. and Liu, H. J., *Org. Synth.*, **57**(1977), 113.

10 This treatment serves two purposes. First, it effects the epimerization of the ring juncture of the initial photoadducts from *trans*-fused to *cis*-fused, and second, it serves to eliminate those photoadducts which possess the undesired regiochemistry, i.e. those resulting from head-to-head addition of vinyl acetate to the enone.

11 Cheng, Y.－S., Liu, W.－L. and Chen, S.－H., *Synthesis,* (1980), 223.

12 Emmons, W. D. and Lucas, G. B., *J. Am. Chem. Soc.*, **77**(1955), 2287.

13 Sun, K. M. and Fraser-Reid, B., *Synthesis,* (1982), 28.

Plenary Lectures

Antioxidant and Prooxidant Activity of Vitamin E in Micelles

LIU Youcheng, LIU Zhongli, HAN Zhengxu and WANG Lijuan

(National Laboratory of Applied Organic Chemistry and Department of Chemistry, Lanzhou University, Lanzhou 730000, China)

α-Tocopherol (VE) is the principal lipid-soluble chain breaking antioxidant present in plasma and erythrocyte membranes which acts to protect lipids from peroxidation[1], a process implicated in aging and a variety of degenerative diseases[2]. Much effort has been made so far to investigate the antioxidant action of VE and its analogues in homogeneous solutions[3], in micelles[4, 5], as well as *in vitro* and *in vivo* biomembranes[1, 6], with the aim of elucidating the mechanism and the activity-microenvironment relationship of the reactions. We wish to report in this article some results on the microenvironmental effects of the antioxidant and prooxidant activity of VE in micelles.

The antioxidant efficiency of VE is reported to be greatly enhanced through a synergistic action of vitamin C(VC) due to the fact that the latter can reduce vitamin E radical ($VE^{\cdot}$) to vitamin E, thereby maintaining the VE level in the system[7]. The key step of the synergism is the reaction between vitamin E radical and vitamin C (Eq. (1)).

$$VE^{\cdot} + VC^{\overline{\cdot}} \rightarrow VE + VC^{\overline{\cdot}}. \qquad (1)$$

The rate constant for this reaction was determined to be $1.55 \times 10^6 M^{-1}s^{-1}$ in homogeneous solution[7], and $2 \times 10^5 M^{-1}s^{-1}$ in soybean phosphatidylcholine liposomes[8], indicating the remarkable effect of the microenvironment. We[9, 10] have reported recently that the antioxidant activity of lipophilic vitamin C derivatives in micelles is dependent on the side-chain length of VC derivatives and the charge type of the micelles, despite the fact that the side-chain length does not significantly influence the reactivity in homogeneous solutions[11]. Therefore, it seems worthwhile to investigate whether the side-chain would affect the synergistic effect of VC derivatives in micelles.

The $VE^{\cdot}$ was generated in cetyl trimethylammonium bromide (CTAB) micelle by oxidizing VE with Fremy's salt ($NO\cdot$) (Eq. (2)). By using a stopped-flow device the $VE^{\cdot}$ was mixed with ascorbic acid (VC), ascorbyl-6-caprylate (VC-8), ascorbyl-6-laurate (VC-12) and ascorbyl-6-palmitate (VC-16) *in situ* respectively and the kinetics was determined by ESR spectroscopy (Figs. 1, 2).

$$VE + (K^+SO_3^-)_2NO\cdot \rightarrow VE\cdot + (K^+SO_3^-)_2NOH \qquad (2)$$

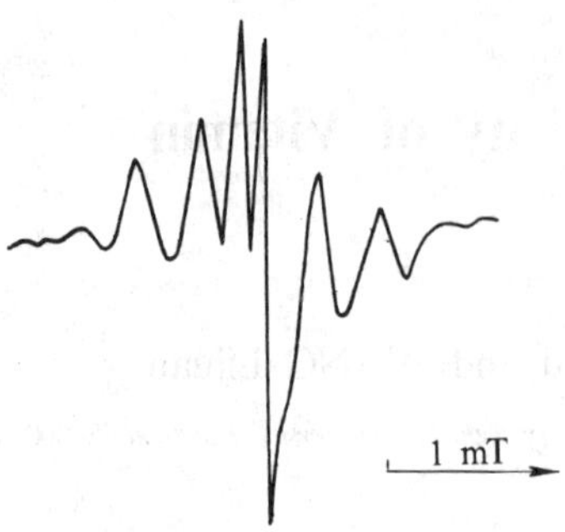

Fig. 1 ESR spectra of $VE^{\cdot}$ and $VC\text{-}16^{\cdot-}$ obtained in 0.015 mol/L CTAB under fast flow, pH 7.2.

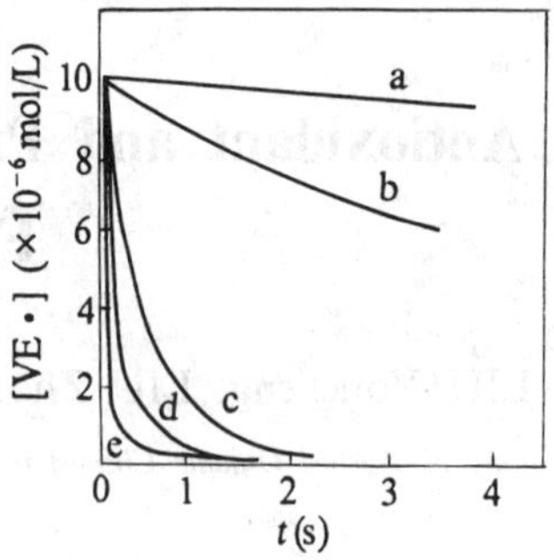

Fig. 2 Decay of $VE^{\cdot}$ in 0.015 mol/L CTAB, pH 7.2. a, $VE^{\cdot}$ alone; b, with VC-16; c, with VC-12; d, with VC-8; e, with VC.

The kinetics of decay for VE· was pseudo-first order in the presence of a large excess of VCs. Plotting the pseudo-first order rate constant versus the initial concentration of VCs gave straight lines from the slope of which the second order rate constants, k_{eff}, were obtained (Table 1). It is seen that the reactivity of VC and its derivatives in CTAB micelle is remarkably influenced by the side-chain length in the order of $VC > VC-8 > VC-12 \gg VC-16$. Clearly, it must be caused by formation of the micelle-$VE^{\cdot}$ and micelle-VCs aggregates. The reaction in micelles may be represented by the following equations:

$$M + VE^{\cdot} \underset{}{\overset{K_1}{\rightleftharpoons}} M - VE^{\cdot} \tag{3}$$

$$M + A \overset{K_2}{\rightleftharpoons} M - A \qquad K_2 = k_2/k_{-2} \tag{4}$$

$$M - VE^{\cdot} + A \xrightarrow{k_3} M - VE + A^{\cdot} \tag{5}$$

$$VE^{\cdot} + A \xrightarrow{k_4} VE + A^{\cdot} \tag{6}$$

$$M - VE^{\cdot} + M - A \xrightarrow{k_5} M - VE + M - A^{\cdot} \tag{7}$$

where M and A represent the micelle and VCs respectively. Since VE and VE· are believed to be located entirely within micelles and the reaction between two micelles carrying similar charge must be difficult to take place due to electrostatic repulsion, reactions 6 and 7 can be neglected. Hence, we have

$$-d[VE\cdot]_T/dt = k_3[VE\cdot]_T[A]_T/(1 + K_2[M]), \tag{8}$$

the subscript T denotes the total concentration of the substrates present in the bulk water and in the micelle. The effective rate constant obtained experimentally may be expressed as

$$k_{eff} = k_3/(1 + K_2[M]). \tag{9}$$

That is, k_{eff} is related to the reaction rate of the aggregated VE· with VCs in the water-phase, and the aggregation ability of VCs with the micelle. If K_2 is known and the entry rate of VCs, K_2, is assumed to be constant and equal to $10^9 M^{-1}s^{-1}$[12], the exit rates, k_{-2}, can be calculated from Eq. (9) and are listed in Table 1.

Table 1 Rate Constants for the Reaction of VE $^{\cdot}$ With VCs in 0.015 mol/L CTAB Micelles

	k_{eff} ($M^{-1}s^{-1}$)	k_3 ($M^{-1}s^{-1}$)	K_2 (M^{-1})	k_{-2} (s^{-1})
VC	$(9.0 \pm 1.4) \times 10^5$	1.1×10^6	9.2×10^2	1.1×10^6
VC−8	$(3.0 \pm 0.6) \times 10^5$	9.2×10^5	9.3×10^3	1.1×10^5
VC−12	$(7.0 \pm 2.0) \times 10^4$	7.9×10^5	4.6×10^4	2.0×10^4
VC−16	$(3.0 \pm 0.8) \times 10^3$	1.2×10^5	1.5×10^5	6.7×10^3

It is seen from Table 1 that the exit rate k_{-2} decreases with the increase of the side-chain length of VC derivatives, and parallels the reactivity sequence of k_{eff}. The k_3 values also change in the same trend, but to a much less extent. These results enable us to depict a mechanism for the reaction in micelles. For a lipophilic VC derivative which shows a strong preference for the micellar environment to react with VE$^{\cdot}$ within another micelle, it must diffuse out from the micelle in which it is located and enter another micelle and does so repeatedly until it encounters a VE$^{\cdot}$ for reaction to occur. In this case the reaction should give second-order kinetics with exit rate being rate-determining. It has been reported that the exit rate, i.e. the intermicellar diffusion rate, is dependent on the side-chain length of the substrate[12]. Moreover, the variation of k_3 with the side-chain length reveals that the rate for intramicellar diffusion of VCs may also contribute to the reactivity.

It is most interesting to note that the microenvironment of the reaction medium is not only effective in changing the antioxidant reactivity of VE, but also renders it possible to alter the reaction pathway, making VE a prooxidant in the autoxidation of linoleic acid. The prooxidant action of VE has been noticed by several investigators[13—15] but its mechanism is not well understood. In the study of the antioxidant reactivity of VE in the peroxidation of linoleic acid we found accidentally that when linoleic acid containing 18% peroxidized linoleic acid (LOOH) was mixed with VE in anhydrous alcohol at 37°C, no significant reaction occurred for a period of several hours but, when they were mixed in SDS micelles, oxygen uptake took place rapidly and linoleic acid was peroxidized[16]. The reaction kinetics was studied by UV, ESR and HPLC techniques and the results indicate that the oxidation product was α-tocopherone (VEQ) with VE$^{\cdot}$ as the intermediate. The sums of concentrations of VE, VE$^{\cdot}$ and VEQ remained constant through the whole course of the reaction, in compliance with a typical consecutive first-order kinetics (Fig. 3). The decay kinetics of VE is first-order with respect to the LOOH. The decay kinetics of VE$^{\cdot}$ depends on the initial concentration of VE and LOOH as shown in Fig. 4. Based on the kinetic analysis the mechanism of reaction between VE and LOOH is proposed as follows:

$$VE + LOOH \xrightarrow{k_6} VE\cdot + LO\cdot + H_2O, \tag{10}$$

$$VE\cdot + LOOH \xrightarrow{k_7} VEQ + LO\cdot\ . \tag{11}$$

The rate constants in 0.1 mol/L SDS micelles and 37°C were evaluated as follows:

$$k_6 = 2.93\ M^{-1}s^{-1},$$
$$k_7 = 6.21\ M^{-1}s^{-1}.$$

The $LO^{\cdot}$ produced in Eqs. (10) and (11) can initiate the peroxidation of linoleic acid, rendering VE a prooxidant. Recently Niki[15] has also reported the prooxidant effect

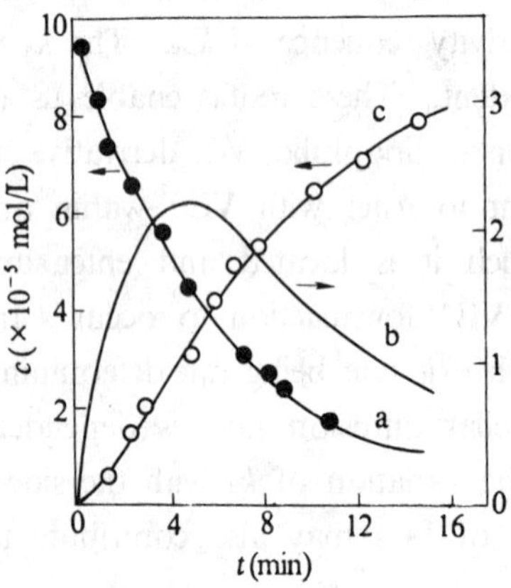

Fig. 3 Kinetics of VE(a), VEQ(b) and VE· (c) during the reaction of VE and LOOH in 0.1 mol/L SDS micelles.

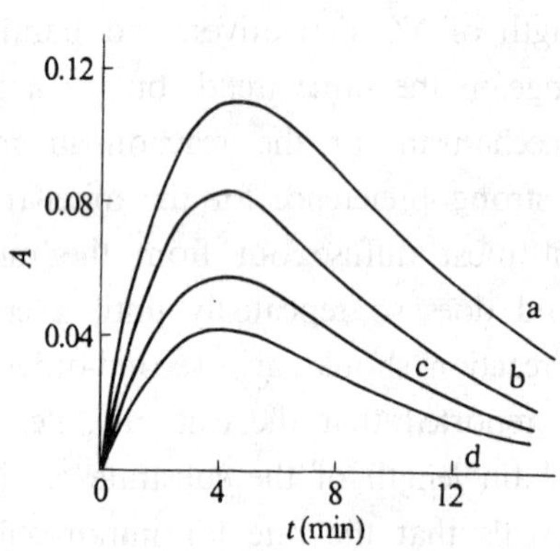

Fig. 4 Relationship between the kinetic behaviour of VE· and $[VE]_0$ during the reaction of VE and LOOH in 0.1 mol/L SDS micelle. $[VE]_0$ decreases in the order of a → d.

of VE on linoleic acid in homogeneous solution with the suggestion that the high concentration of VE and low propagation rate are crucial for VE to be a prooxidant. Our results show, however, that VE can accelerate the peroxidation of linoleic acid in SDS micelles in the presence of LOOH even if the concentration of VE is very low (10^{-4}— 10^{-5}mol/L). This is presumably due to the aggregation of VE and LOOH within the micelle which brings about an increase of the local concentration of the reactive groups around the surface of the micelle and thereby increases the rate for reaction. Furthermore, the formation of hydrogen bond between the head group of the micelle and peroxidized linoleic acid may also facilitate the splitting of the peroxidic linkage.

References

1 Burton, G. W. and Ingold, K. U., *Acc. Chem. Res.*, **19**(1986), 194.

2 Halliwell, B. and Gutteridge, J. M. C., *Free Radicals in Biology and Medicine*, Clarendon, Oxford, 1985.

3 Mukai, K., Kikuchi, S. and Urano, S., *Biochim. Biophys. Acta,* **1035**(1990), 77.

4 Pryor, W. A., Strickland, T. and Church, D. F., *J. Am. Chem. Soc.,* **110**(1988), 2224.

5 Castle, L. and Perkins, M. J., *J. Am. Chem. Soc.,* **108**(1986), 6381.

6 Niki, E., *Br. J. Cancer,* 55, **Suppl. VIII**(1987), 153.

7 Packer, J. E., Slater, T. F. and Willson, R. L., *Nature,* **278**(1979), 737.

8 Scarpa, M., Rigo, A., Maiorini, M. *et al., Biochim. Biophys. Acta,* **801**(1984), 215.

9 Liu, Z. L., Han. Z. X., Chen, P. *et al., Chem. Phys. Lipids,* **56**(1990), 73.

10 Liu, Z. L., Han, Z. X., Chen, P. *et al., Chinese J. Chem.,* **9**(1991), 144.

11 Mukai, K., Nishimura, M., Nagano, A. *et al., Biochim. Biophys. Acta,* **993**(1989), 168.

12 Aniansson, E. A. G. *et al., J. Phys. Chem.,* **80**(1976), 905.

13 Peers, K. and Coxon, P. T., *Chem. Phys. Lipids,* **32**(1983), 49.

14 Cillard, J. and Cillard, P., *J. Am. Oil Chem. Soc.,* **63**(1986), 1165.

15 Takahashi, M., Yoshikawa, Y. and Niki, E., *Bull. Chem. Soc. Jpn.,* **63**(1989), 1885.

Synthesis and Structure-Activity Relationship of Potential Inhibitors of Benzo[a]pyrene Carcinogenesis

David K. Ho, John M. Cassady,

(*Division of Medicinal Chemistry and Pharmacognosy, College of Pharmacy, The Ohio State University, Columbus, Ohio* 43210, *U.S.A.*)

Young H. Chae, Vanessa M. Cook and William M. Baird

(*Department of Medicinal Chemistry and Pharmacognosy, School of Pharmacy and Pharmacal Sciences, Purdue University, West Lafayette, Indiana* 47907, *U.S.A.*)

Abstract A benzo[a]pyrene (B[a]P)-based bioassay in hamster embryo cells has been employed in identifying biochanin A and acacetin as promising potential chemopreventive agents. Current work includes the structure-activity relationship studies of various flavonoid ring systems to determine the best compounds for further testing as potential chemopreventive agents.

I. Background

A bioassay which measures the change of the metabolism of benzo[a]pyrene (B[a]P) to water-soluble metabolites in Syrian hamster embryo cells has been developed in the search for natural and synthetic chemopreventive agents[1]. One of the metabolic pathways of B[a]P leads to formation of B[a]P-7, 8-diol, and then its subsequent conversion to B[a]P-7, 8-diol-9, 10-epoxide, an ultimate carcinogen. Other pathways result in detoxification to water-soluble metabolites. Therefore inhibitors of B[a]P metabolism are potential cancer chemopreventive agents. Systematic screening of edible and medicinal plants using this B[a]P-based bioassay resulted in the identification of biochanin A from red clover, *Trifolium pratense*, flavone from *Feijoa sellowiana*, a series of flavones and flavanones from *Eriodictyon californicum*, and coumarins from *Heracleum lanatum*[2].

II. Mechanism of Action of Biochanin A

The mechanisms of biochanin A action in the inhibition of B[a]P carcinogenesis was further studied in hamster embryo cell cultures[3]. Biochanin A was found to inhibit the metabolism of B[a]P to water-soluble metabolites, B[a]P-9, 10-diol, and B[a]P-7, 8-diol by 44%, 60%, and 52% respectively. Biochanin A reduced the amounts of the glucuronides of 9-hydroxy-B[a]P and 3-hydroxy-B[a]P. It decreased the total B[a]P-DNA binding through the 120-hour incubation and inhibited the formation of both major adducts: (+)-*anti*-BPDE-dGuo and *syn*-BPDE-dGuo. Biochanin A inhibited B[a]P-induced mutagenesis in Chinese hamster V79 cells.

III. Structure-Activity Relationships of Synthetic and Natural Flavonoids

Inhibition of B[a]P Metabolism in Hamster Embryo Cell Cultures

To study the functional group requirements for the inhibition of B[a]P carcinogenesis, a series of synthetic and natural flavonoids were tested in hamster embryo cell cultures (Tables 1 and 2). This structure-activity relationship study showed that the essential features of the best inhibitors include the presence of free hydroxyl groups at positions 5

Table 1 Effects of Isoflavones on B[a]P Metabolism

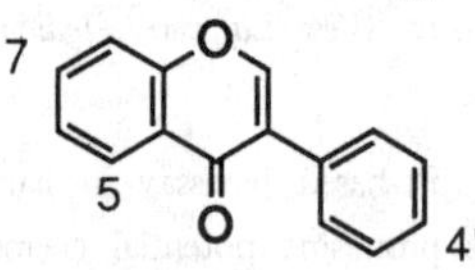

Compound	5-	7-	4'-	ID_{50} [a]	TD [b]
Biochanin A	OH	OH	OMe	21	50
Formononetin	H	OH	OMe	N.E.	N.T.
Daidsein	H	OH	OH	>100	25
4',7-Dimethoxyisoflavone	H	OMe	OMe	N.E.	N.T.
5-Hydroxy-4', 7-dimethoxyisoflavone	OH	OMe	OMe	>100	N.T.
Prunetin	OH	OMe	OH	>100	N.T.
4', 5, 7-Trimethoxyisoflavone	OMe	OMe	OMe	52	25
Genistein	OH	OH	OH	32	5

Note: ID_{50}, the amount of compound to produce 50% inhibition in B[a]P metabolism in μg/ml; TD, the lowest dose in μg/ml to produce toxicity; NT, not toxic; NE, no effect.

Table 2 Effects of Flavones on B[a]P Metabolism

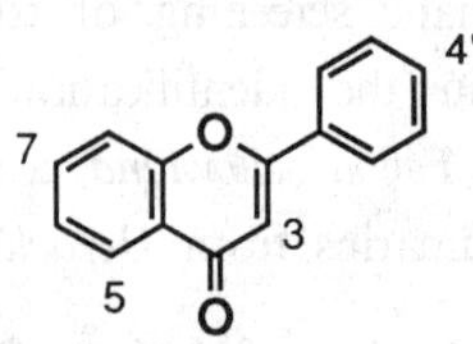

Compound	3-	5-	7-	4'-	ID_{50}	TD
Acacetin	H	OH	OH	OMe	15	N.T.
Apigenin	H	OH	OH	OH	17	25
4',5,7-(OMe)$_3$-flavone	H	OMe	OMe	OMe	12	18
Chrysin	H	OH	OH	H	17	25
Kaempferide	OH	OH	OH	OMe	10	N.T.
Kaempferol	OH	OH	OH	OH	13	18
Galangin	OH	OH	OH	H	8	10
4', 7-Dihydroxyflavone	H	H	OH	OH	66	25

and 7 of the flavonoids. In addition, the double bond at positions 2 and 3 is also critical for the inhibition of B[a]P metabolism. It was also observed that flavones were slightly more active inhibitors than the corresponding isoflavones. The subst tution at the 4′-position with hydroxyl or methoxyl groups did not affect the inhibition greatly. On the other hand, the presence of a hydroxyl group at the 3-position helped enhance activity slightly.

Effects on Mutagenicity of B[a]P

To test their effects on the mutagenicity of B[a]P in the hamster embryo cell-medicated V79 cell mutation assay, several flavonoids were further investigated. It was found that apigenin and acacetin treatments at 10 μg/ml for 24 hour resulted in a large reduction of mutation induction by B[a]P (Table 3). However, biochanin A was effective only at 15 μg/ml or higher doses. Although apigenin was a more effective inhibitor of mutation than acacetin, it was also cytotoxic.

Table 3 Effects of Flavonoids on B[a]P-Induced Mutagenesis (at 10 μg/ml)

Treatment	Test Compound	Cloning Efficiency, %	No. of 6-TG Mutants/Plate	Mutants per 10^5 Viable Cells
Acetone	DMSO	100	0±0	0
B[a]P	DMSO	101	14±4	36
B[a]P	biochanin A	108	12±4	28
B[a]P	apigenin	59	1±0	2
B[a]P	acacetin	88	6±3	11

Effects on B[a]P Metabolism by S-9 Liver Homogenate From Aroclor 1254-Induced Rats

The structure-activity relationships of the flavonoids on cytochrome P450 mediated metabolism of B[a]P were studied. The flavonoids were tested in S-9 homogenate of liver

Table 4 The Effects of Isoflavones on B[a]P Metabolism by S-9 Rat Liver Homogenate

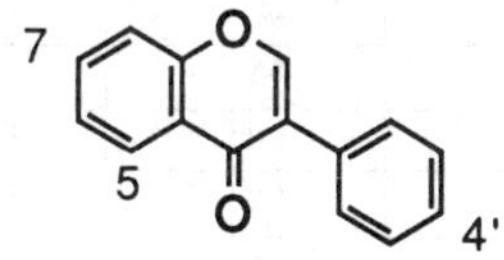

Compound	5-	7-	4′-	IC_{50} (μg/ml)
Biochanin A	OH	OH	OMe	143
Formononetin	H	OH	OMe	>500
Daidzein	H	OH	OH	>500
4′,7-Dimethoxyisoflavone	H	OMe	OMe	>500
5-Hydroxy-4′,7-dimethoxyisoflavone	OH	OMe	OMe	>500
Prunetin	OH	OMe	OH	190
4′,5,7-Trimethoxyisoflavone	OMe	OMe	OMe	80
Genistein	OH	OH	OH	12

from Aroclor 1254-induced rats which contained several P450 isozymes 4. Among the isoflavones (Table 4), the presence of the 5-hydroxyl group was required for the inhibition of B[a]P metabolism. Methylation of the 7-hydroxyl group decreased the inhibition of B[a]P metabolism. However, 4′, 5, 7-trimethoxyisoflavone showed better activity than that of biochanin A, although it has methoxyl groups at both 5 and 7 positions. Genistein is the most active compound in this series.

Similarly, the effects of flavanones and flavones on the metabolism of B[a]P by S-9 rat liver homogenate were studied (Table 5). Flavones were more active than their corresponding isoflavones and flavanones. Flavones with two hydroxyl or two methoxyl groups at 5 and 7 positions were the most active.

Table 5 Effects of Flavanones and Flavones on B[a]P Metabolism by S-9 Rat Liver Homogenate

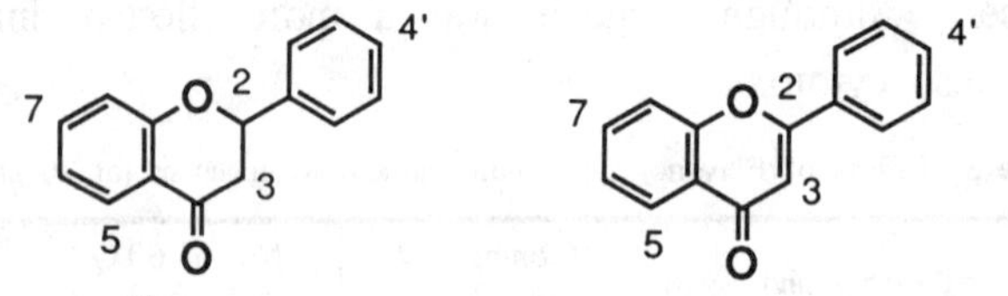

Compound	3-	5-	7-	4′-	IC_{50} (μg/ml)
Naringenin (flavanone)	H	OH	OH	OH	29
Pinocembrin (flavanone)	H	OH	OH	H	10
Acacetin	H	OH	OH	OMe	3.6
Apigenin	H	OH	OH	OH	3.6
Chrysin	H	OH	OH	H	4.6
Kaempferide	OH	OH	OH	OMe	24
Kaempferol	OH	OH	OH	OH	4.7
Galangin	OH	OH	OH	H	3.6
Pratol	H	H	OH	OMe	27
4′, 7-Dihydroxyflavone	H	H	OH	OH	5.3
7-Hydroxy-5-methylflavone	H	Me	OH	H	25
Genkwanin	H	OH	OMe	OH	16
4′, 5-Dihydroxyflavone	H	OH	H	OH	3.2
4′, 5, 7-$(OMe)_3$-flavone	H	OMe	OMe	OMe	3.2
Chrysin dimethyl ether	H	OMe	OMe	H	2.9

Effects on B[a]P Metabolism by Hepatic Microsomes From Rats Induced With Specific Agents

A group of 8 flavonoids with 5, 7-dihydroxy-substitution patterns were tested for their effects on B[a]P metabolism by liver microsomes from rats induced with β-naphthlflavone (βNF) or phenobarbital (PB) (Table 6). All the flavonoids were effective inhibitors of B[a]P metabolism by βNF-induced microsomes (P_{450IA1} or P_{450IA2}), but none were very effective inhibitors of PB-induced microsomes. The most active inhibitors were apigenin, acacetin and kaempferol.

Table 6 Effects of Flavonoids on B[a]P Metabolism by Induced Hepatic Microsomes

4′-Substitution	Isoflavone		Flavone		Flavonol	
H			*Chrysin*		*Galangin*	
			con	3.5	con	2.2
			PB	48	PB	>500
			βNF	1.2	βNF	1.5
OH	*Genistein*		*Apigenin*		*Kaempferol*	
	con	>500	con	>500	con	3.5
	PB	>500	PB	>500	PB	48
	βNF	4.4	βNF	0.7	βNF	1.2
OMe	*Biochanin* A		*Acacetin*		*Kaempferide*	
	con	200	con	>500	con	3.4
	PB	150	PB	>500	PB	150
	βNF	38	βNF	0.9	βNF	2.3

Note: con, Control from non-induced rats; IC_{50}, dose of flavonoid required to inhibit B[a]P metabolism by 50% in μg/ml.

IV. New Ring Systems as Potential Inhibitors of B[a]P Carcinogenesis

Besides the isoflavone and flavone rings, other systems are currently being tested for their potential effectiveness as inhibitors of B[a]P metabolism. Preliminary data showed that some xanthones and coumarins have moderate activities while anthraquinones with proper substitution pattern have slightly stronger activities. Flavones with 5,6- or 6,7-dihydroxyl groups exhibited good inhibition of B[a]P metabolism. Studies of the similarities and differences of the molecular geometries of these systems are underway.

*The financial support of this work by the National Cancer Institute Grant CA*38151 *(JMC and WMB) is appreciated.*

References

1 Cassady, J. M., Zennie, T. M., Chae, Y. −H. *et al., Cancer Research,* **48**(1988), 6257.

2 Cassady, J. M., Wang, X., Liu, Y. L. *et al., Proceedings of the International Symposium on "Recent Advances in Chemistry and Molecular Biology of Cancer Research"*, previous article.

3 Chae, Y. −H., Coffing, S. L., Cook, V. M. *et al., Carcinogenesis,* **12**(1991), 2001.

4 Chae, Y. −H., Marcus, C. B., Ho, D. K. *et al., Cancer Letters,* **60**(1991), 15.

ESR Studies on the Active Oxygen Radicals Produced in the Leukocytes of Malignant Lymphoma Patients and Healthy People

XIN Wenjuan, ZHAO Baolu, LI Xiaojie and HOU Jingwu

(Institute of Biophysics, Academia Sinica, Beijing 100080, China)

I. ESR Studies on Active Oxygen Radicals Produced in the Respiratory Burst of Human Polymorphonuclear Leukocytes

When human polymorphonuclear leukocytes (PMN) are stimulated or when they are in phagocytosis, there will be a respiratory burst, an increase in oxygen uptake, production of active oxygen radicals and activation of the hexose monophosphate shunt. The active oxygen radicals produced in this process play an important role in microbicidal and tumoricidal activity and in protecting the healthy body from diseases. But, if there are excess active oxygen radicals in the body, they will damage the components of cells or even kill the normal cells and cause very serious diseases, such as cancers, heart disease, stroke, atherosclerosis, pulmonary emphysema.

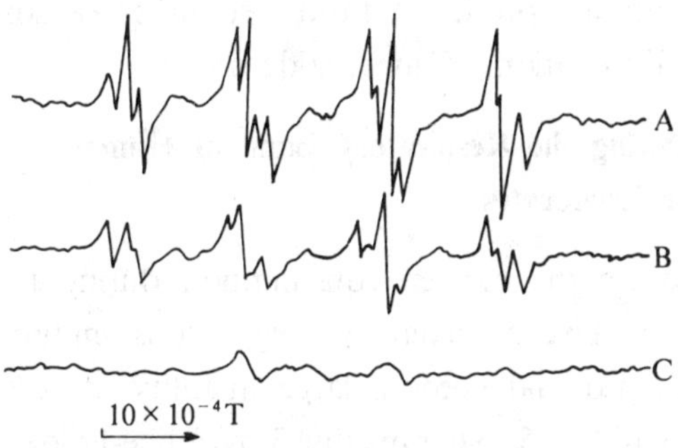

Fig. 1 A. The ESR spectrum resulting from 1.5×10^7/ml PMN stimulated with 100 ng/ml PMA in the presence of 0.1 mmol/L DETAPAC. 0.1mol/L DMPO was added to the mixture after incubation for 2 min at 37°C. B. Conditions were the same as those for A, except that 300 units/ml catalase were present. C. Conditions were the same as those for A, except that 10 μg/ml SOD was present.

Spin trapping of superoxide anions $O_2^{\overline{\cdot}}$. The ESR spectrum of spin adducts resulting from a mixture containing PMN stimulated with PMA and spin trapped with DMPO is shown in Fig. 1A. This is a composite of two distinct products: the superoxide anion spin adduct of DMPO (DMPO-OOH), $g=2.0055$, $a_N=14.3$G, $a_H^B=11.3$G, $A_H^r=1.26$G and the hydroxyl radical spin adduct of DMPO (DMPO-OH), $g=2.0053$, $a_N=a_H=14.9$G. This result is consistent with the spectrum simulated by computor. The size of the DMPO-OOH and DMPO-OH peaks increased with sequential scans, indicating progressive generation of free radicals. In order to identify the source of superoxide anion and hydroxyl radicals in the ESR spectrum, catalase was added to the system. It was found that the signals decreased a little but still contained two components, DMPO-OOH and DMPO-OH (Fig. 1B). After SOD was added to the system, both DMPO-OOH and DMPO-OH spectra were almost eliminated from the spectrum (Fig. 1C), indicating that the ESR spectrum in Fig. 1A came mainly from superoxide anion and hydroxyl radicals resulting from superoxide anion produced from stimulated PMN.

Spin trapping of hydroxyl radicals OH. The ESR spectrum of spin adducts resulting from a mixture containing PMN stimulated with 20 ng/ml PMA, after incubation at 37°C for 2 min and addition of DMPO, is shown in Fig. 1. In contrast to the ESR spectrum in Fig. 1A, it has almost one component of DMPO-OH, indicating that mainly hydroxyl radicals were trapped from PMN when the stimulation was diluted enough. After addition of SOD to the sample, which is twice the concentration in Fig. 1C, the DMPO-OH signals are decreased but not eliminated as in Fig. 1C (Fig. 2B). After addition of catalase to the sample, which doubles the concentration in Fig. 1B, the DMPO-OH signals are decreased a little. The above results indicate that parts of DMPO-OH come from the hydroxyl radicals produced in the dismutation reaction of superoxide radicals of superoxide anions but it is difficult to say that all the DMPO-OH signals in the figure come from the hydroxyl radicals produced from Fenton's reaction utilizing the hydrogen peroxide produced from dismutation of superoxide anions.

II. ESR Studies on Oxygen Consumption During the Respiratory Burst of Human Polymorphonuclear Leckocytes

An oxygen electrode has been used to measure the oxygen consumption during the respiratory burst of PMN. This method can only give an average oxygen consumption, but cannot tell where the oxygen has been consumed and needs a large quantity of cells. In this paper the spin probes CTPO (3-carbamoyl-2, 2, 5, 5-tetramethyl-3-pyrroline-1-yloxy) and TEMPOL (2, 2, 6, 6-tetramethyl piperidine-N-oxyl-4-ol) were used to study oxygen consumption of human PMN stimulated by PMA (phorbol myristate acetate) with ESR spectrometry. It was found that during production of active oxygen radicals, oxygen consumption came from the medium outside the cells. No change of oxygen was found from the medium inside the cells.

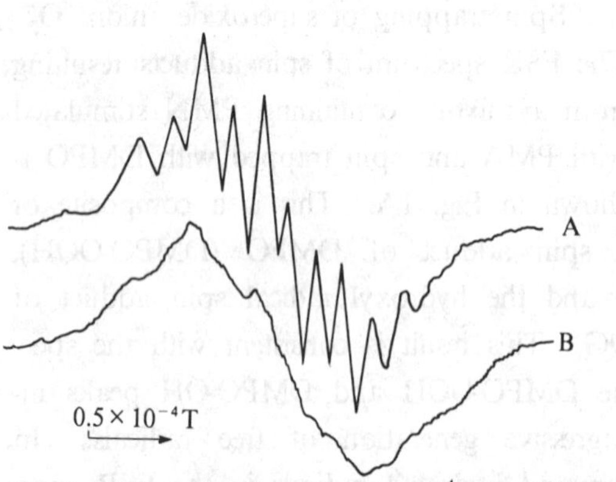

Fig. 2 ESR spectrum resulting from 10^{-4}mol/L CTPO in 2.5×10^7 PMN stimulated with (A) and without (B) 100 ng/ml PMA.

1. *Oxygen Consumption During the Respiratory Burst Process of PMN Stimulated With PMA*

The M_0 component of the ESR spectrum of CTPO in PMN, with and without PMA, incubated at 37°C for 2 min is shown in Fig. 2A, B. The broad peak in Fig. 1B arises from hyperfine splitting of nitrogen because of interaction of the spin moment of nitroxide with the spin moment of oxygen. No obvious change in the spectrum even after 20 min indicated that the respiration of PMN was not strong enough to cause the change of the oxygen concentration in the medium and the change of the ESR spectrum in these conditions.

After stimulation with PMA, the spectrum in Fig. 2A became different from that in Fig. 2B in that it was split into over 10 hyperfine peaks. That is because after stimulation with PMA, the respiratory burst of PMN had produced active oxygen radicals and caused oxygen consumption, the oxygen concentration in the medium had changed and the spin-spin interaction between oxygen and spin probe had decreased, and the superhyperfine structure from hydrogens of 4 methyl groups had appeared. CTPO cannot penetrate the cell membrane during the experiment. So the appearance of hyperfine structure in Fig. 2A simply reflected the oxygen consumption in the intercellular medium during the production of active oxygen radicals by PMN stimulated with PMA.

2. *No Intracellular Oxygen Consumption was Found During the Respiratory Burst of PMN Stimulated With PMA*

The results above indicate intercellular oxygen consumption when PMN were stimulated with PMA. However, it cannot exclude intracellular oxygen consumption in this process. The ESR spectra of 10^{-4}mol/L TEMPOL in PMN stimulated by PMA, with and without CrOX incubated at 37°C for 2 min are shown in Fig. 3A, B. The superhyperfine structure from hydrogens of methyl groups appeared in Fig. 3A, but only a wide peak without any superhyperfine structure splitting appeared in Fig. 3B. The spin probe TEMPOL can penetrate the cell membrane and is present in both intercellular and intracellular media. The ESR spectrum in Fig. 3A should be the overlap of the contributions from the probes in both intercellular and intracellular media. The transition element ion Cr^{+3} with spin moment can widen the ESR spectrum of the spin probe. The straight line in Fig. 3C was the result of 10^{-4}mol/L TEMPOL mixed with 37 mmol/L CrOX in aqueous solution. However, CrOX cannot penetrate the cell membrane and can only widen the ESR spectrum of TEMPOL in the intercellular medium. Furthermore, addition of CrOX to the mixture of CTPO and PMN resulted in a loss of the ESR spectrum showing that both CTPO and CrOX are only in the intercellular medium. So the ESR spectrum in Fig. 3B without any superhyperfine struc-

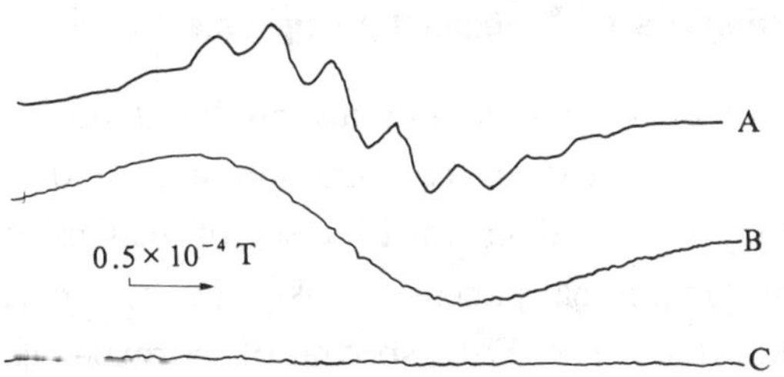

Fig. 3 ESR spectrum resulting from 10^{-4}mol/L TEMPOL in 2.5×10^{7}/ml PMN stimulated with 100ng/ml PMA without (A) and with (B) 37 mmol/L CrOX; (C) ESR spectrum of 10^{-4}mol/L TEMPOL and 37 mmol/L CrOX in PBS.

ture of hydrogens of methyl groups came from the contribution of TEMPOL in the intracellular medium. This indicated that the superhyperfine splitting in Fig. 3A coming from the contribution of TEMPOL in the intercellular medium was due to production of active oxygen radicals and oxygen consumption by PMN stimulated with PMA, and suggested that no oxygen consumption was found in the intracellular medium during production of active oxygen radicals in PMN stimulated with PMA.

3. *Discussion*

PMA stimulates PMN from outside the cells. From the above experiment of oxygen consumption, it is suggested that when active oxygen radicals were produced in PMN stimulated by PMA, the main oxygen consumption was found in the intercellular medium but no change of oxygen concentration was found in the intracellular medium. This means that the location of production of active oxygen radicals is in the cell membrane and may be near the outside layer of the cell membrane. If the location of production of active oxygen radicals was near the inside of the cell membrane, the oxygen inside the cell should be absorbed and the concentration of oxygen should be changed during the respiratory burst. However, this was not found in the experiment. SOD and catalase are macromolecular and cannot penetrate cell membranes. When SOD was added to the PMN and PMA system, the oxygen free radicals were eliminated which further indicated that the oxygen radicals were out of the cells. All of these events connected with the production of active radicals may take place on the cell membrane.

III. Active Oxygen Radicals Produced by Leukocytes of Malignant Lymphoma Patient

The electron spin resonance (ESR) spectra of active oxygen radicals produced during the respiratory burst of PMA-stimulated leukocytes and oxygen consumption were studied by ESR spin trapping and spin probe oxymetry for 31 times in 17 cases of malignant lymphoma. Fig. 4 shows that ESR spectra of lymphoma patients' leukocytes are quite different from those of healthy person's leukocytes. The ESR spectra of normal Leu stimulated by PMA showed an overlapping of DMPO-OOH and DMPO-OH, the DMPO-OOH signals being stronger. In the majority of the lymphoma cases, abnormal ESR spectra showed marked DMPO-OH spectra and decreased or even no DMPO-OOH signals. Fig. 4b shows the ESR spectra of 6 cases which were improved or in remission, their ESR spectra were nearly normal. The ESR spectra were often as in Fig. 4c, d when the patients' condition was severe or progressing. The active oxygen radical signals produced by Leu respiratory burst were very weak, or almost no signals could be detected as shown in Fig. 4e. The patient died within a month. We have observed a predominant DMPO-OH spectrum in normal Leu stimulated with a low concentration of PMA or when the Leu are aged. The spectra of PMA-stimulated Leu during respiratory burst are shown in Fig. 5. It has been reported that a large amount of oxygen is consumed dur-

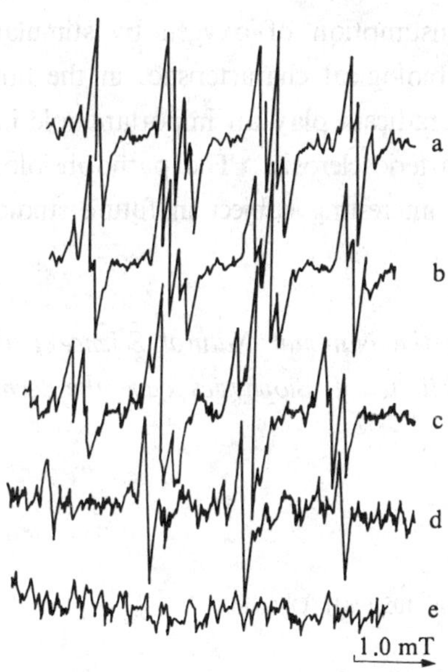

Fig. 4 ESR spectra of DMPO-trapped active oxygen radicals produced from the leukocytes stimulated with PMA, of healthy people and malignant lymphoma patients.
a, Leu of healthy people; b, c, d and e, Leu of malignant lymphoma patients. The time of determination is 4 min after PMA was added at room temperature.

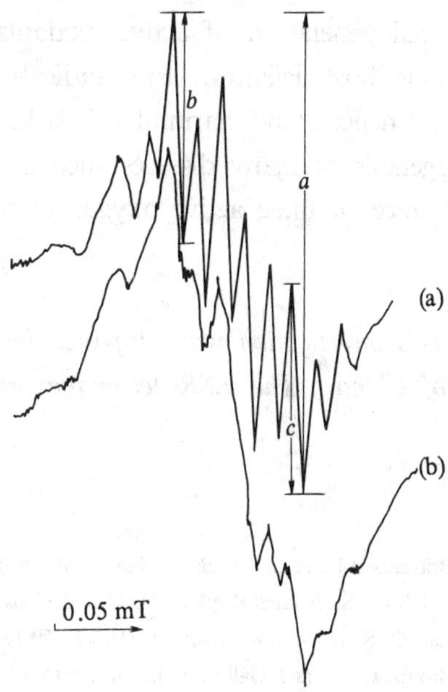

Fig. 5. ESR spectra of oxygen consumption of Leu stimulated with PMA during respiratory burst.
(a) Leu of healthy people; (b) Leu of malignant lymphoma patients. The time of determination is 20 min after PMA was added at room temperature.

ing the production of active oxygen radicals from PMA-stimulated normal Leu, resulting in marked decrease in the oxygen concentration of the media. This can be detected as the 13 superhyperfine splitting ESR spectra produced by the coupling of 13 protons (12 methyl protons plus 1 ring proton). The *K* parameter was used as an empirical parameter for determining O_2 concentration in solution. Therefore, the oxygen consumption was calculated by the formula: $K=(b+c)/2a$; *a*, *b* and *c* are shown in Fig. 5 (a). The *b* and *c* heights are directly proportional to the amount of oxygen consumed in solution, e.g. the larger the *K* value, the greater the amount of oxygen consumed. We found that the *K* value was 0.460 ± 0.047 20 min after respiratory burst in 25 normal persons' Leu. The *K* value was 0.306 ± 0.116 in 25 measurements of patients' Leu. The *K* value varied from 0.20 to 0.28 in 16 (64%) tests. The *K* value varied significantly (*P* 0.001) in patient and normal Leu. It is known that oxygen consumption during respiratory burst of Leu is closely related to membrane bound oxidases. In our study the oxygen consumption of lymphoma patients' Leu was significantly lower than normal. This suggests there are defects of their membrane bound oxidases. It may be that in lymphoma patients the Leu age faster, and a defect in membrane bound oxidases leads to abnormal generation of active oxidants and low consumption of oxygen by stimulation, impairing host defences. Free radicals possess dual biological characteristics in the human body, beneficial and harmful. It is known that free radicals play an important role in the pathogenesis of many diseases such as malignancy, arteriosclerosis. The pathophsiological significance of these active oxygen compounds is an interesting subject in future studies.

This investigation was supported by a grant from the National Natural Science Foundation of China. The ESR technique group of the Institute of Biophysics gave the technical help.

References

1 Britigan, B.E. *et al., J. Biol. Chem.,* **261**(1986), 4426.
2 Colowike, S. P. and Kaplan, N. O., *Methods in Enzymology,* Vol. 105(1984), Orlando.
3 Lai, C. S. *et al., Proc. Nat. Acad. Sci.,* **79**(1982), 1166.
4 Brown, C. C. and Gallin, J. I., *Hemat/Oncol. Clin. Noth. Am.,* **2**(1988), 61.
5 Chandor, S. B. *et al., Clin Lab Med.,* **8**(1989), 273.
6 Fantone, J. C. and Ward, P. A., *Human Pathol.,* **16**(1985), 973.

Flexible and Rigid Chain-linked Bis-pyrimidine and Bis-purine Derivatives as Potential Intercalating Agents

Cyril Párkányi, Hui Liang Yuan, Martha C. Marin-Montes, Meng-Kan M. Tsai, Thomas L. Aung, Hans T. Essoussi

(Department of Chemistry, Florida Atlantic University, P. O. Box 3091, Boca Raton, FL 33431-0991, U.S.A.)

and László von Szentpály

(Department of Chemistry, University of the West Indies, Mona Campus St. Andrew, Kingston 7, Jamaica)

Abstract Various types of organic compounds can bind to DNA by intercalation and thus exhibit anticancer, antiviral, or antiparasitic activity. Some of the interesting novel types of bifunctional intercalators are pyrimidine or purine bases or their analogs with a flexible or rigid chain providing a bridge between two such pyrimidine or purine units. The compounds with a flexible chain are represented by a series of polymethylene chain-bridged (with a varying number of methylene groups in the chain) substituted bis-6-chloropyrimidines, bis-6-chloropurines, and bis-6-hydroxy-8-azapurines. The compounds with conformationally restricted tethers are represented by substituted bis-6-chloropyrimidines and bis-6-chloropurines with -p-$C_6H_4 \cdot CH_2 \cdot$-p-C_6H_4- and -p-$C_6H_4 \cdot O \cdot p$-C_6H_4-bridges. The synthesis, spectral data, and other physical properties of the new compounds will be discussed. The compounds are expected to be biologically active.

I. Introduction

The model of intercalation was first described in 1961 by Lerman[1]. He suggested that organic compounds can bind to DNA by an intercalation mechanism. From the time of that pioneering work, interference with nucleic acid metabolism has been implicated for an increasing number of drugs used as antitumor agents or for the treatment of parasitic diseases[2, 3].

Much of our knowledge of intercalation has come from studies of the DNA binding properties of synthetic molecules, such as ethidium bromide (**1**), proflavine (**2**) and quinacrine (**3**). Recently, Le Pecq *et al.* synthesized dimers containing two moieties of 2-methoxy-6-chloro-9-aminoacridine linked by spermine and showed that these agents were twice as effective in the unwinding and extension of the DNA helix than the corresponding monomeric compound[4]. The Watson-Crick hypothesis for DNA postulates a twin helical structure in which certain purine and pyrimidine bases in each helix are cross-linked by hydrogen bonds. These bonds will be momentarily broken at the time of replication. In our current work, this working hypothesis has been elaborated upon by supposing that purines and pyrimidines, similar to those occurring naturally and joined in a linear fash-

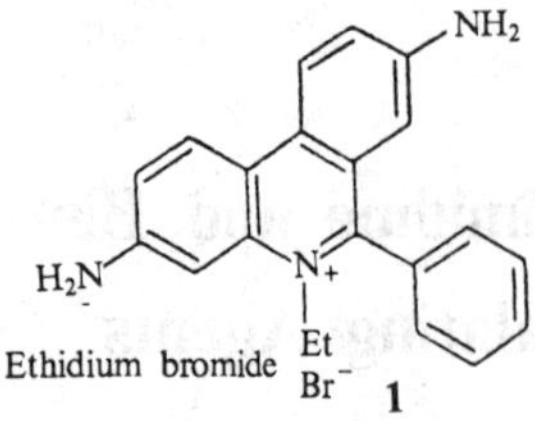

Ethidium bromide 1

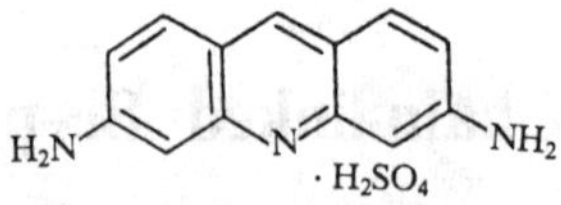

Proflavine (septoflavine) 2

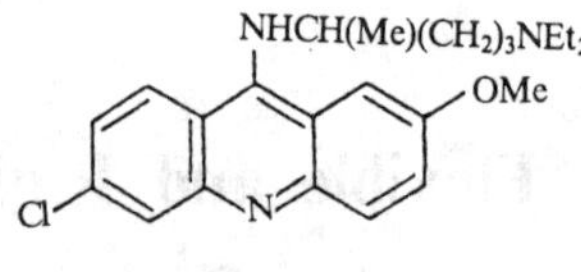

Quinacrine (atabrine) 3

ion, might be effective for this purpose. Several dipurinyl derivatives, such as dipurin-9-ylethane and dipurin-9-ylhexane, have been reported and have shown biological activity[5—7]. It is well known that a number of analogs of these pyrimidine and purine bases and their respective nucleosides are now in use as anticancer drugs. The new intercalators are compounds in which purine or pyrimidine chromophores are connected by various types of linking groups, like polymethylene chains or spermine, that bridge the two chromophores. In one case, the linking chain was chosen in such a way that it has an affinity for DNA and a geometry allowing intercalation in nonadjacent binding sites. A series of compounds of the type **4** have demonstrated that there can be a transition from monofunctional to bifunctional intercalation as the polymethylene chain is increased from six to eight atoms. We are also interested in extending this bifunctional intercalation concept to the design and synthesis of bifunctional intercalating compounds containing bridges more rigid than the polymethylene chains. It was reported that a flexible chain, e.g. a polymethylene bridge may show an intramolecular self-stacking of the two chromophores which may reduce the binding ability of the agents[8]. In order to prevent the self-stacking of the chromophores, more rigid linking chains, e.g. diphenyl ether and diphenylmethane, have been introduced as well.

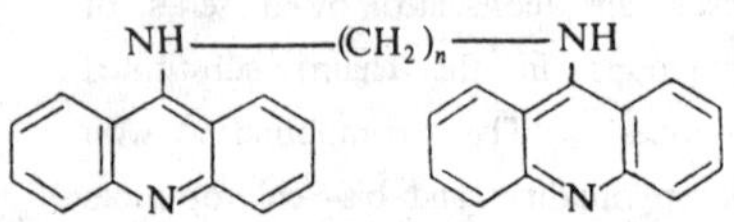

4 $n = 2-12$

By using computer simulation, their molecular stereostructures have been generated. The two purine chromophores lie approximately parallel to each other and are 11 Å apart. The carbon and oxygen-center bridges give the molecules the ability to bend and twist along the long axis in order to fit better into the narrow groove of the DNA helix. The bridge should cover two affinity sites of the DNA sequence. Since a higher binding ability and selectivity of the binding site are most desirable, studies of new types of intercalators have become one of the major issues in the area of cancer research.

II. Experimental

Melting points were determined in capillary tubes heated in a Thomas-Hoover melting point apparatus and are uncorrected. The ^{1}H NMR spectra were obtained on Varian EM-360 (60 MHz) and IBM NR 200 AF (200 MHz) spectrometers using tetramethylsilane as the internal standard. The UV spectra were measured on a Perkin-Elmer Lambda 4C spectrophotometer, with a Perkin-Elmer 7700 professional computer. Their spectra were recorded in pressed potassium bromide disks on a Perkin-Elmer 580B spectrophotometer with a Perkin-Elmer data station. The purity of all the compounds were checked by thin-layer chromatography on silica gel 60 F-254 precoated plates and the spots were located under UV light or iodine vapor. The elemental microanalyses were performed by Desert Analytics, Tucson, AZ.

The syntheses of bis-purinyl and corresponding bis-8-azapurinyl derivatives bridged by polymethylene chains of different lengths (with the number of carbon atoms in the chain, *n*, equal to 3, 8, and 12) are shown in Scheme 1. The N, N′-bis-(4-chloro-5-amino-6-pyrimidyl)-1, 3-diaminopropane (**7**), N, N′-bis-(4-chloro-5-amino-6-pyrimidyl)-1, 8-diaminooctane (**8**), and N, N′-bis-(4-chloro-5-amino-6-pyrimidyl)-1, 12-diaminododecane (**9**) were prepared by condensation of, 4, 6-dichloro-5-aminopyrimidine (**5**) with 1, 3-diaminopropane (**6**, $n=3$), 1, 8-diaminooctane (**6**, $n=8$), and 1, 12-diaminododecane (**6**, $n=12$), in refluxing 1-butanol in the presence of triethylamine by a previously described method[10–12]. The 1, 3-bis-(6-chloro-9-purinyl)propane (**10**), 1, 8-bis-(6-chloro-9-purinyl)octane (**11**), and 1, 12-bis-(6-chloro-9-purinyl)dodecane (**12**) were prepared by acid-catalyzed reaction of 7-9 with triethyl orthoformate in N, N′-dimethylacetamide[10, 13, 14]. The 1, 3-bis-(6-hydroxy-8-aza-9-purinyl)propane (**13**), 1, 8-bis-(6-hydroxy-8-aza-9-purinyl)octane (**14**) and 1, 12-bis-(6-hydroxy-8-aza-9-purinyl) dodecane (**15**) were obtained through diazotization of **7-9**, respectively, with sodium nitrite in aqueous acetic acid. The synthesis of novel bis-(6-chloropurines) bridged by conformationally restricted diphenyl tethers is shown in Scheme

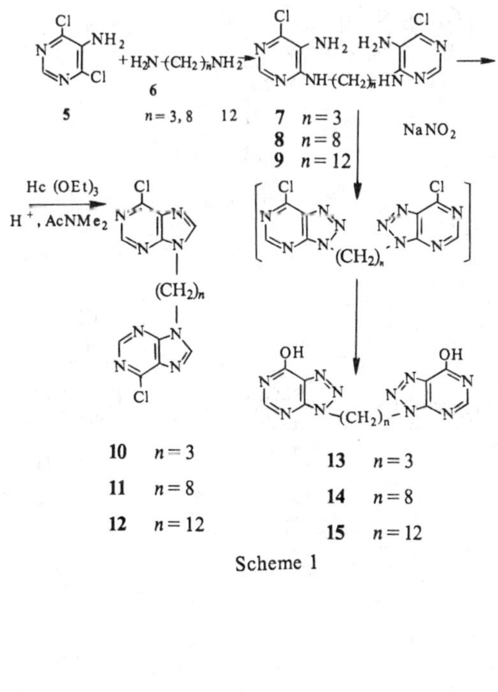

Scheme 1

2. The compounds were synthesized by a straightforward, two-step procedure described herein. 5-amino-4, 6-dichloropyrimidine (**5**) and 4, 4′-diaminodiphenylmethane (**17**) refluxed in 1-butanol in the presence of triethylamine, using a previously described method[10–12], gave bis-[4-(N-5-amino-4-chloro-6-pyrimidyl)aminophenyl]methane (**19**). In an analogous reaction, **5** and bis-(4-aminophenyl)ether(**18**) yielded bis-[4-(N-5-amino-4-chloro-6-pyrimidyl)-aminophenyl]ether (**20**). Subsequent acid-catalyzed condensation of **19** and **20** with triethyl orthoformate carried out in N, N′-dimethylacetamide afforded bis-[4-(6-chloro-9-purinyl)-phenyl]methane (**21**) and bis-[4-(6-chloro-9-purinyl) phenyl] ether (**22**), respectively, in good yield[10, 13]. By the same procedure, the N, N′-bis-(2-amino-4-chloro-6-pyrimidyl)-1, 3-diaminopropane and related compounds with flexible chain bridges were synthesized (Scheme 3).

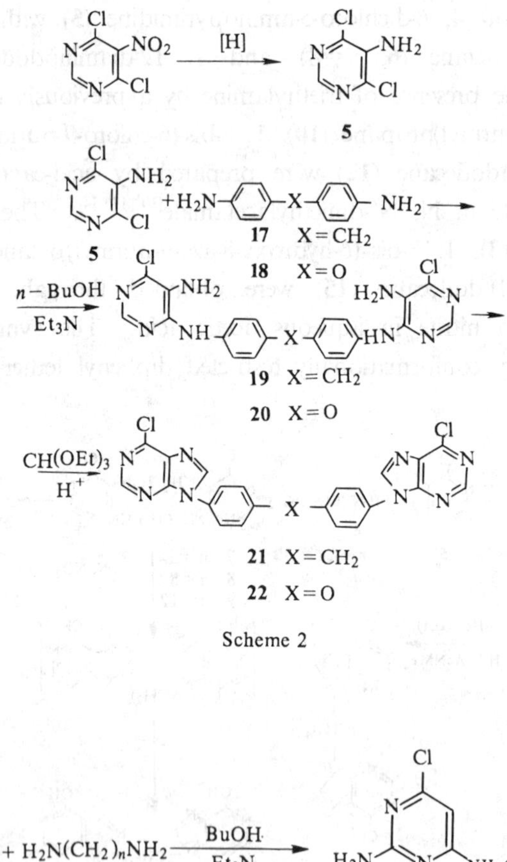

Scheme 2

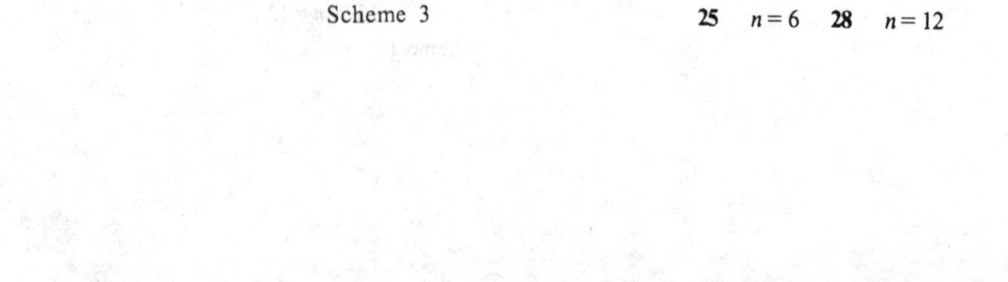

Scheme 3

The structures of these new compounds were established on the basis of their elemental microanalyses and spectral data. For example, their spectra of compounds **19** and **20** contain the characteristic NH stretching frequencies due to the presence of primary and secondary amino groups, 3350—3450 cm^{-1} and around 1650 cm^{-1}. Their spectra of **21** and **22** are as expected, with the primary and secondary amino group frequencies in the 3350—3450 cm^{-1} range while there is no absorption at 1650 cm^{-1}. The ^{1}H NMR spectra of the new compounds measured in dimethyl sulfoxide-d_6 (DMSO-d_6) show the presence of the expected protons, in agreement with the proposed structures. The UV spectrum of 5-amino-4, 6-dichloropyrimidine (**5**) is that of a multiply substituted pyrimidine system[14]. The amino group, acting as an auxochrome, shifts the maxima of the unsubstituted pyrimidine at 210 and 240 nm towards longer wavelengths (260, 320 nm, respectively). The UV spectra of the compounds **19**—**22** contain a maximum at 240 nm due to the presence of benzene rings. An additional maximum at 265 nm[15] can be found in the uv spectra of 6-chloropurines.

III. Biological Activity

The biological activity of the synthesized compounds was tested using the bioluminescent bacterium *Vibrio fischeri*. The intensity of the light emitted by the bacteria corresponds to the activity of the living cells and can be quantitatively measured (Fig. 1 and Fig. 2). In the case of the starting materials themselves, the bacteria were not affect-

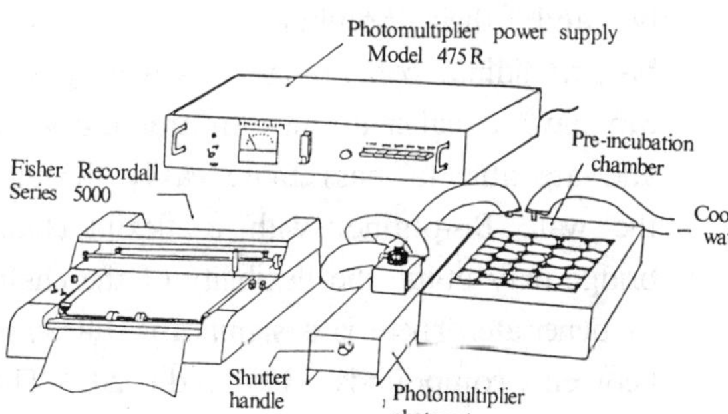

Fig. 1 Photomultiplier photometer assembly.

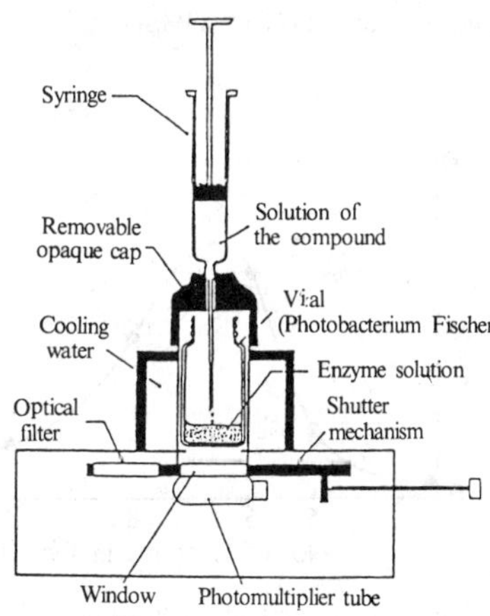

Fig. 2 Cross-sectional view of the photomultiplier photometer assembly for the standard assay of luciferase.

ed until 100 μl of the compound had been added. A significant decrease in the intensity of luminescence was observed when only 1 μl of the bis-pyrimidine was added, and there is an apparent difference in the effects of bis-pyrimidines and bis-purines (Table 1).

Apparently, bis-purines with rigid-chain bridges do not pass through the cell walls easi-

Table 1 Inhibition of *Photobacterium fischeri* by Various Compounds

Compd.	Concn. ($\times 10^{-2}$ mol/L)	Dose (μl) 1	5	10	20	40	100
		Inhibition, %					
DMSO	NEAT	−	−	−	−	ne	50.0
5	1.05	−	−	−	−	ne	50.0
7	1.00	3.5	5.3	8.8	8.8	8.8	−
8	1.13	37.5	66.7	75.0	−	72.5	−
9	1.13	22.9	18.8	12.5	2.1	0.0	−
11	1.01	ne	−	17.8	36.8	56.4	−
14	1.23	ne	5.0	22.5	−	56.7	−
19	1.01	10.0	36.7	45.0	45.0	45.0	−
20	1.22	46.8	73.0	73.7	73.0	−	−
21	1.05	sti	sti	sti	−	−	−
22	1.06	sti	sti	sti	−	−	−
23	1.16	5.0	17.3	20.0	30.7	49.3	−
24	1.09	20.6	38.2	47.1	64.7	79.4	−
25	1.06	67.6	79.4	85.3	91.2	91.2	−
26	1.10	48.1	65.4	61.5	50.0	42.3	−
27	1.14	15.1	13.5	7.5	3.8	5.7	−
28	1.12	4.5	18.2	20.5	36.4	56.8	−
16	1.05	ne	ne	ne	ne	ne	10.0

Inhibition of bioluminescence. Symbols: −, no data; ne, no effect; sti, stimulation (increase of intensity of bioluminescence). Solvent: DMSO.

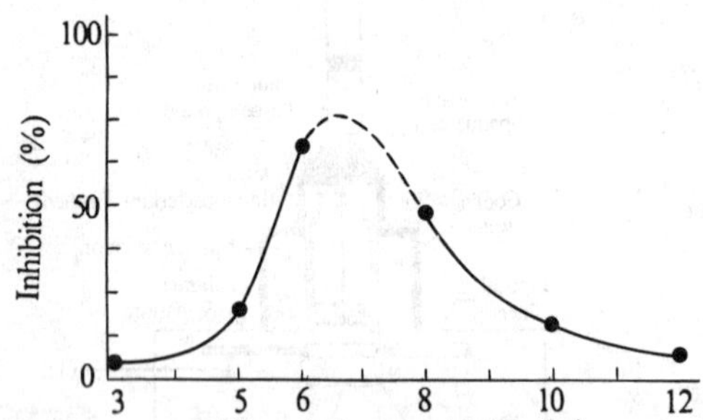

Fig. 3 Inhibition of bacterial luminescence at low concentration (1 μl) by compounds **23**—**28**, as a function of the length of the linking chain.

ly and their solubility is low. The bis-pyrimidines containing an amino group can have a higher affinity towards cell walls and are able to pass more easily through the wall. Bis-purines with a flexible-chain bridge may utilize the flexibility of the chain to penetrate. There is a significant difference between compounds **19** and **20**. The oxygen-center bridged compound, **20**, is much more effective than the carbon-center bridged compound **19**. The hydrogens of the methyl group may restrict the binding and twisting of the bridge and thus make it more rigid than the ether and may lower the inhibiting ability. A comparison of the compounds tested has revealed that the self-stacking effect influences the activity of compounds with a polymethylene bridge of more than 8 carbons, the optimum length of the polymethylene chain being about 6 carbons (approximately 10 Å long) (Fig. 3).

Financial support of this work by the Elsa U. Pardee Foundation (Midland, MI), the Robert A. Welch Foundation (Houston, TX; work done at the University of Texas at El Paso, El Paso, TX), the National Institutes of Health (Bethesda, MD), and Florida Atlantic University (Boca Raton, FL) is gratefully acknowledged. The authors wish to express their sincere thanks to Dr. James E. Becvar for his help with the determination of biological activity.

References

1 Lerman, L. S., *J. Mol. Biol.*, **3**(1961), 18.

2 Gale, E. F., Cundliffe, E., Reynolds, P. E. *et al.*, *The Molecular Basis of Antibiotic Action,* Wiley, New York, 1973, pp. 173—205.

3 Waring, M. J., in *Mechanism of Action of Antimicrobial and Antitumor Agents* (eds. Corcoran, J. W. and Hahn, F. E.), Springer-Verlag, New York, 1975, pp. 141—165.

4 Le Pecq, J. B., Le Bret, M. and Roques, B. P., *Proc. Natl. Acad. Sci. USA,* **72**(1975), 2915.

5 Lister, J. H., *J. Chem. Soc.*, (1963), 2228.

6 Rose, F. L., *J. Chem. Soc.*, (1954), 4116.

7 Lister, J. H., *J. Chem. Soc.*, (1960), 3394.

8 Jaycox, G. D., Gribble, G. W. and Hacker, M. P., *J. Heterocyclic Chem.*, **24**(1987), 1405.

9 Schaeffer, H. J., Vogel, D. and Vince, R., *J. Med. Chem.*, **8**(1965), 502.

10 Schaeffer, H. J. and Bhargava, P. S., *Biochemistry,* **4**(1965), 71.

11 Colla, L., Busson, R., De Clercq, E. *et al.*, *Eur. J. Med. Chem.*, **17**(1982), 569.

12 Shealy, Y. F., O'Dell, C. A., Shannon, W. M. *et al.*, *J. Med. Chem.*, **27**(1984), 1416.

13 Shealy, Y. F., O'Dell, C. A. and Arnett, G., *J. Med. Chem.*, **30**(1987), 1090.

14 Mason, S. F., *J. Chem. Soc.*, (1965), 2071.

15 Clark, L. B. and Tinoco, I., Jr., *J. Am. Chem. Soc.*, **87**(1965), 11.

On Control Strategy of Environmental Carcinogens and the Catalytic Elimination of Carcinogenic Polycyclic Aromatic Hydrocarbons in Combustion Exhaust*

ZHENG Qingying, WANG Shoulan, SHI Xuejun, TAN Jianjun
CHI Guihong and DAI Qianhuan

(*Centre of Chemistry & Bioengineering of Cancer, Beijing Polytechnic University, Beijing* 100022, *China*)

Abstract The hypothesis of the authors is that PAH exhaust is the main reason of increasing cancer incidence ratio along with industrial development and population concentration. Systematic work has been done related to the catalytic elimination of polycyclic aromatic hydrocarbons (PAH) in various combustion exhausts. The elimination ratios of PAH in automobile, diesel engine and coal combustion exhausts, all reach to 95% by catalyses with three economic catalysts.

I. Introduction

It is a common estimation in chemical, environmental, epidemiological and health circles that 75% — 90% of all human cancers are evoked by environmental chemical factors. The World Health Organization was the first to propose this estimation[1]. Boyland estimated that 90% of human cancers are induced by chemical agents[2], and Higginson gave 80— 90% as his estimation for the chemical origin of human cancer[3]. In terms of the epidemiological investigation of cancer mortalities in China[4], some higher mortalities are related to certain environmental chemical factors. The southeast coastal areas of this country, such as Shanghai, Fujian and Guangxi provinces have the highest liver cancer mortality ratios, over 16 per 100,000 population, possibly due to mycotoxin pollution, the higher content of nitrite and nitrate in drinking water. In contrast the plateau and inland province Yunnan is the lowest area of liver cancer mortality, only 4.44 per 100,000 population, and is famous for its mild weather. As in other countries, Shanghai, a developed industrial city, has the highest mortalities of lung cancer which may be related to the higher level of PAH pollution in the atmosphere. The highest lung cancer mortality for women is in Xuanwei county of Yunnan Province, an area rich in bituminous coal. It is known that the combustion of soft coal produces a lot of methylated PAHs which easily induce cancer in the contacted organs of an animal. The incidence of cancer is closely related to the chemical factors in our environment,

* Project supported by the National Natural Science Foundation of China.

making it possible to take preventive measures.

The investigation of cancer incidence has shown what we might call the developmental cancer phenomenon. In undeveloped countries, the total cancer incidence or mortality always is relatively low, however, with industrial development and the improvement of people's living standards, cancer incidence and mortality always show an increase. In 1951, the mortality in Beijing was only 40.1 per hundred thousand population, but along with the development of industry and the increase in population density, the mortality in the same area per hundred thousand reached 93.3 in 1975. In terms of the statistical data in some cities, the total cancer mortality in this country before 1949 is estimated to be only about 30 per hundred thousand population. In 1990 a survey of causes of death was made in 72 counties and 32 cities in 22 provinces and regions around this country. This showed that the mortality rate of Chinese urban residents was 585.8 per 100,000 population, among which, the total cancer mortality rate was 146.45 per 100,000, i.e. about one fourth of all deaths were caused by cancer. Therefore, cancer has replaced cerebral and cardio-vascular diseases as the number one killer in Chinese cities. In the countryside, the mortality rate was 643.3 per 100,000 people, among which the deaths caused by cancer were 128.66, so about one fifth were cancer related. In the countryside, respiratory disease is the number one cause of death, and cancer is listed as the second. In summary, the total cancer mortality rate has been increased by four or five times in the past forty years. All developed countries have undergone the increase of cancer incidence or mortality rate, and now, the cancer incidence ratios have stabilized between 300—400 per 100,000 population.

In the process of development, people's diets usually show a great improvement with increase in protein content and the intake of more vitamins. This should be advantageous for protection against cancer diseases. However, it seems that the increase in cancer incidence and mortality rate is proceeding more quickly than the improvement in people's nutrition. In 1985, in an investigation of cancer mortality rates in China, Dai Qianhuan put forward a hypothesis to explain the environmental cancer phenomenon[5]. Currently social progress is accompanied by two aspects, one is the industrial and technical development, and the other is the population concentration. The results of industry development and population concentration give rise to increasing combustion processes, which produce more and more polycyclic aromatic hydrocarbons from coal combustion, automobile and diesel exhaust gases. Another reason might be related to n-nitroso compounds (NNC) originating from the increase of nitrites or nitrates in drinking water due to the increasing consumption of nitrogen contained food and fertilizer. The conditions under which grain is stored generally improves, so the mycotoxins have a negligible influence on the environmental cancer phenomenon. The development of fast food has not become very popular because of Chinese people's dietary customs, so the influence of PAHs and n-nitroso compounds present in fried meals and sausage type meat, respectively, might be neglected for the developmental cancer phenomenon in this country. Therefore, the PAH pollution exhausted from the increasing combustion processes, and the NNC formation *in vivo* by reaction between nitrite or nitrate in water or food, and nitrogen-containing compounds in more nutritious food, are probably the most important causes of developmental cancer.

Pollution in drinking water by nitrates or nitrites is easy to control through the administration by arousing public concern at least at present in this country. For example, the drinking water in the cities of Beijing and Tianjin is channeled from the neighbouring mountain areas, which not only benefits people's general health but is also advantageous for the protection against the potential risk of NNC. However, the control of PAH cannot be made by administrative measures, the remedy is to eliminate harmful PAH at source.

The exhaust of combustion processes has three main sources, i.e. the combustions of gasoline, diesel and coal. The most important exhausts come from automobiles, engines as well as industrial and domestic coal combustion. In recent years, systematic work relating to catalytic elimination of PAH in the exhausts from automobile, diesel machine and coal combustion, has been done in our laboratory. In this paper, we will briefly introduce this work.

II. Materials and Methods

Sampling: The particular substance is collected using a glass fiber circular cone, the organic substances are extracted with cyclohexane or chloroform, the solvent is concentrated to a given small volume, then chromatography on silica gel is used to collect the fluorescent part and concentrated again to give a small volume[6, 7].

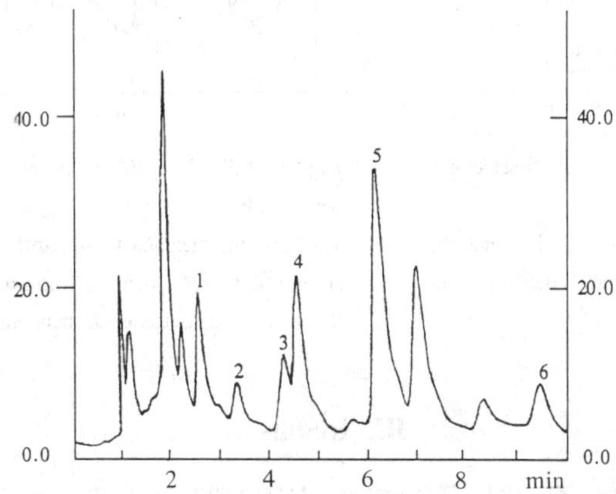

Fig. 1 HPLC of PAH in automobile exhaust before catalysis.
1, fluoranthene; 2, benz[a]pyrene; 3, benzo[b]- and benzo[k]fluoranthene; 4, benz[a]pyrene; 5, benzo[ghi]perylene; 6, coronene.

Analysis: The quantitative analyses of PAH are made on a Varian 8500 HPLC instrument with fluorescence detector[6]. The chromatograms of PAH contained in the exhaust of automobile, diesel engine and coal combustion by HPLC, respectively, before catalysis are listed in Figs. 1— 3.

Catalyst: ZD401 and ZD402 catalysts are cheaper metal oxides containing light rare earth metal oxides produced directly from the ore, and are different from others in the literature or patents. They do not contain precious metals, such as platinum, palladium and rhodium. The ZD403 catalyst is a monolithic honeycomb metallic support covered with suitable metals. One goal was to find the economic catalysts, all of which have possible practical applications.

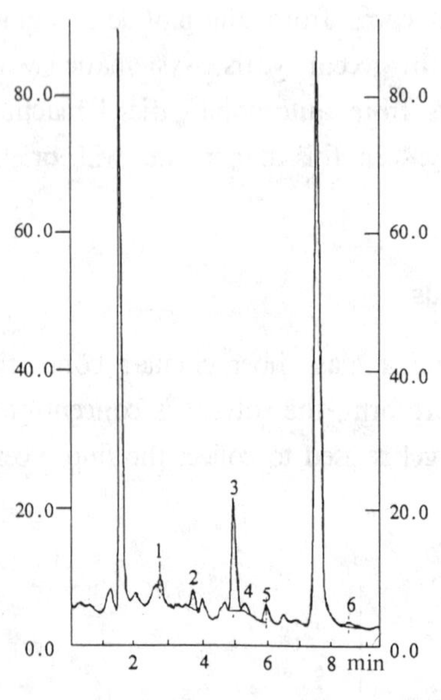

Fig. 2 HPLC of PAH in exhaust of diesel engine before catalysis.
1, fluoranthene; 2, benz[a]anthracene; 3, benzo[b]-fluoranthene; 4, benzo[k]fluoranthene; 5, benz[a]pyrene; 6, benz[ghi]perylene.

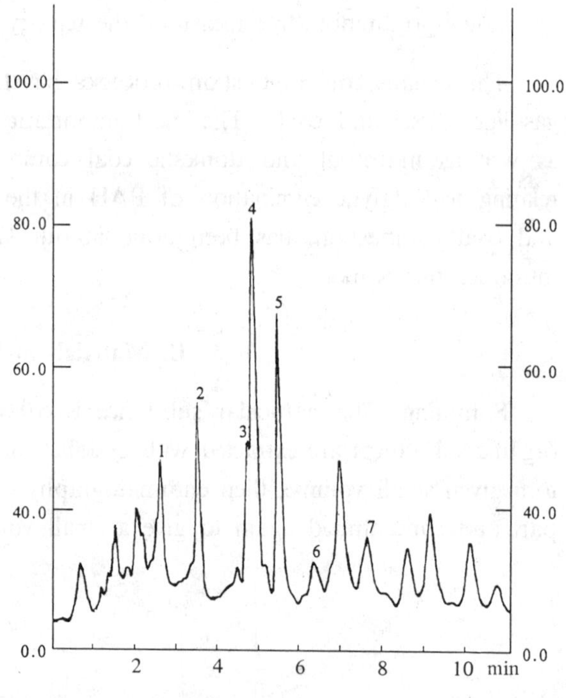

Fig. 3 HPLC of PAH in exhaust of coal combustion before catalysis.
1, fluoranthene; 2, benz[a]anthracene + chrysene; 3, benz[b]-fluoranthene; 4, benzo[k]fluoranthene; 5, benz[a]pyrene; 6, dibenz[a, h]anthracene; 7, benzo[ghi]perylene.

III. Results

The cheaper catalysts, ZD401, ZD402 and ZD403, are designed for the exhausts of automobile, diesel engine and coal combustion, respectively. The experiment on automobile uses the idle run with a Beijing 130 car as the model. The test on diesel engines uses the Beijing type 285 diesel engine as the model under real working conditions. For the exhaust of coal combustion, the honeycomb-form briquet made from coal powder together with the same content of lime and clay is used as the model material for the research. In the north of China, people use this form of briquet for fuel in winter. It is very interesting to note that combining the coal powder with lime and clay can lower the sulfer dioxide content to a level of 4 ppm.

The efficiencies of PAH elimination by all the three catalysts in the three conditions reach up to about 95%, which are almost the same as using not metal catalysts[8] in automobile or diesel engine exhausts. The results are listed in Table 1.

Table 1 Elimination Ratio of PAH in Various Combustion Exhausts

	Automobile Exhaust (idling 75 h.p.)	Diesel Engine (2040 r/min)	Coal Combustion (10.8 m^3 flue gas)
Fluoranthene	96%	96%	91%
Benz[a]anthracene	94%	98%	
Benz[a]anthracene + chrysene			93%
Benzo[b]fluoranthene	93%(with BkF)	99%	97%
Benzo[k]fluoranthene		94%	98%
Benz[a]pyrene	99%	96%	99%
Dibenz[a, h]anthracene			99%
Benzo[ghi]perylene	99%	95%	99%
Carbon monooxide	80%		49%
Low boiling point hydrocarbons	95%		
Smog degree		(0, from 1. 4)	
Sulfur dioxide		(0, from 4ppm)	

IV. Discussion

In the USA, Japan as well as in Europe, a legislation requiring control of emission from automobiles is already in force. This limits the emissions of total hydrocarbons, carbon monoxide and nitrogen oxide exhausted from gasoline and diesel engines of motor vehicles. However, although the PAH from various combustion processes have a potential carcinogenic risk, the legislation neglects PAH control. The reason for this omission might be that the catalytic elimination of PAH must use the noble metals as the catalyst. This paper for the first time demonstrates the possibility of using economic cheaper metal oxides as catalysts to eliminate the PAH. In the catalytic control of coal combustion exhaust, the elimination of PAH as well as sulfur dioxide, if it is only in a low concentration, can be realized simultaneously.

The di-region theory for carcinogenesis put forward in this laboratory[9] summarized that a chemical carcinogen (including PAH) must produce two reactive centers *in vivo*. The catalytic oxidation should destroy at least one of the potential reactive center even though the oxidation is not complete oxidation of the carcinogen to carbon dioxide. For example, benz[a]pyrene through partial chemical oxidation forms the 1, 6-, 3, 6- and 6, 12-quinones by attacking the 6-position with the lowest localization energy and three other positions with lower localization energies than that of other positions. In practice, the above three quinones are non-carcinogens, so it can be estimated that the catalytical oxidation would not cause secondary pollution. This idea in light of the di-region theory encourages our endeavour in the catalytical control of PAH. However, the corresponding mutation tests for the samples in exhausts after the catalyses are now, being undertaken in order to verify the harmlessness of the catalytical control.

It is very interesting to note from Table 1, that the carcinogenic PAHs, such as benz-[a]pyrene, are eliminated more effectively than the non-carcinogens, such as fluoranthene, because the former always possesses the position with lower localization energy which can offer the reactive epoxide *in vivo*, but the latter is often without the position of lower localization energy.

It might not be such an extravagant hope that we can control the discharge of PAH from every combustion exhaust and greatly lower cancer incidence in the not too distant future.

References

1 World Health Organization, *Prevention of Cancer, Technical Report Services,* (1964), pp. 1—53, Geneva.

2 Boyland, F., *Exp. Tumor Res.,* **11**(1969), 222—234.

3 Higginson, H., *Can. Cancer Conf.,* **8**(1969), 40—75.

4 Cancer Prevention Office of National Health Ministry, *The Investigation of Malignant Tumor Mortalities in China,* People's Health Press, Beijing, 1980.

5 Dai Qianhuan, Plenary Lecture on the 2nd Congress of Chinese Association of Environmental Sciences 1985, Beijing.

6 Lee, M. L., Novotny, M. V. and Bartle, K. D., *Analytical Chemistry of Polycyclic Aromatic Compounds,* Academic Press, New York, 1981.

7 George, M. B. *et al., Anal. Lett.,* **17**(1984), 1293—1306.

8 Acres, G. J. K., Harrison, B. and Wyatt. M., in *Mobile Source Emission Including Polycyclic Organic Species* (eds. Rondia, D. *et al.*), D. Reidel Publishing Company, 1983.

9 Dai Qianhuan, *Scientia Sinica,* **23**(1980), 464.

Storage and Active Forms of N-*myc* Oncoprotein in Mammalian Embryos and Their Role in Tumorigenesis and Embryogenesis

Hiroyuki Shimatake, Chizuru Nakagawa, Takahiko Yokoyama and Hiromichi Hemmi

(*Department of Molecular Biology, Toho University School of Medicine, Ohta-Ku, Tokyo 143, Japan*)

Abstract In the human late embryo, N-*myc* positive cells were detected in the brain, the neural crest and the renal tubules of the mesonephros as well as in the corresponding tumors. In contrast to the above "functional" N-*myc* protein, cleavage to blastocyst stage embryos were suggested to contain "storage" type N-*myc* protein in their cytoplasm.

The N-*myc* oncoprotein has never been found physiologically in postnatal tissues except under pathological circumstances such as neuroblastoma[1], retinoblastoma[2] and nephroblastoma. There have been several Northern blot studies to show that the N-*myc* gene is expressed during embryogenesis. These studies, however, have been unable to localize exactly which cells are responsible for the N-*myc* protein production, nor to detect possible storage-type N-*myc* protein in embryos, because of intrinsic limitations of the methods used. The N-*myc* gene is very rarely activated in human postnatal tissues, under pathological circumstances[3]. Although there have been Northern blot or *in situ* hybridization studies to detect the expression of the N-*myc* gene in embryos at mRNA level[4, 5], mere presence of the mRNA does not guarantee the presence of the N-*myc* protein in the embryo. Some species of mRNA are known to stay inactive in embryos[6] and we show evidence that the N-*myc* protein exists as a possible storage form in early mouse embryos.

I. Materials and Methods

The plasmid pTNB 8 that contained exon 2 of the human genomic N-*myc* gene was digested to isolate a DNA fragment that coded for the N-*myc* specific 85 amino acids[7]. The ligation product was transformed into the lysogen, N 4830[8]. Details of the construction procedures is published elsewhere[9]. Human neuroblastoma cells IMR 32 and TNB 1[10, 11] and human promyelocytic leukemia cells HL 60 as well as clinical samples of neuroblastoma, retinoblastoma and Wilms' tumors were examined by Western blotting with 10^{-3} dilution of the anti N-*myc* antibody and by immunohistochemistry with 3×10^{-2} dilution of the antibody.

A human embryo used for the present study was obtained by a legal abortion and the experiment was conducted with full approval of the Standing Advisory Committee on Ethics in Human Experimentation of the Toho University School of Medicine. The human embryo (7 weeks gestation) and early mouse embryos were fixed with Bouin's solution and then embedded in paraffin. The tissue preparations were de-paraffinized by ethanol series. Immunohistochemical examination was done with 3×10^{-2} dilution of the anti human N-*myc* serum for 18 hours. Samples were counter-stained with hematoxylin. Otherwise the Sternberger method was followed[12]. An absorption test done with neighboring sections gave negative immunoreactions. Other bacteriological, immunological and biochemical manipulations were according to the standard procedures[13].

II. Results and Discussion

The human N-*myc* protein was genetically engineered by inserting a human N-*myc* specific DNA clone into the universal gene expression vector, pCA 200 (Fig.1). The purified N-*myc* fusion protein was used to immunize rabbits, which typically reacted with 0.24 ng (6 fmol) of the antigen on dot ELISA at 10^{-4} dilution of the antiserum (data not shown).

Western blot analysis of the human neuroblastoma cell lines, IMR 32 and TNB 1, revealed the presence of two N-*myc* protein bands of 62 and 64 kDa (Fig.2). The antibody against the genetically engineered human N-*myc* fusion protein (anti N-*myc* antibody) reacted only with the N-*myc* protein of tumor cells, either natural or genetically engineered, and not with c-*myc* protein nor with other non N-*myc* proteins of tumor cells (Fig.2; lane C).

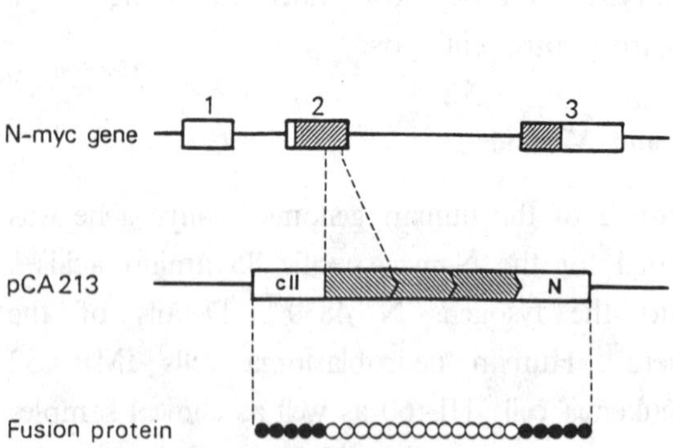

Fig.1 Construction of the N-*myc* expression vector pCA 213. DNA fragment of 225 bp that coded for 85 amino acids in exon-2 of the N-*myc* gene (top) was inserted to creat the N-*myc* expression vector pCA 213 (middle) that expressed a large amount of the human N-*myc* fusion protein (bottom).

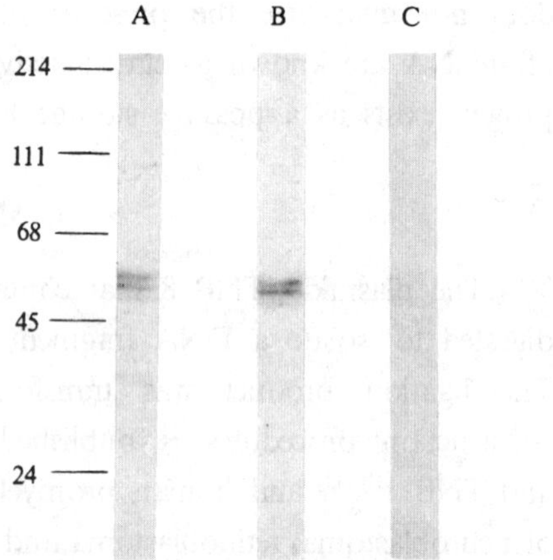

Fig.2. Western blot analysis of human tumor cells with N-*myc* antibody.
A, neuroblastoma IMR 32; B, neuroblastoma TNB 1; C, promyelocytic HL-60. For each strip 1×10^5 cells were loaded.

Clinical samples of human neuroblastoma and retinoblastoma (Figs. 3A and 3B, respectively) were examined by immunohistochemistry. Both of these pediatric tumor cells showed that the N-*myc* protein was localized in the nucleus. These tumors also showed the presence of the N-*myc* protein on Western blot analysis (data not shown). On immunohistochemical examination, the in ensity of the staining reaction differed from cell to cell. Neuroblastoma cells showed that various amounts of the N-*myc* protein were present among the same cell population on histological preparation (Fig. 3) as well as on fluorescence-activated cell sorting analysis (data not shown). This "heterogeneity" of N-*myc* protein staining could be partly explained by the fact that the amount of the N-*myc* protein in tumor cells fluctuated according to cell cycle progression. Even within the same phase of the cell cycle, however, greater fluctuation of the amount of the N-*myc* protein was observed (see accompanying paper; H. Shindo, CN, HH, SO, HS). Examination of Wilms' tumor by immunohistochemistry failed to detect the N-*myc* protein in our lab. Western blotting, however, was able to detect the N-*myc* protein in the tumor (data not shown). It was obvious that a smaller amount of the N-*myc* protein was expressed in the tumor than in neuroblastoma or in retinoblastoma (unpublished observation; CN, TT, HS). Summarized in Table 1 are the tissues that were examined for the expression of the N-*myc* protein.

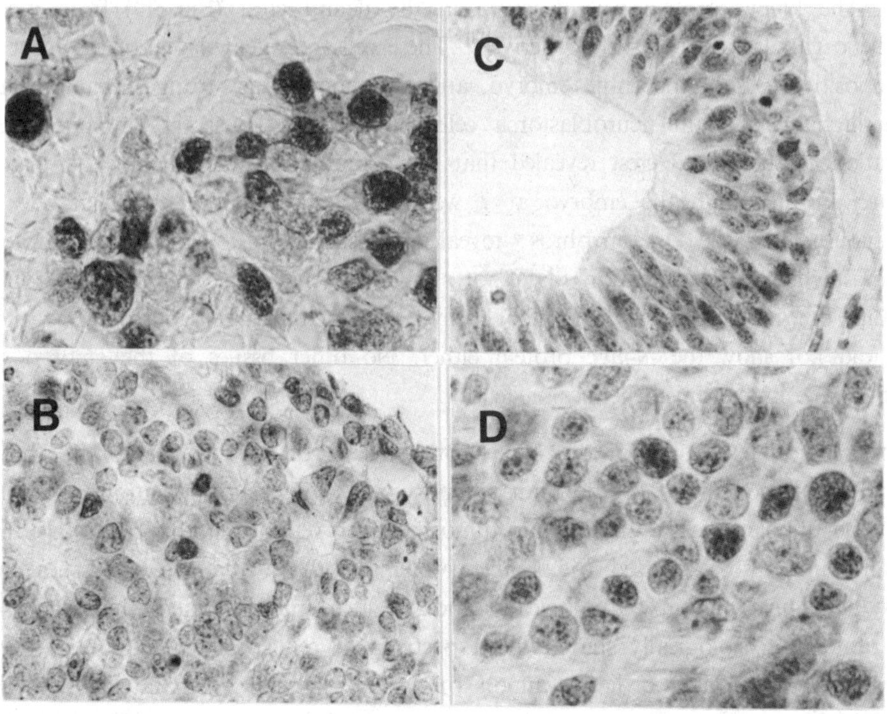

Fig.3 Immunohistochemical determination of the N-*myc* protein in clinical tumors (A, B) and human embryo (C, D).

A, human neuroblastoma; B, human retinoblastoma; C, brain near the optic stalk; D, neural crest.

Table 1 Identification of N-*myc* Protein With Anti-N-*myc* Antibody

	Western Blotting	Immunohistochemistry
Positive	**Neuroblastoma**	**Neuroblastoma**
	cell line: IMR 32, TNB 1	cell line: IMR32, TNB1
	xenograft: TNB9	xenograft: TNB9
	surgical samples	surgical samples
	Retinoblastoma	**Retinoblastoma**
	cell line: Y79	cell line: Y79
	surgical samples	surgical samples
	Others	**Others**
	Wilm's tumor cultured cell	embryonal cells
	mouse pre B cell line: 70Z3	(human and mouse)
Negative	leukemia cell line: HL-60	leukemia cell line: HL-60
	glioblastoma cell line: A-7	acoustic Schwannoma
	fibroblast	adult mouse tissue

Distribution of the N-*myc* protein through the whole embryo was examined by immunohistochemical procedures using the anti N-*myc* antibody. The N-*myc* protein was detected in neural cells of the mantle zone near the third ventricle of the brain where the optic stalk branched out (Fig.3C). Other areas of the brain were not immunoreactive. There was no immunoreaction in the optic cup nor in the optical stalk at this stage of the late embryo. The N-*myc* protein was observed in the neural crest (Fig. 3D) from where the sympathetic ganglia are believed to derive[14]. These cells represented one of the most intense immunopositive cells of the entire embryo, and they showed as strong immunoreaction as did the highly malignant neuroblastoma cells (see Fig. 3). Thus, the immunohistological examination of the neural crest revealed that the neural crest was one of the major sites of N-*myc* production in the embryo at 7 weeks of gestation. The epithelial cells of the renal tubules of the mesonephros revealed existence of the N-*myc* protein by immunohistochemical examination (data not shown). There was no immunoreaction in the glomerulus nor in the duct of the mesonephros. Mesenchymal cells surrounding the renal tubules did not show the N-*myc* protein either. No other tissues of the embryo showed positive N-*myc* immunohistochemical reaction.

Physiological expression of the N-*myc* protein was detected in the brain, the neural crest and the mesonephros of the human embryo of 7 weeks of gestation. Examinations of pediatric tumors revealed that certain tumors such as retinoblastoma, neuroblastoma and nephroblastoma also expressed the N-*myc* protein. Both of the tumors tissues that expressed the N-*myc* protein pathologically and the late embryo tissues that expressed the N-*myc* protein physiologically shared their spectrum of cell specificities. Only those tissues from which N-*myc* related pediatric tumors originate[15] later in postnatal life were the major sites of N-*myc* protein expression in the human embryo at 7 weeks of gestation (Table 2). It would be possible to postulate that the N-*myc* protein is an embryonal version of the c-*myc* protein, and further that the persistent expression of the N-*myc* protein beyond the

Table 2 N-*myc* Positive Tissues

Tumor	Late Embryo
Retinoblastoma	brain
Neuroblastoma	neural crest
Nephroblastoma	mesonephros

Table 3 Two Types of N-*myc* Protein

	"Functional" Type	"Storage" Type
Localization	necleus	cytoplasm
Distribution	heterogeneous	homogeneous
Tissue	late embryo tumor	early embryo

childbirth may be a cause of childhood N-*myc* tumors such as neuroblastoma. In addition, both tumors and late embryo tissues shared cytological features of N-*myc* protein expression: 1, The localization of the N-*myc* protein was confined inside the cell nucleus in both tissues; 2, the N-*myc* protein expressing cells were distributed not uniformly among tissues but "heterogeneous" expression of the N-*myc* protein was the common feature (see accompanying paper; H. Shindo, CN, HH, SO, HS).

We, then, examined early mouse embryos to trace the earliest stage of the embryo where the N-*myc* protein can be detected. Immunohistochemistry of the blastocyst stage mouse embryos revealed the presence of the N-*myc* protein in extra-embryonic and embryonic ectoderms. Surprisingly, however, the N-*myc* protein was located in the cytoplasmic compartment instead of the cell nucleus. Also, the distribution of the protein was uniform among the same tissue cells rather than "heterogeneous". Every blastomere of the 4-cell stage mouse cleavage embryo showed strong positive reaction of the N-*myc* protein. Again, intracellular localization was cytoplasmic and intercellular distribution was uniform. Negative control experiments where the antibody was pre-absorbed with the N-*myc* antigen gave very weak immunoreactions. Although the unfertilized mature eggs showed moderate immunohistological staining, western blot analysis revealed that the immuno-positive materials of the mature eggs run with the same mobility as the N-*myc* protein from neuroblastoma cells at 64 kD on SDS-PAGE (data not shown). The function of the cytoplasmic N-*myc* protein in the early embryos is not clear. Intracellular localization of the protein, however, suggests that the N-*myc* protein in the early embryos may not be a functional one but a "storage" form for later use during cleavage, blastoderm formation and organogenesis (Table 3). *Mos* oncoprotein is known to be present in unfertilized eggs and involved in meiosis[16]. The N-*myc* protein was more abundant in cleavage embryos rather than in unfertilized eggs, suggesting that the N-*myc* protein accumulates during cleavage to blastoderm formation stage of the embryogenesis in order to play its role for later organogenesis.

We gratefully acknowledge the excellent assistance of Hideki Fujii and Tetsuo Tsukahara.

References

1 Seeger, R. C., Brodeur, G. M., Sather, H. *et al.*, *New Engl. J. Med.*, **313**(1985), 1111.

2 Yokoyama, T., Tsukahara, T., Nakagawa, C. *et al.*, *Cancer*, **63**(1989), 2134.

3 Schwab, M., Ellison, J., Busch, M. *et al.*, *Proc. Natl. Acad. Sci. USA*, **81**(1984), 4940.

4 Grady, F. E., Schwab, M. and Rosenau, W., *Cancer Res.*, **4** (1987), 2931.

5 Mugrauer, G., Alt, F. W. and Ekblom, P., *J. Cell. Biol.*, **107**(1988), 1325.

6 Cascio, S. M. and Wasserman, P. M., *Develop. Biol.*, **89**(1982), 397.

7 Nakagawa, C., Kikuchi, T., Tsukahara, T. *et al.*, *J. Med. Soc. Toho Univ.* (Tokyo), **36**(1989), 199.

8 Shimatake, H. and Rosenberg, M., *Nature*, **292**(1981), 128.

9 Nakagawa, C., Tsukahara, T. and Shimatake, H., *J. Med. Soc. Toho Univ.* (Tokyo), **36**(1989), 207.

10 Shimatake, H., Kikuchi, T., Abe-Nakagawa, C. *et al.*, In *Advances in Neuroblastoma Research*, 2, (eds. Evans, A. E., *et al.*), Alan R Liss, New York, 1988, pp. 121—131.

11 Tsuchida, Y., Kanda, N., Shimatake, H. *et al.*, *Exp. Cell Biol.*, **56**(1988), 277.

12 Sternberger, L. A., Hgardy, P. H. Jr., Cuculis, J. J. *et al.*, *J. Histochem. Cytochem.*, **18**(1970), 315.

13 Maniatis, T., Fritsch, E. F. and Sambrook, J., *Mol. Cloning*, Cold Spring Harbor Lab., New York, 1982.

14 Hamilton, W. J. and Mossman, H. W., *Human Embryology, Prenatal Development of Form and Function*, Heffer, Cambridge, 1972.

15 Rudolph, A. M., *Pediatrics*, Appleton Lange, Norwark, 1987.

16 Sagata, N., Daar, I., Oskarsson, M. *et al.*, *Science*, **245**(1989), 643.

Synergism Between Environmental Ester Carcinogens

R. Schoental

(Department of Veterinary Pathology, The Royal Veterinary College, University of London, Royal College Street, London NW1 OTU, UK)

I. Introduction

I am grateful to the Organisers for their kind invitation to give a talk at this International Symposium on Recent Advances in Chemistry and Molecular Biology of Cancer in Beijing, and thank them for it.

Though unable to speak in person, I accepted the invitation because I wish to share with you my recent views, based on more than half a century of experimental research into various aspects of chemical carcinogenesis, mostly using lipophilic ester-compounds.

When I started my cancer studies, the prevailing accepted views were that cancer is mainly spontaneous, and possibly genetically predetermined. However, the fact that great differences exist in the incidence of certain cancers in specific geographical areas—— but disappear when people move to other countries, pointed to the existence of environmental factors which influence the incidence of cancer.

Concentrating on liver cancer, its particularly frequent incidence in countries which retained traditional treatment of diseases with herbal remedies, indicated involvement of toxic plants. Toxic plants belonging to the genus *Senecio* were known to cause liver damage when consumed by livestock, yet have been recommended as a remedy for a variety of disorders, by all the herbal books consulted, including a Chinese one[1, 2].

From a local herbalist we were able to obtain supplies of dried plants of the common ragwort, *Senecio jacobaea*. Using crude plant extracts, or isolated pure alkaloids (now known as pyrrolizidine alkaloids) tumours of the liver were induced in white rats treated intragastrically, even with only one, or a few doses. Young suckling rats developed liver damage when their lactating mothers received the alkaloids, while the mothers appeared mostly not affected by the treatment.

Results obtained using a number of other pyrrolizidine alkaloids, (some received as gifts from Roger Adams, D. H. G. Crout, C. C. J. Culvenor, J. R. Price and F. L. Warren) showed (a) that many of these toxic plant constituents can cause cancer (of the liver and of certain other organs); (b) that exposure to the alkaloids does not need to be continuous for the induction of tumours——a few, or even a single dose, may be sufficient; and (c) that the very young animals are significantly more susceptible to the toxic and carcinogenic action of these substances, than adults[3—5].

This work demonstrated that liver tumours are not necessarily `spontaneous' or predestined, but can be induced by environmental agents. A film was made partly in Ethiopia, and partly at the MRC Toxicology Research Unit, by Mr. R. F. Legg, in which are depicted some of the toxic plants used as herbal remedies, and the lesions produced in rats in comparison with those described in children suffering from kwashiorkor.

In subsequent studies of other types of naturally occurring substances, I selected certain mycotoxins[6], in particular certain secondary metabolites of the common, and almost ubiquitous soil microfungi, the *Fusaria*, namely T-2 toxin and zearalenone. Fusarial mycotoxins were known to have been the cause of much morbidity and mortality among the starving people in the Orienburg district of the USSR during World War II in the 1940s, who had to use, for making bread, mouldy cereals left in the fields, unharvested over the winter[7].

Tumours of various organs, especially of the stomach, developed in a number of rats given intragastrically a few doses of T-2 toxin, alone[8, 9] or in conjunction with zearalenone[10]; animals treated during the perinatal period were more often affected than when the initial dose was given to adult rats.

Other types of natural products, which are of importance in relation to animal and human health and cancer, are α, β unsaturated lactones[11] which include the mycotoxins, aflatoxins[12] and zearalenone[10]; azoxy compounds like cycasin[13] and elaiomycin[14, 15], and many others.

In this communication I propose to consider certain enzyme systems, which are likely to be involved in the detoxication of some of these toxic and carcinogenic substances.

II. The Role of Carboxylesterases/Amidases

In recent years the importance of the enzymes and isoenzymes, knwon as carboxylesterases/amidases, received much attention[16], particularly in relation to pesticides[17].

These types of enzymes, present in most animal tissues, especially in the liver and the brain, catalyse the hydrolysis (and esterification) of ester-, amide- and thioester-groups, replacing these by the more hydrophilic hydroxyls. Though in the past this aspect was little stressed, it is obvious that carcinogenic compounds must possess some degree of lipophilicity in order to be able to pass through a number of lipid membranes[18] in order to reach the critical target(s) in the cellular micro-organelles, whichever these may be.

Indeed, most of the carcinogens, which are known to act locally, at the site of application, are lipophilic, including the polycyclic aromatic hydrocarbons[19, 20], certain organo-halogen compounds[21], mycotoxins[6], certain nitroso compounds[22] and the co-carcinogen from croton oil, phorbol myristate acetate[23]. Certain other carcinogenic agents, e. g. aromatic amines, appear to be metabolically transformed by esterifying liver enzymes to more lipophilic derivatives, which then act locally and induce liver tumours; similar derivatives prepared synthetically induce sarcomas on subcutaneous injection[24].

III. Pyrrolizidine Alkaloids

The pyrrolizidine alkaloids, now known to be carcinogenic, are cyclic di-esters, like retrorsine (Fig. 1A) in which the sterically hindered ester groups are less readily hydrolysable than those of the open-di-ester alkaloids, like lasiocarpine (Fig.1B), and this is reflected in their respective toxicities (Table 1).

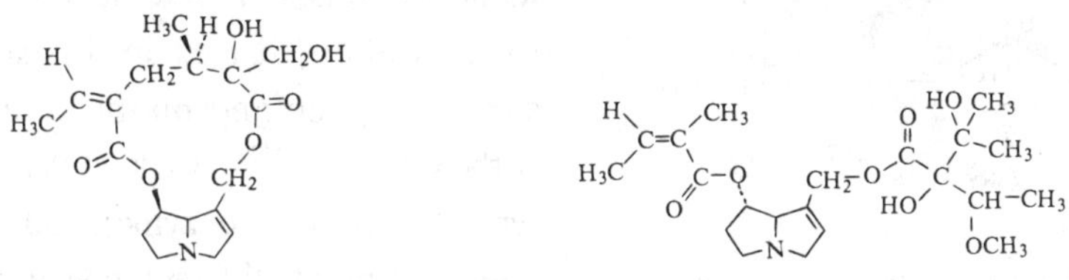

(A) Retrorsine (B) Lasiocarpine

Fig.1 Structures of pyrrolizidine alkaloids: retrorsine and lasiocarpine.

Table 1 Toxicity of Pyrrolizidine Alkaloids in Relation to Their Numbers of Ester Groups

Compound	Toxicity	No. of Ester Groups
Retrorsine	++++	2 (cyclic di-ester of retronecine)
Lasiocarpine	+++	2 (open di-ester of heliotridine)
Heliotrine	++	1 (mono-ester of heliotridine)
Heliotridine	±	0 (heliotridine-no ester groups)

Hydrolysis of one of the two ester groups in lasiocarpine yields heliotrine, which is about three times less toxic, while the hydrolysis of both the ester groups gives heliotridine, of hardly any activity (Table 1). It is not yet known whether the di-hydroxy-pyrrolizidine moieties can become esterified in the mammalian body by the tissues' carboxylesterases in accordance with the law of mass action, as the esterases under appropriate conditions can catalyse esterification[16].

The detoxication of pyrrolizidine alkaloids in the body is critically dependent on the respective carboxylesterases; during the perinatal period and early in life, young animals have yet to develop their full endowment of the carboxylesterases, hence their great susceptibility to the toxic (and carcinogenic) action of the pyrrolizidine alkaloids. Similar explanation applies to the variations in susceptibility of different animal species, e.g. guinea pigs, known to possess very effective systems of esterases, are more resistant than rats to the action of pyrrolizidine alkaloids.

Moreover, animals exposed to tri-*ortho*-cresyl phosphate, the known inhibitor of carboxylesterases, became more sensitive, and doses smaller than LD_{50} were sufficient to kill them[25].

IV. Trichothecenes

Among other natural carcinogenic esters, the trichothecene mycotoxin, the tri-ester T-2 toxin (Fig. 2) is indeed very toxic (its LD_{50} for rodents is less than 5 mg/kg body weight). On consecutive hydrolysis of its ester groups, the hydroxy-derivatives become significantly less toxic (Table 2) and less carcinogenic; T-2 tetraol is almost non-toxic. The LD_{50} of T-2 toxin is about halved in animals exposed to some organo-phosphorus inhibitors of carboxylesterases[26]. Cells differ in their content of esterase iso-enzymes, and may hydrolyse ester groups at different positions[27, 28].

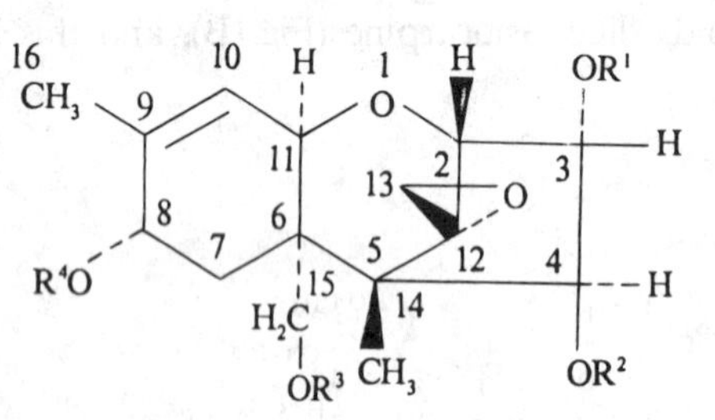

Fig. 2 Structure of T-2 toxin (4β, 15-diacetoxy-8-α (3-methylbutyryloxy)-12, 13-epoxytrichothec-9-en-3α-ol), a secondary metabolite of certain *Fusarium* microfungi. ($R^1=H$; $R^2=R^3=CH_3CO$; $R^4=(CH_3)_2CHCH_2CO$.)

It is fortunate that trichothecenes found to contaminate most frequently the staple cereals worldwide[29, 30] (including China[31, 32]), such as deoxynivalenol (DON), nivalenol (NIV), and zearalenone (which often accompanies the trichothecenes) are not as toxic as is T-2 toxin. However, the presence of mixtures may occasionally result in potentiation of toxicity; this we found using crude extracts of *Fusarium* cultures, which induced various tumours including oesophageal cancer[33].

Table 2 Toxicity of T-2 Toxi and Other Trichothecenes in Relation to the Number of Free Hydroxyls in Their Structures

Trichothecene	No. of Free HO-Groups	Toxicity
T-2 toxin	1	++++
HT-2 toxin	2	+++
T-2 triol	3	++
DON	3	+
T-2 tetraol	4	±

Synergistic effects have been reported between T-2 toxin and aflatoxin in skin tumours induction[34] and when combinations of *Fusarium* toxins were used[35]. Pyrrolizidine alkaloids and aflatoxin can also act synergistically in causing liver tumours[36].

V. Pesticides

Instances have been reported which indicate that certain organo-phosphorus compounds can potentiate the toxicity of other organo-phosphorus compounds about 2—5-fold. However, in the case of malathion more than 100-fold increase of its toxicity by tri-*ortho*-cresylphosphate was reported. This was considered exceptional by Hayes[37] who said: "Whether potentiation will be of any practical importance depends on its degree and on the chance a person or animal may have of simultaneous exposures to adequate amounts of two potentiating compounds. Potentiation as high as four- or five-fold, such as that seen with some organic phosphorus insecticides is of limited toxicological importance. The chance that a person or animal will encounter both members of a potentiating pair is smaller than the chance of encountering either one separately …. Potentiation may be of critical importance in isolated instances, but it is virtually impossible to predict them, partly because there may be no apparent —— and therefore predictive —— pharmacological relationship between the two compounds involved and also because the mechanismof their interaction may not be known initially …[37]".

In expressing these views, Hayes did not take into consideration the existence of mycotoxins, which under certain environmental conditions, can be present in agricultural products at high levels, just at a time when the farmers will be using pesticides more liberally in an effort to save their crops from further deterioration. Such conditions are not infrequent. One has then a difficult decision to make: whether to use pesticides at very high levels that would eliminate all pests, but may present serious hazards to animal and human health, (consuming the treated agricultural products), or to use levels of pesticides which only inhibit the visible growth. In the case of e.g. moulds, the latter will then tend to sporulate, and at this stage they may actually produce more mycotoxins than under less stressful conditions. Stimulation of the production of aflatoxins and of T-2 toxin by sorbic acid has been reported[38]. Similar production of more significant levels of toxic metabolites can occur when toxic plants are treated with herbicides; at present the outcome cannot be predicted[39—41].

Unexpected results have sometimes been reported after using organo-phosphorus compounds against warble-fly by skin application. Though this treatment is usually safe, occasionally individual animals, mostly calves, may develop paralysis and even die; apparently this may happen after the animals are exposed to ragwort (*Senecio jacobaea*), or other toxic agents[42]. However, as pyrethroids have recently been used in cowsheds, could this be a case of potentiation of their toxicity by organo-phosphorus inhibitors of carboxylesterase? Hydrolysis of the ester group in pyrethroids is critical for their detoxication in the mammalian body[43]. Examples of potentiation of the toxicity of pyrethroids by certain organo-phosphorus compounds have indeed been observed[44].

Cases of pyrethroid poisoning in China have been reported among agricultural workers using pyrethroids[45]. These pesticides are considered very safe but as yet no data are available of appropriate long-term tests for potential carcinogenicity. It would therefore be advisable and instructive to follow up the health of the Chinese workers who recovered from acute episodes of poisoning with pyrethroids.

VI. Summary

Attention is drawn to the prevailing disregard of the existence in the environment of natural toxic and carcinogenic agents produced by plants and by micro-organisms. These may increase the health hazards of individuals exposed concurrently to the modern pesticides, medicines and industrial chemicals. A number of mould products, known as mycotoxins (the aflatoxins, the trichothecenes and zearalenone; the ergot alkaloids, ochratoxin A, etc.) are lipophilic lactone- or ester-compounds, and as such can penetrate cellular membranes and reach the targets critical for the development of cancer. Among the primary defence mechanisms against these deleterious substances are tissue carboxylesterases/amidases, which catalyse hydrolysis of the respective ester or amide groups, and transform the xenobiotics into more hydrophilic and less toxic derivatives, readily degraded further, and eliminated in the urine. A number of the modern pesticides, notably some of the organo-phosphorus compounds, are known inhibitors of the carboxylesterases/amidases enzyme systems; accordingly, they prevent or delay the detoxication of the natural carcinogens, when acting concurrently, as occasionally can occur, and may act synergistically.

It is suggested that some of the unexpected results encountered in experimental and epidemiological studies of cancer (and of certain other disorders) may have been due to such synergism between chemically unrelated compounds, which, however, engage the same enzyme systems, and exhaust their potential for detoxication.

I thank Ms. Anna John for excellent secretarial help.

References

1 Schoental, R., In *Potential Carcinogenic Hazards from Drugs*, UICC Monograph Ser. 7 (ed. Truhaut, R.), 1967, pp. 152—161. Springer-Verlag, New York.

2 Read, B. E., *Chinese Medicinal Plants*, 3rd ed, Peking, 1936.

3 Schoental, R., *Israel J. Med. Sci.*, 4(1968), 1135—1145.

4 Schoental, R., in *Chemical Carcinogens, ACS Monograph* 173 (ed. Searle, C. E.), Washington DC, 1976, pp. 626—689.

5 World Health Organization, *Pyrrolizidine Alkaloids, Environmental Health Criteria* 80, WHO, 1988, Geneva.

6 Rodricks, J. V., Hesseltine, C. W. and Mehlman, M. A., *Mycotoxins in Human and Animal Health*, Pathotox, Park Forest South, 1977, I11.

7 Joffe, A. Z., *Fusarium Species, Their Biology and Toxicology*, Wiley Interscience, New York, 1986.

8 Schoental, R., Joffe, A. Z. and Yagen, B., *Cancer Res.*, **39**(1979), 2179—2189.

9 Schoental, R., *Front. Gastrointes. Res.*, **4**(1979), 17—24.

10 Schoental, R., *Adv. Cancer Res.*, **45**(1985), 217—290.

11 Dickens, F., in *Potential Carcinogenic Hazards from Drugs*, UICC Monographs Series 7 (ed. Truhaut, R.), Springer-Verlag, New York, 1967, pp. 144—151.

12 Busby, W. F. and Wogan, G. N., in *Chemical Carcinogens*, 2nd ed, ACS Monograph 182 (ed. Searle, C. E.), Washington DC, 1984, pp. 945—136.

13 Laqueur, G. L. and Matsumoto, H., in *Dietary Influences on Cancer, Traditional and Modern* (eds. Schoental, R. & Connors, T. A.), 1981, pp. 61—89, CRC Press, Boca Raton, Florida.

14 Schoental, R., *Nature*, **221**(1969), 761—766.

15 Schoental, R., in *Toxins of Animal and Plant Origin* (eds. de Vries, A. & Kochva, E.), Gordon and Breach, NY, 1972, pp. 781—789.

16 Heymann, E., in *Metabolic Basis of Detoxication, Metabolism of Functional Groups* (eds. Jacoby, W. B., Bend, J. R. & Caldwell, J.), Academic Press, New York, 1982, pp. 229—245.

17 Reiner, E., Aldridge, W. N. and Hoskin, F. C. G., eds., *Enzymes Hydrolysing Organophosphorus Compounds*, Ellis Horwood Ltd., Chichester, 1989.

18 Gurr, M. I. and Harwood, J. L., *Lipid Biochemistry: An Introduction*, 4th ed, 1991, Chapman Hall, London.

19 Schoental, R., in *Polycyclic Hydrocarbons* (ed. Clar, E.), Academic Press, London, 1964, pp. 133—160.

20 Dipple, A., Moschel, R. C. and Bigger, A. H., in *Chemical Carcinogens*, 2nd ed. ACS Monograph 182 (ed. Searie, C. E.), Washington DC, 1984, pp. 41—162.

21 Greim, H., and Wolff, T., in *Chemical Carcinogens*, 2nd ed. ACS Monograph 182 (ed. Searle, C. E), Washington DC, 1984, pp. 525—575.

22 Magee, P. N., Montesano, R. and Preussmann, R., in *Chemical Carcinogens*, ACS Monograph 173 (ed. Searle, C. E.), Washington DC, 1976, pp. 491—625.

23 van Duuren, B. L., in *Chemical Carcinogens*, ACS Monograph 173(ed. Searle, C. E.), Washingon DC, 1976, pp. 24—51.

24 Garner, R. C., Martin, C. N. and Clayson, D. B., in *Chemical Carcinogens*, ACS Monograph 182 (ed. Searle, C. E.), Washingon DC, 1984, pp. 175—276.

25 Bull, L. B., Culvenor, C. C. J. and Dick, A. J., *The Pyrrolizidine Alkaloids*, 1968, North-Holland, Amsterdam.

26 Johnsen, H., Odden, E., Lie, O. *et al.*, *Biochem. Pharmacol.*, **35**(1986), 1469—1473.

27 Johnsen, H., Odden, E., Lie, O. *et al.*, *Biochem. Pharmacol.*, **37**(1988), 3139—3197.

28 Schoental, R., *Biochem. Soc. Trans.*, **17**(1989), 475—476.

29 World Health Organization, *Selected Mycotoxins: Ochratoxins, Trichothecenes, Ergot*, Environmental Health Criteria 105, WHO, 1990, Geneva.

30 Tanaka, T., Hasegawa, A., Yamamoto, S. *et al.*, *J. Agric. Food. Chem.*, **36**(1988), 979—983.

31 Ueno, Y., Lee, U. S., Tanaka, T. *et al.*, *Toxicon*, **24**(1986), 18—21.

32 Qiujie, X., Xiaoqiu, L., Jianli, W. *et al.*, *Zhonghuazhongliuzazi*, **10**(1988), 4—8, quoted in *WHO Environmental Health Criteria* 105, WHO, Geneva.

33 Schoental, R. and Joffe, A. Z., *J. Path.*, **112**(1974), 37—42.

34 Lindenfelser, L. A., Lillehoj, E. B. and Burmeister, H. R., *JNCI*, **52**(1974), 113—116.

35 Bhavanishankar, T. R., Ramesh, H. P. and Shantha, T., *Arch Toxicol.*, **61**(1988), 241—244.

36 Newberne, P. M. and Rogers, A. E., *Plant Foods Man.*, **1**(1973), 23—31.

37 Hayes, H. J. Jr.., in *Handbook of Pesticide Toxicology* (eds. Hayes, H. J. Jr. & Laws, E. R. Jr.), Academic Press, San Diego, California, 1991, pp. 39—105.

38 Garcia, M., Bauer, J., Von Montgelas, A. *et al.*, *Appl. Environ. Microbiol.*, **47**(1984), 416—418.

39 Williams, M. C. and James, L. F., *Amer. J. Vet. Res.*, **44**(1983), 2420—2422.

40 Lydon, J. and Duke, S. O., *Pestic. Sci.*, **25**(1989), 361—373.
41 Schoental, R., *J. Appl. Toxicol.*, **11**(1991), 75.
42 Andrews, A. H., *Vet Rec.*, **109**(1981), 171—175.
43 Ray, D. E., in *Handbook of Pesticide Toxicology* (eds. Hayes, W. J. Jr. & Laws, E. R. Jr.), Academic Press, NY, pp. 585—636.
44 Gaughan, L. C., Engel J. L. and Casida, J. E., *Pestic. Biochem. Physiol.*, **14**(1980), 81—85.
45 He, F., Wang, S., Liu, L. *et al.*, *Arch. Toxicol.*, **63**(1989), 54—58.

Study on Cyclonucleotides

ZHANG Lihe

(*Research Laboratories of Natural and Biomimetic Drugs, Beijing Medical University, Beijing* 100083, *China*)

Abstract New methods have been developed for synthesizing Cyclic Nucleotides and the stereochemistry of the cyclophosphorylation of nucleosides has been investigated. It is reported that modification of the cyclophosphate moiety in cyclonucleotides is significant for developing new drugs.

Recently there has been considerable attention given to 3′, 5′-cyclic nucleotides because of their important biological and biochemical activities. There is solid evidence that c-AMP and c-GMP do have a role in regulation of cellular proliferation in mammalian cells.

A number of papers have appeared which reported the syntheses of analogues and derivatives of 3′, 5′-cyclic nucleotides, the interaction of cyclic nucleotide analogues with isolated enzymes, and the activities of these analogues *in vivo* and *in vitro*. Some analogues of cyclic nucleotides have been used as targets for developing new drugs. It was reported that site-selective cyclic AMP analogues inhibit growth and induce changes in morphology in a spectrum of human cancer cell lines. Differential regulation of type I versus type II protein kinase is involved in the inhibition of human cancer cell growth by site-selective cAMP analogues. 8-Cl-cAMP, the most potent site-selective cAMP analogue, is now in preclinical Phase I studies at the National Cancer Institute[1]. If some analogues of cyclic nucleotides are to be used as drugs, these compounds would have to have penetrability, stability to phosphodiesterase and specific activity to protein kinase. Modification of the cyclic phosphate ring is the target of this research. The chemistry and biological activities of cyclic nucleotides modified on the cyclic phosphate ring are reported here.

I. Chemistry of Cyclic Nucleotides

It was found that the phosphate moiety of cyclic nucleotides was low in chemical reactivity and the P—O bond was not easily cleaved by reagents during the synthesis of nucleoside 3′, 5′-cyclic phosphotriesters and phosphoramidates[2]. On the other hand, the solubility of cyclic nucleotides in organic solvents limits the syntheses of phosphotriesters and phosphoramidates in good yields. Some new synthetic methods have been investigated[3—13].

Starting from c-AMP, c-AMP phosphotriesters and phosphoramidates were obtained by esterification or amidation, but the products were a mixture of stereoisomers. Protected nucleosides reacted with trivalent or pentavalent phosphorus reagents to give nucleoside 3′, 5′-cyclic phosphites or nucleoside 3′, 5′-cyclic phosphates by cyclophosphorylation in very good yield. Nucleoside 3′, 5′-cyclic phosphites could be converted to the corresponding cyclic phosphates or cyclic thiophosphates by reacting with iodine or sulfur. The reaction occurred stereospecifically. The configuration of phosphorus in these derivatives can be inverted by treatment of base or F^-.

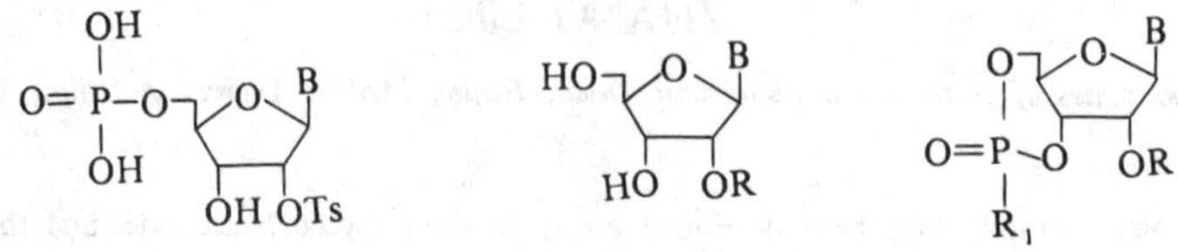

B = Adenine, Guanine, Cytosine, Uracil

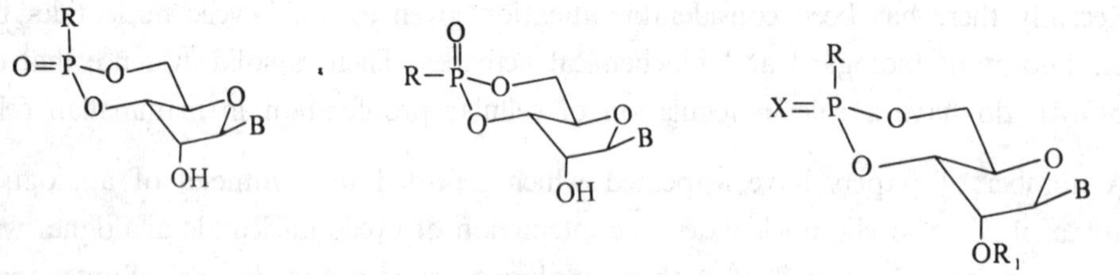

1 $R=OC_4H_9$-*n*, B=A
3 $R=OCH_2Ph$, B=A
5 R=Cyclohexylamino, B=A
7 $R=OC_4H_9$-*n*, $B=G^{DMF}$

2 $R=OC_4H_9$-*n*, B=A
4 $R=OCH_2Ph$, B=A
6 R=Cyclohexylamino, B=A
8 $R=OC_4H_9$-*n*, $B=G^{DMF}$

9 X=S, $R=N(C_2H_5)_2$
R_1=H, B=A

II. Biological Activities of Cyclonucleotides

1. *Effects of Adenosine 3′, 5′-cyclophosphotriesters and Adenosine 3′, 5′-cyclophosphoramidates on the Growth of Tumor Cells*

At the concentrations of 3.3×10^{-7}—3.3×10^{-13} mol/ml, c-AMP, c-GMP and adenosine 3′, 5′-cyclophosphotriesters showed no effect on the activity of DNA polymerase α of isolated Ehrlish ascites tumor cells. But at a concentration of 5×10^{-7}mol/ml, c-AMP and its triesters inhibited the activity of DNA polymerase α from intact Ehrlish ascites tumor cells. No effect was observed in the case of adenosine 3′5′-cyclophosphoramidates[14](Table 1).

Table 1 Effects of Derivatives of c-AMP on DNA Polymerase α From Intact Ehrlich Ascites Tumor Cells

Compd.	Conc. (mol/ml)	Case	Inhibition (%) ($\overline{x}\pm S_{\overline{x}}$)	$P^{a)}$
c-AMP	5×10^{-7}	6	3.33±8.9	<0.02
c-GMP	″	6	−9 ±6.1	
1	″	6	30.04±6.56	<0.01
2	″	6	33.65±6.88	<0.01
3	″	5	41.6 ±9.73	<0.02
4	″	10	38.64±5.29	<0.01
5	″	8	7.6 ±5.82	>0.02
6	″	6	6.3 ±6.1	>0.02

a) Compared with control (100%).

Gohil *et al.* suggested that c-AMP phosphotriesters might be easily transported into cells and then they might liberate c-AMP. These analogues could be used as prodrugs or drug-delivery forms. On the contrary, it was found that compound **4** can be transported into cell but cannot liberate c-AMP in the cell. Compound **4** was labeled with ^{3}H on the benzyl moiety, ^{3}H l beled **4** was cultured with Ehrlish ascites tumor cells for 4 h. The tumor cells were washed thoroughly to remove ^{3}H labeled **4** then the cells were crushed and extracted. The extract was purified on silica gel TLC to give ^{3}H labeled **4**. This result showed that compound **4** was stable in the cell under the culture conditions for 4 h. The effects on the activities of liver phosphodiesterase by compounds **3**, **4**, **5**, **6**, were investigated. It showed that compounds **3** and **4** can inhibit significantly the activities of liver phosphodiesterase but compounds **5** and **6** have no effect (Table 2).

Table 2 The Effects on the Activities of Liver Phosphodiesterase by Derivatives of c-AMP

Compound (20 n mol)	Inhibition of Liver Phosphodiesterase (%)	
	normal mice	hepatoma
4	66.5	79.5
3	68.0	72
6	27	29
5	26	32.5

c-AMP has long been considered to have a role in the control of cell growth and differentiation in a variety of cell types. c-AMP exerts its effect in eukaryötes by binding to the regulatory subunits of either type I or type II c-AMP-dependent protein kinase. Mayer reported that substitution of or on the phosphate itself was deleterious to its activity in stimulating c-AMP dependent protein kinases. Jastoff suggested that the lack of activity of all cyclic phosphate ring modified analogues was due to a steric effect. We found that compounds **4**, **3** had an effect very similar to c-AMP on the activities of protein kinases[15] (Table 3).

Table 3 The Effects on Activities of Protein Kinases by Derivatives of c-AMP

Compd.	Compd. I_{50}/c-AMP I_{50}		
	Protein kinase from rabbit skeleton muscle	Protein kinase from normal mice liver	Protein kinase from mice hepatoma
c-AMP	1	1	1
2	60.2	412	737
1	210	441	50
4	1	1.5	0.93
3	0.71	1	0.75
6	>8000	>8000	>8000
5	>8000	>8000	>8000

From experimental data of Table 3, it can be seen that the cyclic phosphate ring was extremely sensitive to modification. But it seems there is no effect on the activity of the protein kinase whether the benzyl group is axial (**3**) or equatorial (**4**). All things considered, some site-selective c-AMP analogues could be found from the cyclic phosphate ring modified analogues.

2. *Effects on the Growth of Tumor Cells by c-UMP*

c-UMP was synthesized by a known method and its effect on growth of Ehrlich ascites tumor cells was investigated. The data showed that c-UMP can inhibit the syntheses of DNA and RNA in Ehrlish ascites tumor cells, the inhibition depended on the concentration of c-UMP (Table 4).

Table 4 Effects on the Syntheses of DNA and RNA in Ehrlish Ascites Tumor Cell

Conc. of c-UMP ($mol \cdot L^{-1}/10^6$ cells)	Inhibition of Synthesis of DNA		Inhibition of Synthesis of RNA	
	cases	%	cases	%
10^{-6}	10	89.2	6	90.5
10^{-7}	10	47.1	6	47.3
10^{-8}	10	24.2	6	30.1
10^{-9}	10	9.3	6	16.7
10^{-10}	10	1.7	4	3.1
10^{-11}	5	0	3	0

After Ehrlish ascites tumor cells had been incubated with c-UMP (10^{-7} $mol \cdot L^{-1}/10^6$ cells) no effect on the level of c-AMP in the cells was observed, but the level of c-GMP in the cells was increased significantly (38.3%, $P < 0.005$). The mechanism suggested was that c-UMP can inhibit the activity of c-GMP-dependent phosphodiesterase but has no effect on c-AMP-dependent phosphodiesterase (Table 5).

Table 5 Effect on the Activities of c-AMP-dependent Phosphodiesterase and c-GMP-dependent Phosphodiesterase by c-UMP

Conc. of c-UMP (mol/L)	Rate of Hydrolysis (%) c-AMP	Rate of Hydrolysis (%) c-GMP
10^{-6}	60.2	13.6
10^{-7}	62.7	34.1
10^{-8}	64.3	52.0
10^{-10}	63.5	55.1
10^{-12}	62.9	58.2
0	63.1	59.6

Although the level of c-GMP was increased in tumor cells, it was lower than the level which could cause the proliferation of the cell cycle. Previous studies showing growth inhibition by c-AMP have tended to use higher concentrations of dibutyryl-c-AMP or other agents which could increase the level of c-AMP in cells. The effect of c-UMP may not be mediated through c-AMP. Experimental data showed that c-UMP could competitively combine with c-AMP-dependent protein kinase (Table 6).

Table 6 Competitive Combination With c-AMP-dependent Protein Kinase by c-UMP in Ehrlish Ascite Tumor Cells

Conc. of c-UMP (mol/L)	10^{-6}	10^{-7}	10^{-8}	10^{-9}	10^{-10}	10^{-11}	10^{-12}
Combination rate of c-AMP-dependent PK by c-AMP (%)	2.4	2.7	11.7	35.2	55.5	83.9	85.6
Combination rate of c-AMP-dependent PK by c-UMP (%)	97.6	97.3	88.3	64.8	44.5	16.1	14.4

This study might open a way to the synthesis of some c-UMP derivatives which could mimic the effects of c-AMP as intracellular regulatory agent.

3. *The Effect of Cyclonucleotides on Adenylate Cyclase Activity*

Rat osteosarcoma clonal cell line (ROS 17/2.8) is a target cell of parathyroid hormone (PTH). The binding of PTH with its receptor on ROS cell will stimulate adenylate cyclase activity. The effects of different kinds of nucleotides on adenylate cyclase activity were examined. The results showed that AMP, GMP, UMP, CMP or adenosine alone had no significant effect on adenylate cyclase activity, but they might inhibit the stimulating effect of PTH. On the other hand, derivatives of c-GMP did increase the response of adenylate cyclase activity to PTH significantly (Table 7).

Table 7 Compounds **7** and **8** on the Activity of Adenylate Cyclase in Osteoblastic Cell ROS 17/2.8

Compd.	Conc. (μmol/L)	^{3}H c-AMP (dpm)	Compd.	Conc. (μmol/L)	^{3}H c-AMP (dpm)
Control		727±106	Control		845±275
PTH	10	4232±205	PTH	10	6557±803
7	150	3257±30	8	150	1471±288
PTH+7	10+150	11857±1100	PTH+8	10+150	9470±1394

The result suggested that the derivatives of c-GMP might stimulate G protein and increase the activity of adenylate cyclase[10].

4. *Effect of c-GMP, c-AMP and Their Derivatives on the Transcription System of Isolated Rat Liver Nuclei*

In order to estimate the relative transcription activities of RNA polymerase I and II, two transcription systems were set up from isolated rat liver nuclei with or without added amanitin and with reduced concentration of KCl as inhibitors to RNase I and II.

The effects of four cyclic nucleotides on different RNA polymerase were observed. The result showed that c-GMP might increase the activity of polymerase I, while c-AMP could increase the activity of RNA polymerase II. These effects could be intensified by using compounds **1**, **2** or **9**.

In summary, the biological activities of cyclonucleotides were investigated, and it was found that the cyclic phosphate ring was extremely sensitive to modification. Compounds **3** and **4** can penetrate the cell membrane, inhibit the activities of phosphodiesterase in mice liver and stimulate the activities of protein kinase from different sources. c-UMP could mimic the activities of c-AMP by combining with the protein kinase and inhibit the growth of tumor cells. The derivatives of c-GMP could increase the response of adenylate cyclase activity to PTH significantly. The result suggested that compounds **7** and **8** might stimulate G protein and increase the activity of adenylate cyclase. Compounds, **1**, **2** and **9** could increase the activity of RNA polymerase II.

References

1 Ally, A. *et al.*, *Proc. Natl. Acad. Sci. USA*, **85**(1988), 6319.
2 a. Bentrude, W. G. and Tomasz, J., *Synthesis*, **1**(1984), 27.
b. Beres, J. *et al.*, *J. Org. Chem.*, **50**(1985), 1271.
3 Wang Xu and Zhang Li-he, *Acta Pharmaceutica Sinica*, **15**(1980), 7: 396.
4 Zhang Li-he and Ma Ling-tai, *Chemistry* (in Chinese), **12**(1980), 14.
5 Chen Tian-rong, Zhang Yong-min and Zhang Li-he, *J. of Beijing Medical University*, **20**(1988), 5: 351.
6 Zhang Li-he *et al.*, *Chemical J. of Chinese Universities*, **6**(1985), 10: 903.
7 Wang Cong-hui *et al.*, *Acta Chimica Sinica*, **41**(1983), 5: 435.
8 Wu Jin-chang, Wang Chun-guang and Zhang Li-he, *Acta Chimica Sinica*, **44**(1986), 635.
9 Xu Chen and Zhang Li-he, *Chemical J. of Chinese Universities*, **10**(1989), **5**: 549.
10 Cai Hai-ying and Zhang Li-he, *Acta Pharmaceutical Sinica*, **24**(1989), 10: 726.
11 Wang Chun-guang, Dai Yuan-peng, Zhang Li-he, *Acta Pharmaceutical Sinica*, **24**(1989), 11: 872.
12 Chen Xi, Zhang Jun-dong and Zhang Li-he, *Synthesis*, **5**(1989), 383.
13 Zhang Li-he *et al.*, *Pharmaceutical Industry* (in Chinese), **19**(1988), 4: 154.
14 Ge Yun-qin *et al.*, *J. of Beijing Medical University*, **18**(1986), 1: 7.
15 Zhang Li-he *et al.*, *Kexue Tongbao*, **29**(1984), 820.

The Cross-linking Ability Between DNA Double Strands as a New Method for the Identification of Carcinogens

PEI Shu, ZHU Xujing, XIANG Mang, ZHANG Liguo, YANG Lixin

(Beijing Institute of Labor Hygiene and Occupational Disease, Beijing 100020, *China)*

and DAI Qianhuan

(Centre of Chemistry & Bioengineering of Cancer, Beijing Polytechnic University, Beijing 100022, *China)*

Abstract It has been evidenced by alkaline elution method that four carcinogenic aromatic amines, 2-aminofluorene, 2-naphthylamine, 4-aminobiplenyl and benzidine, offer significant cross-linking products between DNA and DNA/protein in cell cultures and show positive dose-correlation between 5 mole and 100 mole concentrations. However, no cross-linking products can be detected in the cultures with three non-carcinogenic aromatic amines, m-toluidine, 1-naphthylamine and 2-aminobiphenyl, from 100 μmole even to 1000 μmole concentrations. These experiments evidence the mechanism of carcinogenesis summarized by di-region theory, which discovered for the first time the importance of the cross-linking between complementary base pairs in DNA as well as the mutation of transcription control genes for the carcinogenesis or oncogenesis. The cross-linking method formulated in this paper might be a new experimental method for the short-term predictive screening of chemical carcinogens.

In recent years, the use of the relationship between chemical structure and carcinogenic activity to predict chemical carcinogenesis has been widely studied. Based upon this relationship, Dai Qianhuan put forward di-region theory[1], which was based on the discovery that the key step to carcinogenesis is the cross-linking between the DNA complementary base pairs. This type of cross-linking would induce a complementary frameshift mutation. Once this mutation transfers even very remote transcription genes into reverse transcription genes after a long incubation period, normal cells would become cancer cells through reverse transcription. Therefore the measurement of the cross-linking effect on DNA is a crux for the identification of carcinogens. In this research, the cross-linking abilities of aromatic amines have been measured *in vitro* to verify the relationship between the theoretical calculations and the experimental results.

I. Materials and Method

The method of Kohn[2] and Erickson was used[3]. The procedure includes the techniques of alkaline elution and fluorimetric analysis of DNA.

Culture of cells. L_{1210} mouse leukemia cells were maintained in a suspension culture in

RPMI 1640 medium, supplemented with 10 — 20% heat-inactivated fetal calf serum, penicillin and streptomycin. During the exponential growth phase when the cells were doubling every 12 h, the solution was diluted to a concentration of 1.0×10^6 cells/ml. These cells were used for the treatment with the drugs.

Drug treatment. The drugs used were the following 7 aromatic amines: 2-aminofluorene (2-AF), 4-aminobiphenyl (4-AB), 2-naphthylamine (2-NA), benzidine, m-toluidine (M-T), 2-aminobiphenyl (2-AB) and 1-naphthylamine (1-NA). They were added to the cultures of L_{1210} cells and shaken with an S9 mixed solution for 3.5 h. Drug exposure was terminated by centrifuging it twice, resuspending in fresh 1640 medium, and culturing for 12h.

Irradiation. Cells were chilled on ice and irradiated with 1000-R of γ-rays.

Alkaline elution. Following the irradiation, the cells were deposited by a mild suction on a filter of pore size 1.2 μm, and washed with ice-cold PBS (Phosphate Buffer Solution). The cells were lysed immediately with Triton X-100 and then an alkaline solution of pH 12.1 was added and pumped through the filter at a rate of 0.04 ml/min. Three 5ml fractions were collected. At the end of the elution, the filter was soaked in alkali solution at 56°C for 3.5h to extract the DNA.

Fluorescence measurement. In the eluted fraction and the extracted solution, the DNA was recovered by adding fetal calf serum albumin and trichloroacetic acid. The samples were mixed and chilled at 4°C overnight. The DNA was collected by centrifugation and washed with absolute ethanol. The precipitate was dried at 70°C. Following drying, diaminobenzoic acid (DABA) was added and the mixture heated at 60°C for 30 min. After being cooled, perchloric acid was added and the mixture centrifuged. The fluoresence was determined at an excitation wavelength of 408 nm and an emission wavelength of 495 nm.

Calculation of results. The DNA cross-linking ability was calculated from the following formula:

$$R=\frac{R_1-R_2}{R_1}\times 100\%,$$

where R_1 is the retention rate of DNA on the filter for drug treated cells. R_2 is the retention rate of DNA on the filter for untreated cell. R is the relative retention rate of DNA on the filter. If the value of R is dose-dependent, the drug can then damage the DNA by cross-linking.

II. Results

The results of the study of the cross-linking effect on DNA of the 7 amines are as follows.

1. 2-AF. The results of the treatment of cells with 2-AF are presented in Table 1.

Table 1 Relative Retention of DNA on the Filter for 2-AF Treated Cells

Concentration (μmol/L)	10	50	80	100
Cross-linking ratio R (%)	10.74	15.80	21.40	45.93
ln (R)	2.37	2.76	3.06	3.82

Table 1 shows that the R values increased significantly, especially at high concentrations (100 μmol/L). Statistically, this result indicates that the cross-linking ability of 2-AF is dose-dependent with correlation coefficient, $\gamma=0.9408$, standard error, $S=0.1807$, $P<0.05$ and $Y=2.1185+0.0148X$, where Y was natural logarithmic.

2. 2-NA

Table 2 Relative Retention of DNA for Various Concentrations of 2-NA Treated Cells

Concentration (μmol/L)	10	50	80	100
Cross-linking ratio R (%)	2.37	19.76	42.29	50.20
ln (R)	0.86	2.98	3.71	3.91

Table 2 shows that a statistically significant correlation exists between the cross-linking effect and the concentration of 2-NA with $\gamma=0.9623$, $S=0.3299$ and $Y=0.8087+0.0345X$. There is a good linear relationship.

3. 4-AB

Table 3 Relative Retention of DNA for Various Concentrations of 4-AB

Concentration (μmol/L)	5	10	50	100
Cross-linking ratio R (%)	13.44	18.75	23.20	31.38
ln (R)	2.59	2.93	3.14	3.44

Table 3 shows that the R values increased along the concentration with $\gamma=0.9367$, $S=0.1082$, $P<0.05$ and $Y=2.7167+0.0076X$.

4. Benzidine

Table 4 Relative Retention of DNA for Various Concentrations of Benzidine Treated Cells

Concentration (μmol/L)	10	25	50	100
R (%)	18.71	20.21	40.20	48.8
ln (R)	2.92	3.00	3.69	3.88

Statistically, the R values for benzidine treated cells show $\gamma=0.9232$, $S=0.1606$, $P<0.05$ and $Y=2.8566+0.0133X$. However, at concentration of 100 μmol/L, the R value did not increase so markedly as with a concentration of 50 μmol/L.

5. The other three aromatic amines did not show a cross-linking effect even at a concentration of 1000 μmol/L for m-toluidine or at concentration of 100 μmol/L for 2-AB (an isomer of 4-AB) and for 1-NA (an isomer of 2-NA).

The correlations between dose and cross-linking ratio of DNA in L_{1210} culture for four carcinogenic aromatic amines are illustrated in Fig.1.

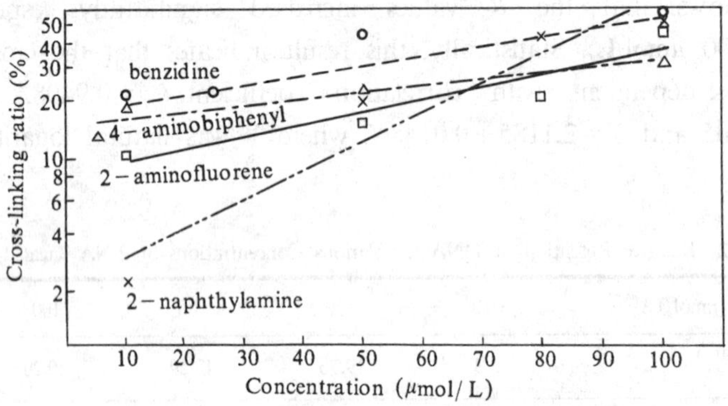

Fig.1 The correlations between concentration and inducing cross-linking ratio in DNA for four carcinogenic aromatic amines, 2-naphthylamine (×), 2-aminofluorene (□), 4-aminobiphenyl (△) and benzidine (○) after being cultivated.

III. Discussion

It is known that after the cultivation of bifunctional alkylation agent in normal mammal cell culture, such as with embryo cell, only the cross-linking product between histone and DNA single strand can be detected. However, in the cultures of cancer cell and prokaryotic cell, the cross-linking products between DNA double strands induced by bifunctional alkylation agent always occur in certain degree, which implies that the normal cell has much better protecting capacity for itself than that of cancer or prokaryotic cell through histone rampart. Therefore, mouse leukemia cell L_{1210} has been selected as a model for the research on cross-linking ability of chemical carcinogens.

Until now, most studies related to chemical induced DNA interstrand cross-linking, are limited only in the bifunctional alkylation antitumor drugs, especially in cisplatin congeners, by suspecting the importance of bifunctional alkylation on DNA for cancer cell killing ability[4]. However, the investigation on interstrand cross-linking in DNA induced by chemical carcinogens has been ignored surprisingly as yet, the researches on interactions between DNA and carcinogen or on metabolism of carcinogens are only within the confines of the discovery of monoalkylation species[5]. Di-region theory discovered the importance of cross-linking between DNA complementary base pairs, for the carcinogenesis, which enlighten us for the first time on systematic research of DNA interstrand cross-linking induced by chemical carcinogens using the aromatic amine as example.

Based upon the epidemiologic investigation and animal test[6−8], 2-aminofluorene is a potent carcinogen (+++), 2-naphthylamine and 4-aminobiphenyl both are marked carcinogens (++), and benzidine is certainly a carcinogen(+), but the pure compounds of 1-naphthylamine, m-toluidine and 2-aminobiphenyl all are non-carcinogens. Obviously, it should not happen by chance, all the above carcinogens induce high ratio of interstrand cross-linking products in culture, but all the non-carcinogens cannot offer any interstrand cross-linking in the detectable level, which is completely consistent with the crucial importance of interstrand bifunctional alkylation on DNA for the chemical carcinogenesis emphasized by di-region theory. It might be expected that most of the chemical carcinogens other than the hormones, including the carcinogenic polycyclic aromatic hydrocarbons, would induce the DNA interstrand cross-linking in cell culture, which would be evidenced by coming experiments.

It is a pity that the monofunctional alkylation on DNA through the nitrenium ion, the so-called "ultimate" carcinogen of aromatic amine, is still thought as the key step for the carcinogenesis of aromatic amine in literature[9, 10]. Perhaps, this experiment will promote the attention of metabolic research on bifunctional alkylation of chemical carcinogen *in vitro* or *in vivo*. For the carcinogenesis by aromatic amine, di-region theory indicated that the epoxidation on the other ring without the amino substitute would form another alkylating species in the bifunctional alkylation[11]. Recently, Dai Qianhuan, Zheng Qingying *et al*. have discussed the quantitative structure-carcinogenic activity relationship (QSCAR) of 63 aromatic amines. In terms of experimental facts and theoretical analyses, they discovered that the QSCAR of aromatic amines can be explained reasonably if both the nitrenium ion and the carbonium ion formed by the epoxide are considered as the two alkylation species. The detoxication of aromatic amine occurs synchroneously with its activation. The pathways of metabolic activation and detoxication on the other ring amino substitute, summarized in their paper may be cited in Fig.2. In terms of mlecular bond localization energies (MBLE) and cation atom localization energies calculated by Hückel molecular theory, the formation trend of epoxides on the bonds in the another ring would be 7, 8- $>$5, 6- $\gg$ 6, 7 bond (cf. Fig. 2). The hydrxyl group would be localized preferentially on the atom with lower cation atom localization energy (CALE) during the NIH shift of the corresponding epoxide. The relative yield of both phenols on the same bond is decided by the difference of their CALEs. Thus, the formation trend would be 8- $\gg$ 7- position ($\Delta\Delta E=0.1289$) and 5- $>$6- position ($\Delta\Delta E=0.1154$). By combining the formation trends, both of epoxides and phenols, the preferential sequence would be 8- $>$ 5- $>$ 6 $>$ 7- phenol. In Dai's

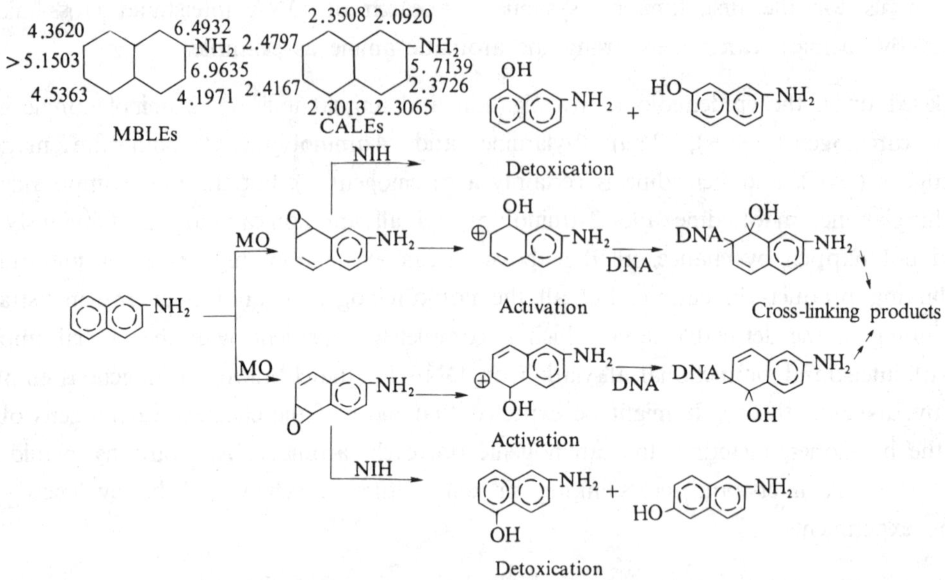

Fig. 2 Possible metabolic activation and detoxication through the ring without amino group in 2-naphthylamine. MO: Monooxygenase; NIH: NIH shift.

laboratory, Li Tingshu *et al.*[13] incubated 2-naphthylamine with rat liver microsome S9 preparation, the determined relative contents of 2-amino-8-, -5-, -6- and -7-naphthol are 52.6%, 28.5%, 14.0% and 4.9% respectively, which show completely consistent with the theoretical prediction. Therefore, the above metabolic model has been evidenced by metabolic experiment. The activation and detoxication through amino group in 2-naphthylamine may be summarized in Fig. 3, and the cross-linking positions of the covalent bridges would be 2-N with 7-C>6-C>5-C>8-C, the concrete contents would be changed in different systems within this sequence, however, in rat liver microsome S9 culture, the relative content of the cross-linking products would approach the above relative ratio.

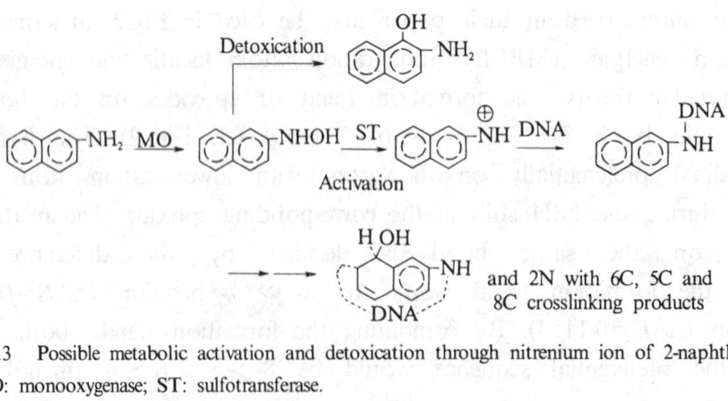

Fig.3 Possible metabolic activation and detoxication through nitrenium ion of 2-naphthylamine. MO: monooxygenase; ST: sulfotransferase.

Therefore, the pathways of the cross-linking are very complex, and among which the latter schema may be more important than the former. In the theoretical treatment[12], as the approximation, only the cross-linking between nitrenium ion and 7-position carbonium ion as in Fig. 3 has been considered. As for the concrete pathways of 2-aminofluorene, 4-aminobiphenyl and benzidine, a detailed predictions might be made based upon Dai and Zheng's model and their calculated data[12], but because of the limited space, we only emphasize their complexity and their analogies with the metabolic pathway of 2-naphthylamine.

The excitation and emission fluorescence spectra of the four cross-linking products have not been recorded. However, from their maximal absorptions and emissions, a conjugated system with amino substituted benzene ring consistent with the above metabolic models might be as the cross-linking bridges in all investigated cases. However, a more rigorous experiment is waiting to be done.

At the low concentrations in Fig. 1, the formed monoalkylation and the successively formed bifunctional alkylation species will react immediately with the excessive DNA, and the parallel detoxication reactions occurring synchronously may be neglected under this condition, both steps are pseudo first order kinetics, if A-B is the amine, which may be summarized as follows:

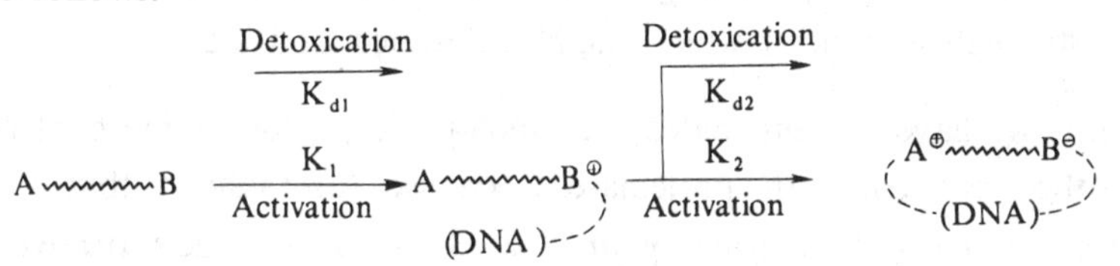

Fig.4 Pseudo first order kinetics of bifunctional alkylation in low concentration.

So, the cross-linking ratio will be decided only by $k_1 \cdot k_2 \cdot [AB]$. Because of the geometric advantage, the rates of catalytic oxidation in assembly biphenyl system, i. e. benzidine and 4-aminobiphenyl, should be certainly higher than in condensed ring system, i. e. 2-aminofluorene and 2-naphthylamine, thus assume that the total rate of cross-linking induced by biphenyl is 0.07 higher than that of condensed aromatic amines. Now, the decisive factor for the combining rate between DNA and the cation is the stability of the related cation, so $k_1 \cdot k_2$ of the amines are direct proportion to the product of the delocalization energies of the successively produced cations, i.e. $\Delta E_1 \cdot \Delta E_2$. In terms of the data of the published papers[12] the $\Delta E_1 \cdot \Delta E_2$ of benzidine, 4-aminobiphenyl, 2-aminofluorene and 2-naphthylamine are 1.8732, 1.8079, 1.7719 and 1.5250, which correlate well with the observed cross-linking ratios at low concentration as in Fig.1.

In Fig. 1, the slopes of the four amines have roughly negative correlation with detoxication trend summarized in the published paper[12], in which the biphenyl systems have been assumed to be detoxified more quickly than the condensed systems through the diphenoquinone with an extended conjugated system. At the high concentration (100 μmole) of the tested amines except the certain lowering of 4-aminobiphenyl, they approach the same about 50%. The log$P$ reflecting the permeabilities[14] should be calculated according to the following sequence, i.e. that of 4-aminobiphenyl > 2-aminofluorene > 2-naphthylamine > benzedine, so it seems that the permeability is not the decisive factor to induce cross-linking tested with L_{1210} cell, but the higher lipophilic property of 4-aminobiphenyl inhibits its approaching to the surface of hydrophilic enzyme.

As for the three non-carcinogenic amines, theoretical treatments[12] have predicted that they would be very easily detoxified through the formation of para-quinone, and further degraded to form the water soluble products through the oxidation on their unoccupied para positions. So, these three non-carcinogenic amines cannot induce the cross-linking between DNA double strands or DNA and protein.

This experimental method put forward by us for the first time might become an excellent measure for the short-term predictive screening of chemical carcinogens, which discriminates the carcinogens among these 7 aromatic amines from arbitrary selection, in a perfect correct manner. Based upon these encouraging results, it might be expected that this cross-linking method should distinguish the chemical carcinogens from the chemicals in other classes with high accuracies which might be waited and seen.

At this time we have not eliminated the DNA-protein cross-linking content in the products through the treatment with proteinase, even we can assume that the DNA-DNA interstrand cross-linking will be roughly at a level in the products treated with different amines. However, a problem with the present alkaline elution method is that it cannot differentiate the interstrand cross-linking between DNA complementary base pairs from that between the non-complementary ones, but the cross-linking between DNA complementary base pairs should be the key step of carcinogenesis according to the di-region theory. If a method can distinguish the complementary cross-linking from the non-complementary one, it ought to determine quantitatively the carcinogenic activity of a chemical and not stop at the qualitative level as in the current method in hand. However, the theoretical calculation based upon di-region theory can give us some interesting information about the quantitative carcinogenic activity. In terms of Ref. [12] and the unpublished calculation data, the major cross-linking in 2-aminofluorene(+++), 2-naphthylamine(++), 4-aminobiphenyl(++) and benzidine(+), would be between 2N-8C, 2N-7C, 4N-3′C and 4N-4′N, respectively. Therefore, the distances between their reactive centers approach 5.05, 6.22, 7.75 and 9.75 Å respectively. The differences with 3.00 Å, the twin negative atoms in complementary base pair, are 2.05, 3.22, 4.75 and 6.75 Å respectively. It might be expected that the smaller the difference from 3.00 Å, the higher the content of the complementary cross-linking in the interstrand cross-linking product would be. At the high concentrations (100

μmole) of the tested carcinogens in Fig. 1, all the cross-linking ratios appear almost the same, so the theoretical estimation complementary cross-linking ratios are just consistent with the carcinogenic potentials of the four carcinogens. Additionally, the distance between two reactive centers in benzidine seems too large for the complementary cross-linking, perhaps, the effective cross-linking occurring at the 2- or 3-position may be more important, but of course, it occurs only at a much lower level.

Now, the extension of this method to other compound classes, the observation of the excitation and emission fluorescence spectra of the interstrand cross-linking products, the formulation of the cross-linking method having the capacity to distinguish the complementary cross-linking, are undertaken in this laboratory through cooperation with Dai's group under the guidance of di-region theory. Di-region theory is an essential conceptional change in the mechanism of carcinogenesis or oncogenesis. We hope that these experiments will call the attention to this theory, which ought to have a valuable influence on cancer research in the coming years.

Project supported by the National Natural Science Foundation of China.

References

1 Dai Qinhuan, *Scientia Sinica*, **23**(1980), 453—470.
2 Kohn, V.W. *et al.*, *Cancer Res.*, **33**(1973), 1849.
3 Erickson, L. C. *et al.*, *Anal. Biochem.*, **106**(1980), 169.
4 cf. Neidle, S. and Waring, M. J. (eds.), *Molecular Aspects of Anti-Cancer Drug Action*, Macmillan, London, 1983.
5 cf. Hathway, D. E., *Mechanism of Chemical Carcinogenesis*, Butterworth & Co Ltd., 1986.
6 Parkes, H. G. and Evans, A. E. J., in *Chemical Carcinogens*, Sec. Ed., Ed. Searle, C. E., Vol. I, Amer. Chem. Soc., 1984, pp. 277—301.
7 Garner, R. C., Marthin, C. N. and Clayson D. B., *ibid.*, 1984, pp. 175—276.
8 Arcos, J. C. and Argus, M. F., *Chemical Induction of Cancer*, Vol. IIB, Academic Press, 1974.
9 Gorrod, J. W. and Manson, D., *Xenobiotica*, **16**(1986), 10—11: 933—955.
10 Miller, J. A. and Miller, E. C., *Environmental Health Perspectives*, **49**(1983), 3—12.
11 Dai Qianhuan, in *Polynucleur Aromatic Hydrocarbons: Mechanisms, Methods and Metabolism* (Eds. Cooke, M. and Dennis, A.), Battelle Press, Columbus, 1984, pp. 1045—1073.
12 Dai Qianhuan, Zheng Qingying and Wang Zhongyi, *Science in China*, **34**(1991), 5: 547—559, and the unpublished calculation data related to the same paper.
13 Li Tingshu, Dai Tianyou, Pei Shu *et al.*, *J. Envir. Science* (in Chinese), **3**(1990), 1: 101—108.
14 cf. Hansch, C. and Leo, A., *Substituent Constant for Correlation Analysis in Chemistry and Biology*, Chapter IV, Wiley, 1979.

Nucleic Acid Biosynthesis and Repair Errors Induced by Mispair Formation as a Pathway of Mutations and Carcinogenesis

V. I. Poltev, N. V. Shulyupina and V. I. Bruskov

(*Institute of Biological Physics, Russia Academy of Sciences, Pushchino, Moscow Region*, 142292, *Russia*)

Abstract Distortions of genetic information, such as single base substitutions, can result in carcinogenesis. Using molecular mechanics calculations we have investigated the mechanisms of such errors, both spontaneous and induced by some environmental factors such as radiation and chemicals.

I. Introduction

Base substitution errors in template directed nucleic acid biosynthesis leading to mutations can result in carcinogenesis. This rather general proposal has now an experimental support in the investigations of the structure of oncogens and proto-oncogens. Unambiguous evidence was obtained that base substitutions lead to ras-oncogen activation in human tumors[1]. The possibility of errors in biosynthesis is intrinsic to the structure of nucleic acids consisting of rigid heterocyclic bases and a flexible sugar-phosphate backbone. Investigation of the pathways of base substitutions could help us to understand on the molecular level the reasons of cancer arising, to predict the influence of unfavourable environmental factors as well as to reveal pathways of decreasing the probability of primary carcinogenic events. During the last two decades we performed a number of theoretical investigations of the molecular mechanisms of base substitution errors, both spontaneous and induced by environmental factors such as radiation and chemicals[2—7]. Here we summarize and discuss the most important ones for carcinogenesis results. Our computations and analysis of the experimental data permitted us to suggest the structure of nucleotide mispairs responsible for all the spontaneous base substitutions and errors caused by some modified base analogs in DNA.

II. Methods of Calculations

Our method suggests the estimation of and search for minima of energy of intermolecular and intramolecular nonbonded interactions via atom-atom potential functions of a simple form. The choice of potential functions is based on the theoretical (quantum-mechanical) considerations and summarizing a large body of experimental data as well as on comparing calculation results with experimentally obtained values. This method has been described in detail earlier and extensively used in several of our studies (see e.g.[2—7]) as well as of other authors.

III. Results and Discussion

1. *Possible Pathways of Spontaneous Base Substitutions*

Various kinds of mispairs could be considered as intermediates for spontaneous base substitutions: (1) the transition of bases into the ionized state, (2) the existence of bases as different tautomers, and (3) the format on of non-Watson-Crick hydrogen-bonded pairs of neutral bases in normal tautomeric forms. The formation of rare tautomer mispairs has been suggested by Watson and Crick[8] as a pathway of transitions and then extended by Topal and Fresco[9] to transversions. But some experimental facts on nucleic acid biosynthesis errors cannot be explained within this mechanism of mispair formation. Among these facts are (1) nucleotide replacements having pyrimidine-pyrimidine mispairs as intermediate stages, (2) the higher error frequency in some systems than the probability of rare tautomer formation, (3) the incorporation into DNA and RNA of base analogs that cannot form rare tautomer mispairs.

Our calculations of and search for minima of interaction energy between normal tautomer nucleic acid bases suggest a mutual in-plane arrangement of bases which may be responsible for every spontaneous base substitution error[2]. Such arrangements correspond to the wobble pairs, to the pairs with syn-orientation of one of bases and to mispairs with single N-H···O or N-H···N H-bond and C-H···O or C-H···N hydrogen bonding[2]. Examples of such mispairs are presented in Fig.1. At least one of such pairs for every pairwise combination could be incorporated into the DNA duplex without short interatom contacts arising, large energy increase and drastic distortion of the sugar-phosphate backbone

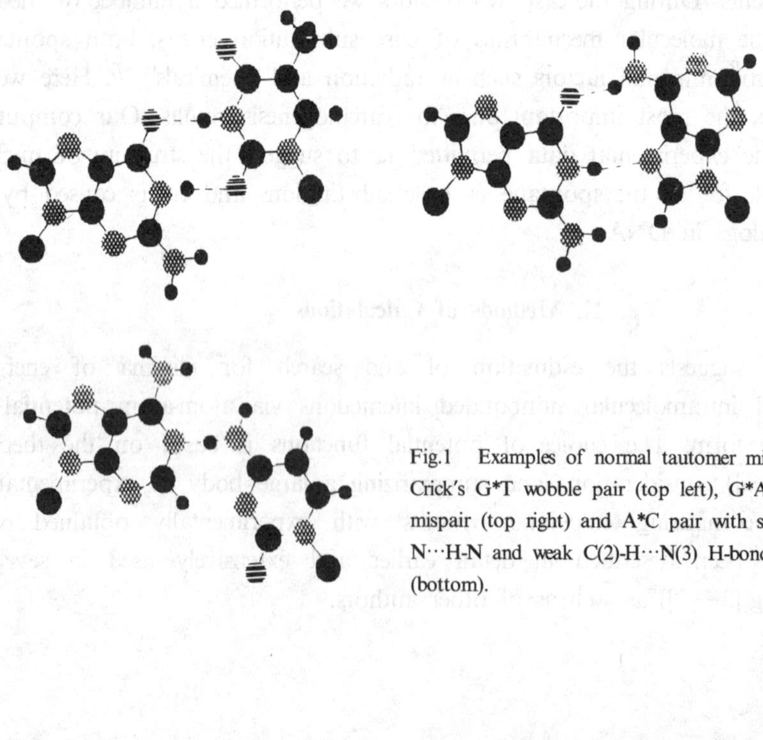

Fig.1 Examples of normal tautomer mispairs. Crick's G*T wobble pair (top left), G*A (syn) mispair (top right) and A*C pair with single N···H-N and weak C(2)-H···N(3) H-bond (bottom).

conformation[3]. The calculated geometry of some nucleotide mispairs has been later experimentally confirmed by crystal[10] and solution[11] investigations of DNA duplexes.

For some pairwise combination of bases, the water-bridged mispairs are favourable from the energy and geometry viewpoint[4]. These mispairs are linked via one interbase H-bond and one or two water bridges. The incorporation of some of such mispairs into the duplex results in a less pronounced distortion of the conformation of the sugar-phosphate backbone than it is the case for the mispairs corresponding to the minimum of interbase interaction energy. Particularly it concerns the pyrimidine-pyrimidine mispairs.

2. *Rare Tautomer Mispairs*

Thus, the appearance of spontaneous errors during the nucleic acid biosynthesis could be explained by the formation of mispairs composed of normal tautomeric forms of the bases. It is also the case for the guanine-thymine mispairs which are found in the crystalline state[10] and in solution[11] in wobble configuration. But the recent experimental infrared studies of nucleic acid bases[12] show that N9-methyl guanine isolated in a low-temperature inert matrix exists as a mixture of two tautomers, amino-oxo and amino-hydroxy. It means that rare tautomer mispairing is probable for guanine containing pairs. Our Monte Carlo simulation data[7] suggest that the wobble guanine: thymine (uracil) mispair in duplexes is a result of interactions of bases with water molecules, water bridging. Consequently, the 'normal' and 'rare' tautomers are possible for guanine containing mispairs during nucleic acid biosynthesis.

3. *Enzyme-Nucleotide Recognition in Nucleic Acid Biosynthesis*

Calculations show that several nucleotide mispairs (e.g. G*T, G*A, G*A (syn)) have an energy close to the Watson-Crick A-T pair. It means that the great accuracy in the coding of genetic information and prevention of the base mispair formation are attained by enzymes of template directed biosynthesis and repair of DNA. The analysis of experimental data and the results of calculations led us to formulate a concept of enzyme-nucleotide recognition in the processes of nucleic acid biosynthesis[7]. According to this concept, the interaction of the enzyme recognition site with the structural invariants of complementary nucleotide pairs increases the probability of such pair formations and prevents mispairing. These invariants are the position and conformation of the sugar-phosphate backbone, as well as N3 atoms of purines and O2 atoms of pyrimidines in complementary pairs[2].

4. *Pathways of Alkylation-Induced Mutagenesis and Carcinogenesis*

Some modifications of the nucleic acid bases under the influence of internal and environmental factors lead to altered and ambiguous coding properties. The alkylating agents are well known mutagens and carcinogens[13]. Series of alkylated bases cause nucleic acid biosynthesis errors. We calculated the possible structures of base pairs containing methylated bases[5] which could be considered as intermediates for mutations. The most important promutagenic base is 6-methylguanine (6MeG) which can form a base pair with both C (like G) and T. The minimum of interaction energy between 6MeG and T corresponds to two H-bonds (Fig.2, top left) and the energy value close to that in the A:T pair[5]. The mutual position of bases is practically the same as in Watson-Crick pairs. Thus 6MeG can initiate transitions via such a pathway: G:C->6MeG:C->6MeG:T->A:T. These transitions can explain mechanism of carcinogenesis by 6MeG formation in DNA. According to NMR data for oligonucleotide duplex in solution[9], the 6MeG: T pair has a single H-bond (N2-H···O2). The configuration of such a pair is presented in Fig.2, top right. It is possible to propose[4] another 6MeG:T pair configuration, stabilized by a single H-bond and a water bridge (Fig.2, bottom).

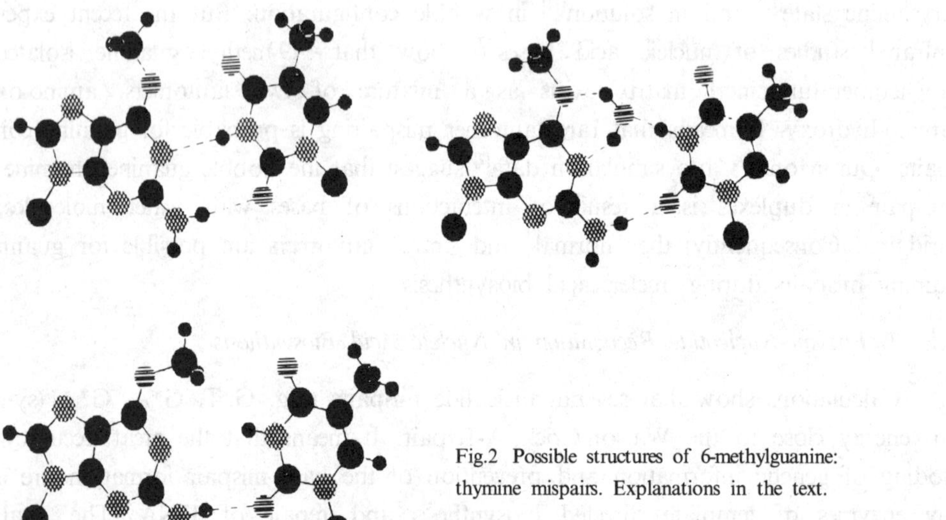

Fig.2 Possible structures of 6-methylguanine: thymine mispairs. Explanations in the text.

5. 8-*Oxoguanine Containing Mispairs as an Intermediate for Carcinogenesis Induced by Irradiation and Oxidation*

8-oxoguanine (8OG) is one of the most important products of DNA damage by irradiation and oxidation. The mutagenecity and carcinogenecity of this product has been confirmed in several investigations (see e.g.[14]). Calculations of interbase interaction energy for pairwise combinations of natural bases with 8OG[6] allows us to reveal several minima. Some examples of these minima are presented in Fig.3. The base position and the minimal interaction energy in the 8OG*C pair (Fig.3) practically coincide with those for the G*C pair. The preferable conformation of 8OG containing nucleotides is the syn-conformation. Calculations suggest that mutual arrangements of glycosyl bonds in the

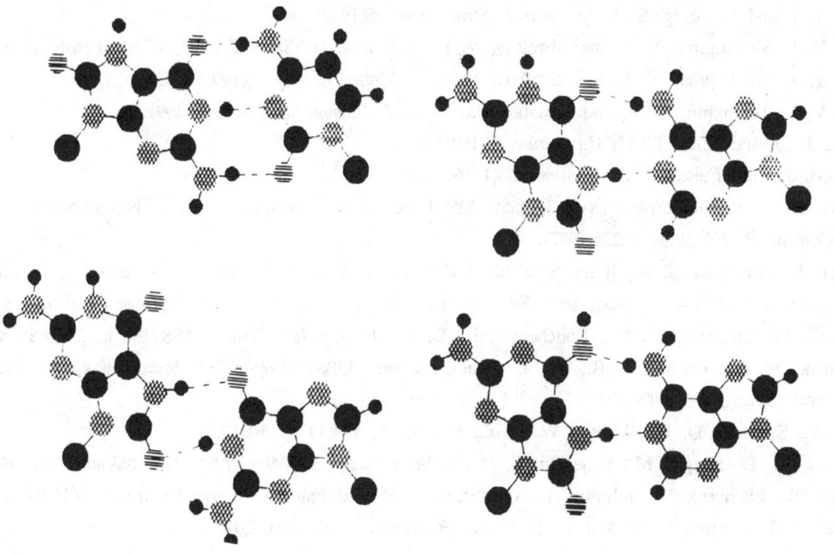

Fig.3 8OG-containing base pairs.

interaction energy minima of 8OG(syn) with A and G do not differ appreciably from those for Watson-Crick pairs. Moreover, the relative positions of N3 atom of the natural base and O8 atom of 8OG in these minima correspond to the invariant arrangement of purine N3 and pyrimidine O2 atoms in Watson-Crick pairs. Thus, the interaction of the recognition site of enzymes of template directed biosynthesis cannot prevent 8OG(syn)* purine mispair incorporation into the duplex. That is why 8OG is a highly mutagenic and carcinogenic substance. The calculation results predict the following base substitution pathways, G*C→8OG*C→8OG(syn)*G→C*G and G*C→8OG*C→8OG(syn)*A→T*A, which correspond to the most frequent G*C→C*G and G*C→T*A transversions arising under the influence of irradiation[14]. Although base replacements induced by oxidation could have other intermediates[15] the relative probabilities of various irradiation induced nucleotide substitutions can be predicted from our computation results[7]. Some probability of 8OG to exist as 6-hydroxytautomer does not create new 8OG-purine mispairs. The arrangements of bases in the 8OG(oxo)-purine and 8OG-(oxy)-purine mispairs practically coincide (Fig.3).

References

1 Nishimura, S. and Sakiya, T., *Biochem. J.*, **243**(1987), 313.

2 Poltev, V. I. and Bruskov, V. I., *J. Theor. Biol.*, **70**(1978), 69; Bruskov, V. I. and Poltev, V. I., *J. Theor. Biol.*, **78**(1978), 29.

3 Chuprina, V. P. and Poltev, V. I., *Nucleic Acids Res.*, **13**(1985), 141; Poltev, V, I. and Chuprina, V. P., *Structure and Motion: Membranes, Nucleic Acids and Protein* (eds. Clementi, E., Corongiu, G., Sarma, M., Sarma, R. H.), Adenine Press, Guilderland, N. Y., 1985.

4 Poltev, V. I. and Steinberg, S. V., *J. Biomol. Struct. Dyn.*, **5**(1987), 307.

5 Poltev, V. I., Shulyupina, N. V. and Bruskov, V, I., *Mol. Biol.* (USSR), **15**(1981), 1276; English ed., **15**(1981), 993.

6 Poltev, V. I., Shulyupina, N. V. and Bruskov, V. I., *J. Molec. Recogn.*, **3**(1990), 45.

7 Poltev, V. I., Teplukhin, A. V. and Kwiatkowski, J. S., *J. Biomol. Struct. Dyn.*, 1991.

8 Watson, J. D. and Crick, F. H. C., *Nature,* **171**(1953), 964.

9 Topal, M. D. and Fresco, J. R., *Nature,* **263**(1976), 285.

10 Kennard, O., *J. Biomol. Struct. Dyn.*, **3**(1985), 205; Prive, G. G., Heinemann, U., Chandrasegaran, S. Kan, L-S and Dickerson, R. E., *Science*, **238**(1987), 498.

11 Patel, D. J., Kozlowski, S. A., Ikuta, S. *et al.*, *Fed Proc.*, **43**(1984), 2663; Patel, D. J., Shapiro, L. and Hare, D., *Nucleic Acids and Molecular Biology* (eds. Eckstein, F., Lilley, D. M. J.), Vol. 1, Springer, Berlin, 1987.

12 Sheina, G. G., Stepanian, S. G., Radchenko, E. D. *et al., J. Mol. Struct.,* **158** (1987), 275; Szczepaniak, K., Szczensniak, M. and Person, W. B., *Int. J. Quantum Chem.*, **QBS13**(1986), 287; Szczepaniak, K. and Szczesniak, M., *J. Mol. Struct.*, **156**(1987), 29.

13 Frei, J. V., Swenson, D. H., Warren, W. *et al.*, *Biocem. J.*, **174**(1978), 1031.

14 Wood, M. L., Dizdaroglu, M., Gajewski, E. *et al.*, *Biochemistry*, **29**(1990), 7024; Kouchakjian, M., Bodepudi, V., Shibutani, S., Eisenberg, M., Johnson, F., Grollman, A. P. and Patel, D. J., *Biochemistry*, **30**(1991), 1403.

15 McBride, T. J., Preston, B. D. and Loeb, L. A., *Biochemistry*, **30**(1991), 207.

Structure-Activity Studies of Some Methyl and Phenyl Derivatives of the Food Mutagen 2-Amino-3-methylimidazo-[4, 5-*f*]quinoxaline (IQx) in the Ames Test

Spiros Grivas,

(*Department of Chemistry, Swedish University of Agricultural Sciences, Box* 7016, *S*-750 07 *Uppsala, Sweden*)

Rose Vikse, Anne Knapstad, B. Bålsrud Mjelva and Leiv Klungsøyr

(*Stabekk College, Ringstabekkv.* 105, *N*-1340 *Bekkestua, Norway*)

Abstract Synthetically produced methyl and phenyl derivatives of food carcinogens in the IQx series have been tested by the Ames *Salmonella typhimurium* assay with TA98 and S9 mix. Their structure-activity relationship is presented.

Several carcinogenic heteroaromatic amines, also called aminoimidazo-azaarenes (AIA), are formed in the crust of fried or grilled proteinaceous foods[1]. These substances display high mutagenic activity in the *Salmonella* mutagenesis assay (Ames test), with the frameshift mutants TA98 and TA1538 as the preferred test organism, but they are also detected with base substitution mutants, such as TA100[1, 2]. The AIA compounds are not direct mutagens, but must first be activated by, e.g. the cytocrome P-450 oxidase system. The ultimate mutagens, which are extremely electrophilic species with limited stability, are thought to be nitrenium ions arising from activated amino groups in the form of hydroxylamines. Sulfuryl, acetyl or other acyl groups bound as the amides or esters of these hydroxylamines are probably intermediates in the nitrenium ion formation[3, 4]. Many different AIA compounds have been isolated, and their structures have been unambiguously determined or confirmed after obtaining sufficient quantities by synthesis[1, 5]. No doubt, food preparation processes lead to other, still unknown compounds, with similar structures and activities. Preparation of such unknown derivatives in this family of mutagenic compounds is of great importance for three reasons: a) the synthesis may precede the analysis of foods, making isolation and identification easier and unambiguous; b) for structure-activity studies which may be useful in understanding the molecular basis for the activity of the ultimate mutagen able to attach itself to DNA[6] and in predicting risk from related chemicals; c) long-term animal feeding studies required large amounts of these substances which can only be produced synthetically[7].

The number and position of the methyl groups in the IQx series and in some other toxic heteroaromatic amines (e.g. IQ and PhIP) found in cooked foods have been shown to be important[8]. In continuation of our previous studies on the roles of the imidazole moiety and the 2-amino group[9], the replacement of the 3-methyl by an ethyl group[10] and the exchange of a 4-methyl by a 5-methyl group[11], we have prepared fifteen possible mono-, di-, tri- and tetramethyl derivatives of the title food mutagen IQx, including three phenyl derivatives of 5-MeIQx. We then subjected them to the Ames test with TA98 as the test organism. A closely related study on the structure-activity relationships of some of the AIA compounds was very recently reported[12]. Generally, for the compounds tested previously, our specific mutagenicity ranking order was in good agreement with other published data[1, 2, 7, 12].

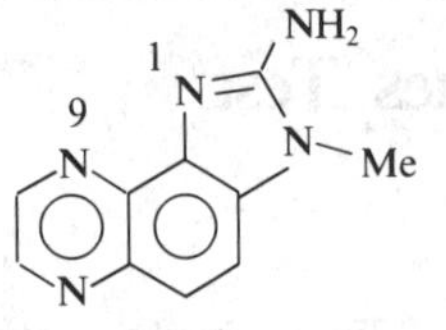

IQx

I. Materials and Methods

Chemicals: The test compounds were >98% pure. They were synthesized via 2, 1, 3-benzoselenadiazoles leading exclusively to the desired isomer[13]. Glucose-6-phosphate and NADP were obtained from Sigma Chemical Company. All the other chemicals and bacteriological media were of the best quality from standard sources.

Mutation assay: Mutagenicity was measured as described[14], and care was taken to follow the procedure as closely as possible, also with respect to the agar volume, which was kept at 30 ml except when the influence of this parameter was checked in a few experiments. The S9 extract was prepared for us from Aroclor 1254 treated rats as described[14] at the Norwegian Veterinary College, Oslo by Drs. Aune and Joner who also supplied us with the TA98 *Salmonella typhimurium* mutant. The S9 mix contained 2 mg protein per dish. A solution of each test compound was made at a concentration of 1 mg/ml in DMSO. After an initial screening of activities, dilutions were made with DMSO, so that the number of revertants per plate would be between 500 and 1500. Triplicate determinations were made at 3 mutagen concentrations in each experiment. The activities presented represent averages from the linear portion of the dose-response curve. The standard deviation values $(n-1)$ presented refer to all the points included in the calculations (usually the two lowest concentrations in each experiment). The mutagenicities are given as the number of revertants per microgram of mutagen (rev/μg).

II. Results and Discussion

As the results accumulated in this study, we realized that our values are low, compared to those of other workers. However, the relative rank of the substances previously tested in other laboratories was identical to this found by us, with two exceptions. We had reasons to believe that the volume of agar in each assay dish was important (P. E. Joner, personal communication), but the study was planned to be carried out as much as possible in accordance with the procedures given[14]. We believed that this would give results which could be the best compared to those from other laboratories, although inter- and even intra-laboratory variations in mutagenicity are very common[2, 15].

After completing our main study we determined the mutagenicity of some of the test substances with an agar volume that was lower than the 30 ml prescribed[14]. The results are illustrated in Table 1, for example 8-MeIQx yields revertants within the range published by others[1, 2, 7, 12] at both 20 ml and 15 ml agar. The relative rank between mutagenicities remains the same, with both 15 ml and 30 ml agar in the dish.

Table 1 (Rev/μg)[a)]

Compound	15 ml agar	20 ml agar	30 ml agar
8-MeIQx	73 800	39 400	22 600
7-MeIQx	381 000		176 000
4-MeIQx	398 000	260 000	183 000
4, 7-DiMeIQx	508 000		200 000
4, 7, 8-TriMeIQx	133 600		67 600

a) Average of triplicate determinations.

We therefore feel confident that our relative ranking order of mutagenicity between test substances is correct within the margin of error expected. The results are presented in Table 2, and are in good agreement with those recently published[12], with two exceptions: in the published results, 4-MeIQx had the highest activity, while we find an activity of the

Table 2

Compound	Rev/μg	Std. dev.	n[a)]
IQx	21 144	3 878	4
8-MeIQx	22 571	2 782	6
7-MeIQx	176 383	18 412	6
7, 8-DiMeIQx	141 180	13 637	5
4-MeIQx	183 067	8 687	6
4, 7-DiMeIQx	199 650	14 019	6
4, 8-DiMeIQx	97 750	6 376	4
4, 7, 8-TriMeIQx	67 633	8 642	6
5-MeIQx	124 288	13 582	8
5, 8-DiMeIQx	23 594	4 639	4
5, 7-DiMeIQx	60 447	3 596	5
5, 7, 8-TriMeIQx	3 773	295	4
4, 5-DiMeIQx	55 580	9 329	5
4, 5, 8-TriMeIQx	17 904	3 235	4
4, 5, 7-TriMeIQx	17 231	774	4
4, 5, 7, 8-TetraMeIQx	3 840	732	4
7, 8-DiPhIQx	1	1	3
8-Ph-5-MeIQx	5 650	1 560	6
7-Ph-5-MeIQx	331	100	4

a) Number of triplicate determinations from which the average was calculated.

same level as 7-MeIQx and 4, 7-DiMeIQx; further, 4, 7, 8-TriMeIQx had a quite low activity, while we find a value not much lower than that of 4, 8-DiMeIQx.

With the first methyl group fixed in position 3 (parent IQx), the mutagenicity remains unchanged with another methyl group in position 8 (8-MeIQx); it is increased by a factor of five when a methyl group enters position 5 (5-MeIQx), and by a factor of seven when a methyl group is in position 4 (4-MeIQx) or position 7 (7-MeIQx).

In the dimethylated IQx series of isomers, the activity pattern is rather complex. The activity of 7-MeIQx is only slightly reduced by methylating position 8 (7, 8-DiMeIQx), it is unchanged or slightly increased by methylation of position 4 (4, 7-DiMeIQx), and it is reduced to almost one third by methylation at 5 (5, 7-DiMeIQx). The activity of 4-MeIQx is more or less halved by methylation of position 8 (4, 8-DiMeIQx, cf. 4, 7-DiMeIQx above), and it is reduced to less than one third by methylation of position 5 (4, 5-DiMeIQx). The activity of 5-MeIQx is reduced to one fifth by methylation of position 8 (5, 8-DiMeIQx), and halved by methylation of position 4 (4, 5-DiMeIQx) or position 7 (5, 7-DiMeIQx).

Of the trimethylated IQx isomers, the 4, 7, 8-TriMeIQx gives the highest activity, about one third of the 4, 7-DiMeIQx, while the equally active 4, 5, 7- and 4, 5, 8-isomers are a little less mutagenic than the parent IQx. The lowest activity among the TriMeIQx isomers is possessed by the 5, 7, 8-compound, which has an activity only about one sixth of the parent IQx.

The 4, 5, 7, 8-TetraMeIQx homologue is identical in activity to 5, 7, 8-TriMeIQx.

Phenylation of 5-MeIQx at the 7-position (7-Ph-5-MeIQx) results in a quite low activity, about 0.25% of the parent 5-MeIQx. The isomeric 8-Ph-5-MeIQx is nearly twenty times more active than the 7-Ph-isomer. Finally, 7, 8-DiPh-5-MeIQx is inactive.

There is probably a number of factors that determine the mutagenic potency of the mutagens, such as the electrophilicity of the attacking group, its life time, the rate of detoxification processes and the steric arrangement of the molecule which in turn might determine its transmembrane transportation and interaction with DNA. The charge distribution charts of the resonance hybrids of the nitrenium ion derived from MeIQx derivatives[12], might explain why the 7- and 4-isomers are more active than the 8- and 5-isomers of MeIQx: In positions 4 and 7 the inductive effect of the methyl group contributes electron density to the ring, and stabilizes the ion. Since the 7- and 8-phenyl derivatives are equally bulky, the explanation for why the 7-isomer is less active than the 8-isomer may be that the phenyl group in position 8 has charge-receiving ability and considerable stabilizing effect on the nitrenium ion. With two phenyl groups in these positions, the molecule may be too bulky to approach the points of attack on DNA.

References

1 Felton, J. S. and Knize, M. G., *Mutation Res.*, **259**(1991), 205.

2 de Meester, C., *Mutation Res.*, **221**(1989), 235.

3 Nagao, M., Fujita, Y., Wakabayashi, K. *et al.*, *Biochem. Biophys. Res. Commun.*, **114**(1983), 626.

4 Abu-Zeid, M, Staiano, N., Yamazoe, Y. *et al.*, *Jpn. J. Cancer. Res.*, **81**(1990), 653.

5 Jägerstad, M., Skog, K., Grivas, S. *et al.*, *Mutation Res.*, **259**(1991), 219.

6 Shahin, M. M., *Mutation Res.*, **221**(1989), 165.

7 Sugimura, T., *Mutation Res.*, **205**(1988), 33.

8 Felton, J. S. and Knize, M. G., In: Cooper, C. S. and Grover, P. L. (eds) *Handbook of Experimental Pharmacology*, Springer, Berlin Heidelberg New York, 1990.

9 Grivas, S. and Jägerstad, M., *Mutation Res.*, **137**(1984), 29.

10 Jägerstad, M. and Grivas, S., *Mutation Res.*, **144**(1985), 131.

11 Nyhammar, T., Grivas, S., Olsson, K. *et al.*, *Mutation Res.*, **174**(1986), 5.

12 Hatch, F. T., Knize, M. G. and Felton, J. S., *Environ Mol. Mutagen*, **17**(1991), 4.

13 Grivas, S., in *Heterocyclic Amines: Mutagens and Carcinogens in Cooked and Pyrolysed Foods* (eds. Sugimura, T. and Takayama, S.) (in press), Cambridge University Press, Cambridge.

14 Maron, D. M. and Ames, B. N., *Mutation Res.*, **113**(1983), 173.

15 Myers, L. E., Adams, N. H., Hughes, T. J. *et al.*, *Mutation Res.*, **182**(1987), 121.

Unwound States of DNA in Gene Control

Frida Shimron and Gad Yagil

(*Department of Cell Biology, The Weizmann Institute of Science, Rehovot 76100, Israel*)

The two basic cellular processes of DNA replication and DNA transcription cannot proceed without being accompanied by at least a certain extent of DNA unwinding. Malfunctioning of the unwinding step can therefore be a significant cause for uncontrolled replication, a primary defect of malignantly transformed cells. The chemotherapeutic effect of several topoisomerases inhibitors[1] supports this notion. Many details of the DNA unwinding process, such as the length and extent of the unwound regions or the conformations DNA assumes in these regions are still incompletely known. The intermediary existence of an unwound region during the prepriming step of DNA replication at *E. coli* Ori C has been demonstrated by using single strand nuclease P1[2] as well as by 2-dimensional topoisomer analysis[3]. Similar information comes from studies of the pBR322[4] of phage lambda[5] and of the mammalian virus SV40[6].

There is ample evidence for the participation of an unwound DNA region of some length in the transcription of DNA (for a review see [7]). An important way to detect unwound regions experimentally became available when Larsen and Weintraub demonstrated[8] that β-globin genes in mature chicken erythrocytes genes become sensitive to single strand specific nucleases (SSN) when nuclei expressing the gene are incubated with a nuclease like S1. To be in a susceptible single stranded state, two DNA strands have to unwind first. Susceptibility to single strand nucleases, in particular in supercoiled plasmids, is therefore a strong indication that a DNA region in the plasmid, or in the nuclear genome, is in a state which from the topological view is unwound, but not necessarily actually in a single stranded state.

As an example for the identification of an unwound region, the cleavage pattern of a β-globin carrying plasmid is shown in Fig.1, and compared with the cutting pattern of the vector plasmid. In pBSTN1 470 bases of the chicken β-globin gene promoter region is inserted into vector pUC8[9]. To obtain the cutting patterns, the isolated supercoiled plasmids were incubated with P1 nuclease for 30 min at 30°. The plasmids were subsequently cleaved with restriction enzyme BamH1 at position 419 (pUC8), or 897 (pBSTN1), end labeled and analyzed on an agarose gel. Two prominent bands are apparent in pUC8, the sum of the length of which (obtained by a linear regression of a mobility plot) is close to the length of the intact plasmid, 2665 bases. This places a nuclease sensitive site in one of two alternate positions on the plasmid. An experiment with a second cut (Taq I), or with an appropriate hybridization probe (Fig. 4) places the cleavage in a region previously documented to be sensitive to mung bean nuclease in plasmid pBR322[10].

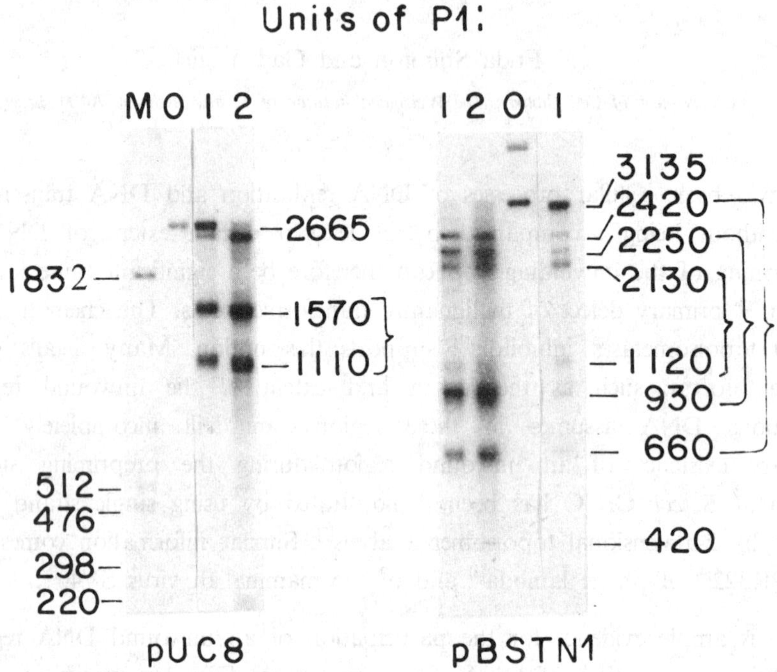

Fig. 1 P1 digestion patterns of plasmids pUC8 and pBSTN1. Supercoiled, CsCl and agarose purified plasmids were incubated with P1, at the concentration shown on top, in 10 mmol/L Tris, 1 mmol/L EDTA, pH 7, for 90 min at 37°. The mixture was deproteinized, ethanol precipitated, and recleaved with BamH1 (at position 419 of pUC8 and 889 of pBSTN1). The fragments were end labelled with ^{32}-P γATP and analyzed on a 1.4% agarose gel. An HinfI digest of a marker plasmid (M) as well as a Hind 3 digest of phage lambda were run in parallel. pBSTN1, which contains the β-globin insert, -303 — $+161$, was kindly provided by Dr. G. Felsenfeld.

The pattern obtained for pBSTN1 contains three prominent pairs of bands, the sum of the fragment size of each pair again being equal to the size of the intact plasmid. The innermost pair maps to the same mung bean sensitive region as the vector plasmid. The two adjoining pairs map to the major and minor cruciform of pBR322 related plasmids around positions 3063 and 3122 of pBR322 (1377 and 1436 of pUC8), known for a long time to be nuclease S1 sensitive[11]. Only at the bottom of the gel was a weak band mapping to the globin promoter region visible. Analysis on acrylamide (not shown) showed this band to be located exactly at the 16+3 G region which is the most sensitive to S1 in the β-globin promoter[12]. Unwound sequences in the vector seem thus to dominate potentially sensitive sites in the globin promoter at physiological pH. The unwinding of a region in the vector is of interest, because the sensitive tracts are in a plasmid region important for plasmid replication. The two cruciforms within the region are transcribed into RNA species I and II, involved in the control of plasmid replication[13, 14]. The main P1 sensitive tract may well serve as an unwinding element as proposed by Kowalski and Eddy[3].

A more formal way to assess the degree of winding of a DNA region inserted into a supercoiled plasmid is by two-dimensional (2-d) topoisomer analysis[15]. By this technique a mixture of topoisomers is analyzed on an agarose gel, at a defined set of conditions. When no region is unwound, the well known regular topoisomer ladder results. In case unwinding occurs at some section of the plasmid, an irregular ladder results. The ladder is best resolved by incubating the gel in chloroquine, which reverts all topoisomers to the right handed form, and rerunning the gel in a direction perpendicular to the first one. An unwound section is manifested then as a break or "jump" in the otherwise continuous arc of topoisomers. From the position of the jump both the number of turns unwound, and the free energy required can be evaluated[16].

The 2-d topoisomer pattern obtained by inserting the origin of replication of SV40 into a vector is seen in Fig. 2a. A jump occurs at topoisomer 12; topoisomer 13 can be seen to have migrated in the first dimension to the same distance as topoisomer 10. Similar mobilities of the two topoisomers mean that they have a similar number of superturns, or, in other words, that nearly 3 turns of the primary helix, close to 30 bases, have opened. This figure is close to the number of bases found to be opened by Borowiec and Hurwitz[6] by applying $KMnO_4$ to a T antigen-SV40 complex.

The 2-d topoisomer patterns formed by pUC8 and pBSTN1 were investigated in greater detail. The pattern obtained under standard conditions (Tris borate 90 mmol/L, EDTA 1 mmol/L, pH 8.3. "TBE") is shown in Fig. 2b. No transition is evident. However, when spermine is added to the concentration of 20 mmol/L (Fig.2c), a clear jump is evident in both vector and the inserted globin region. It can be seen that close to three turns of the plasmid have been opened in both the globin carrying plasmid and the vector. We can therefore not conclude at this stage that unwinding has taken place within the globin promoter region. The P1 digestion data (Fig. 1) also suggest that most unwinding occurs in vector regions.

The transitions observed for both pUC8 and pBSTN1 under a range of conditions are summarized in Table 1. It can be seen that at pH 7.2 the transition is taking place even without addition of spermine, while at pH 9.3 no transition is observed even in the presence of spermine, at a concentration effective at pH 8.3. This may be either due to a change in the protonation of spermine or to the now fully charged phosphate of the DNA backbone.

The effects of spermine and of Mg on the P1 cleavage pattern of pUC8 are shown

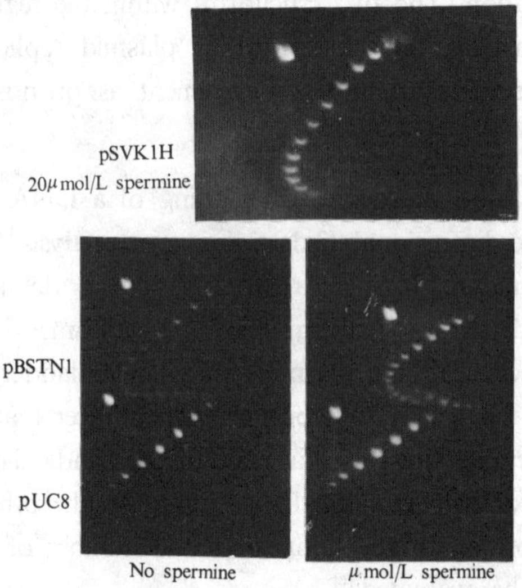

Fig. 2 a, Two-dimensional topoisomer pattern of plasmid pSVK1H. This plasmid contains bases −67— +161 of SV40, i.e., the origin of the replication region, 55 bases into the first 72 base enhancer region[17] (kindly provided by Dr. E. Winocour). A mixture of topoisomers was prepared by topoisomerase treatment of the supercoiled plasmid as described by Wang *et al.*[18]. The mixture was analyzed on a 16×16cm 1.4% agarose gel, cast in TBE containing 20 μmol/L spermine. The same buffer was used for loading (6.6% sucrose added) and as electrophoresis buffer. The gel was run in TBE for 20 h at room temperature at 60 volt. The gel was then shaken for 5 h with 5 μg/ml chloroquine, and run under the same condition in a perpendicular direction, in 50 mmol/L Tris-phosphate, 1 mmol/L EDTA, pH 7.2. The gel was stained with EtBr and photographed under UV light. The topmost band is numbered 0, the next band to the left −1, and so on. b, c, Topoisomer pattern of plasmids pUC8 and pBSTN 1. Fig. 2b contains no spermine in the TBE buffer. In Fig.2c 20 μmol/L spermine were present. The lower arc on each gel represents pUC8, while the upper arc represents pBSTN1. Procedure and running conditions are similar to those of Fig.2a.

Table 1 Topoisomer Analysis: Effect of pH and Polyamines

pH [a]	Spermine (μmol/L)	pUC8		pBSTN1	
		Bases [b] opened	At topo-isomer	Bases [b] opened	At topo-isomer
7.2	0	30—40	−16	30—40	−17
7.2	20	30—40	−17	30—40	−17
8.3	0	0	0	0	0
8.3	5	0	0	0	0
8.3	20	32	−13	32	−12
8.3	50	26	−13	30	−12
8.3	50[c]	+	−12	+	−13
9.4	0	0	0	0	0
9.4	20	0	0	0	0

a) All at 23° in Tris-borate 90 mmol/L, EDTA 1 mmol/L, adjusted to the pH listed with Tris or H_3BO_3.

b) Based on the mobility change of the first topoisomer undergoing transition (listed in the next column).

c) Spermidine.

in Fig.3. It is evident that in the absence of spermine, the main P1 cutting site is in the inner band pair, mapping within the sensitive region between bases 3210 and 3290 of pBR322. With spermine, or magnesium, the main transition shifts to the major cruciform, which from the topological standpoint can be regarded as an unwound structure. It is thus reasonable to assume that the effect of spermine at pH 8.3 is to stabilize the unwound state, and preferentially in the cruciform form. This is in line with the observation of McClellan and Lilley[19] that spermine tends to shift the equilibrium between a cruciform and a proposed U form, presumably unwound, in favor of the cruciform.

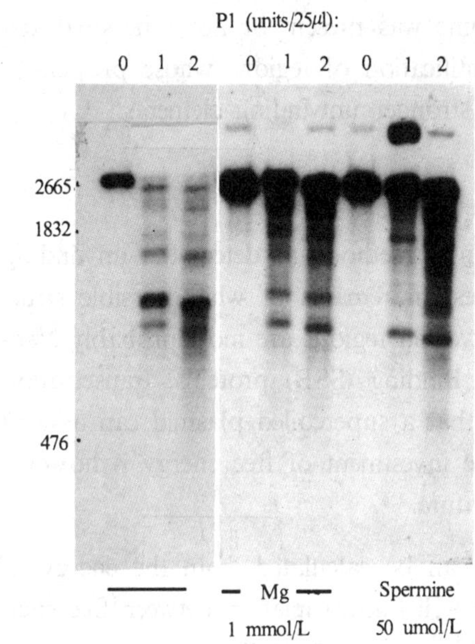

Fig.3 The effect of spermine and magnesium on the cutting pattern of pUC8 by P1 nuclease. Most experimental details are as in Fig.1, except that bands are detected by hybridization with a radioactive probe obtained by random priming of a 680 bp fragment (419—1099) of pUC8. By this probe only the clockwise member of each band pair is visible (unless cleaved in the probe region).

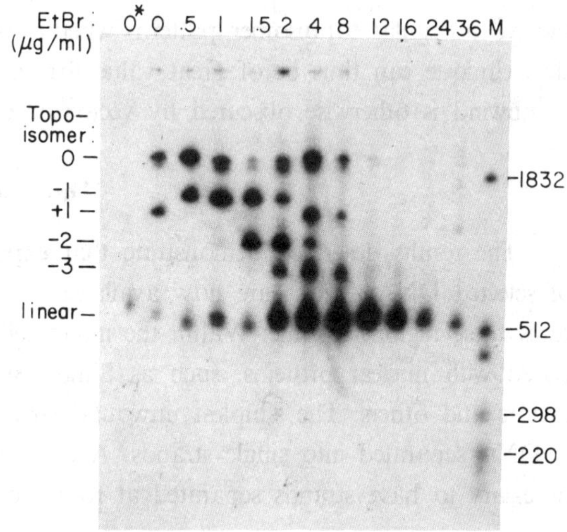

Fig.4 Topoisomer pattern of a 57369 circularized DNA of pBSTN1, containing the 470 base globin promoter region. The fragment was prepared by Hinf1 and BamH1 digestion of the plasmid, end labeled with ^{32}P γATP and circularized by addition of DNA ligase (1 u/25 μl for 30 min at 37°) in the presence of varying amounts of EtBr, as described by Nordheim and Meese[20]. The circularized samples were loaded on a composite gel (3.5% acrylamide and 0.5% agarose) and run in 0.5×TBE for 7h at 23°C. The leftmost sample was not treated with ligase. The suggested topoisomer numbers are indicated on the left of the gel. The rightmost lane shows size markers.

It seems thus that a transition in the globin promoter region, even if it occurs, is obscured by the unwinding of vector regions. To obtain information on vector independent transitions of the globin promoter in the neutral range, we have utilized the small circle method introduced by Nordheim and Meese[20]. By this technique, a linear subfragment of the promoter region, with matching ends, is circularized by the addition of DNA ligase, in the presence of increasing amounts of ethidium bromide (EtBr). Ligase is then removed and upon extraction of EtBr, various topoisomers, some possibly unwound, do appear on an agarose gel. The pattern obtained by a circularized 573 bp Hinfl fragment of pBSTN1, containing the promoter region of β-globin is shown in Fig.4. When no EtBr is present, the only topoisomers formed are 0 and +1. With increasing EtBr concentration, topoisomers −1, −2 and −3 appear. At 4 and 8 μg/ml EtBr, the topoisomer −3 band is weakened, but instead of topoisomer −4, topoisomer +1 reappears. This serves as a strong indication, that nearly 4 turns of the circularized DNA helix, mostly derived from the β-globin promoter region, have been unwound upon removal of EtBr. Control fragments, which contained either the S1 sensitive region, or other regions of pBSTN1, showed a regular topoisomer pattern, whether spermine was present or not. The small circle technique can thus be of great value for the identification of regions whose propensity to unwind is otherwise obscured by vector or other stronger unwinding elements.

Discussion

The results described demonstrate that experimental methods to detect the unwinding of selected DNA regions are now available. The question remains of what possible structures these regions assume. Within the intact cell, unwound regions are most probably associated with nuclear proteins, such as Single Strand Binding (SSB) proteins, transcription factors and others. The simplest unwound structure that a supercoiled plasmid can assume is DNA separated into single strands. A considerable investment of free energy is however necessary to have strands separated at room temperature.

For a supercoiled plasmid, the energy involved can be calculated from the energy of supercoiling before and after the transition, using the well known relation between free energy of supercoiling and linking difference, $\Delta G=(K/N)\tau^2$, where N is the number of bases in the plasmid, K a constant equal to 660 kcal at 25°, and τ the linking difference (cf. Ref.[18]). It can be seen on Figs.2a, 2c that the transition in the presence of spermine at pH 8.3 requires at least $\tau=-13$ superhelical turns, and that 3 superturns are opened, to compensate for the 3 primary turns unwound, so that,

$$\Delta\Delta G=(K/N)(\tau_1^2-\tau_2^2)=(660/2665)(169-100)=17\,\text{kcal}.$$

The free energy required for unwinding is 17 kcal at 25°, or 0.57 kcal per base unwound. This is significantly less than the energy of melting of even an A.T. base pair (0.9—1.9 kcal/bp; Breslauer *et al.*, 1986). This means that unwinding is most probably not accompanied by complete strand separation and that some partially stacked structure is formed.

The main S1 sensitive region in the chicken β-globin promoter has been mapped to a very G rich region[12, 21]. Studies with the conformation-specific reagent bromoacetaldehyde[22,23] are in favor of the formation of a G.C.G triplex structure by the oligo G.C tract. Such a triplex structure is also an unwound structure, as a detailed examination of the H DNA triplex proposed by Lyamichev *et al.*[24] clearly shows (see Ref.[25]). The formation of a triplex requires nevertheless a high degree of mirror symmetry, which is not found in the pUC8 plasmid, certainly not in the S1 or P1 sensitive region. A triplex can therefore not explain the main transition observed in Fig.2b, or the main band in Fig.1.

Another structure which is unwound from the topological standpoint (i.e. cannot form in a closed structure without strand opening) is the cruciform structure. The data in Fig.4 show that cruciforms are formed in the vector, when conditions (Mg, spermine) are favorable. It is thus tempting to speculate, that a primary role of spermine in nuclear activation is the promotion of the unwound, or paranemic, state in its cruciform version.

Cruciforms can however be formed only from dyad symmetric DNA regions, and these are rather rare in genomes. This is in contrast to polypurine stretches like poly G, the prime S1 sensitive motive of DNA, which are exceptionally abundant, in particular in highly transcribed genes[26]. Many of the single strand-specific nuclease sensitive regions have at most very short symmetric regions[7]. If the existence of DNA in the unwound state turns out to be a widespread phenomenon, then we shall have to assume that nonsymmetric unwound DNA structures can be formed. One example can be the paranemic duplex we have proposed[27]. Such paranemic structures can offer a mechanistic solution for the old dilemma how DNA strands are kept unwound for efficient transcription or replication. The unwound structures of the various types discussed may also offer potential targets for the action of cytostatic agents.

This project was carried out with the financial support of the Helen and Milton Kimmelman Center for Biomolecular Research.

References

1 Liu, L. F., *Ann. Rev. Bioch.*, **58**(1989), 358.
2 Baker, T. A., Bertsch, L. L., Bramhill, D. *et al.*, *Cancer Cells*, **6**(1988), 19.
3 Kowalski, D. and Eddy, M. J., *EMBO J.*, **8**(1989), 4335.
4 Tomizawa, J., *J. Mol. Biol.*, **212**(1990), 695.
5 Dodson, M., McMacken, R. and Echols, H., *J. Biol. Chem.*, **264**(1989), 10719.
6 Borowiec, J. A. and Hurwitz, J., *EMBO J.*, **7**(1988), 3149.
7 Yagil, G., *Critical Revs. Bioch. Mol. Biol.*, **26**(1991), 475.
8 Larsen, A. and Weinbtraub, H., *Cell*, **29**(1982), 609.
9 Emerson, B. M., Lewis, C. D. and Felsenfeld, G., *Cell*, **41**(1985), 21.
10 Sheflin, L. G. and Kowalski, D., *Nucl. Acids Res.*, **12**(1984), 7081.
11 Lilley, D. M. J., *Proc. Natl. Acad. Sci. USA*, **77**(1980), 6468.
12 Nickol, J. M. and Felsenfeld, G., *Cell*, **35**(1983), 467.
13 Parada, C. A. and Marians, K. J., *J. Biol. Chem.*, **264**(1989), 15120.
14 Eguchi, Y. and Tomizawa, J., *Cell*, **60**(1990), 199.

15 Lee, C.-H., Mizusawa, H. and Kakefuda, T., *Proc. Natl. Acad. Sci. USA*, **78**(1981), 2838.
16 Peck, L. J. and Wang, J. C., *Proc. Natl. Acad. Sci. USA*, **80**(1983), 6206.
17 Dorsett, D., Dechaite, I. and Winocour, E., *Mol. Cell. Biol.*, **5**(1985), 869.
18 Wang, J. C., Peck, L. J. and Becherer, K., *Cold Spring Harbor Symp.*, **47**(1983), 85.
19 McClellan, J. A. and Lilley, D. M. J., *J. Mol. Biol.*, **197**(1987), 707.
20 Nordheim, A. and Meese, K., *Nucl. Acids Res.*, **16**(1988), 21.
21 Wang, J. N. C. and Hogan, M., *J. Biol. Chem.*, **260**(1985), 8194.
22 Kohwi, Y. and Kohwi-Shigematsu, T., *Proc. Natl. Acad. Sci. USA*, **85**(1988), 3781.
23 Kohwi-Shigematsu, T., Gelinas, R. and Weintraub, H., *Proc. Natl. Acad. Sci. USA*, **80**(1983), 4389.
24 Lyamichev, V. I., Mirkin, S. M. and Frank-Kamenetskii, M. D., *J. Biomol. Struct. Dynam.*, **3**(1986), 667.
25 Htun, H. and Dahlberg, J. E., *Science*, **243**(1989), 1571.
26 Bucher, P. and Yagil, G., *DNA Sequence*, **1**(1990), 157.
27 Yagil, G. and Sussman, J. L., *EMBO J.*, **5**(1986), 1719.

Transgenic Mice Aberrantly Expressing Human Ornithine Decarboxylase, a Growth-related Enzyme

J. Jänne, L. Alhonen, M. Halmekytö, J.-M. Hyttinen and J. Wahlfors

(*Department of Biochemistry & Biotechnology, University of Kuopio, P. O. Box 1627, SF-70211 Kuopio, Finland*)

Abstract We have generated several transgenic mouse lines overexpressing the human ornithine decarboxylase gene. The ectopic expression of the transgene was most striking in the testis and brain. A dramatic overaccumulation of putrescine apparently led to a damage of the testicular germinal epithelium and decrease in brain of free magnesium ions. Owing to the grossly elevated ornithine decarboxylase activity, indicative of accelerated growth, these animals offer an excellent model for carcinogenesis studies.

I. Introduction

Mammalian ornithine decarboxylase (ODC; EC 4.1.1.17) represents an enzyme, the expression of which is tightly coupled to cell growth[1]. This view is supported by a vast number of publications showing an enhanced ODC activity following anabolic stimuli, and, even more convincingly, by a large number of observations indicating that a specific inhibition of ODC inevitably leads to growth arrest of mammalian cells[1]. The requirement of polyamine biosynthesis for growth has established ODC as a meaningful target for cancer chemotherapy.

1. *Molecular Genetics of Mammalian ODC*

The structure and chromosomal localization of mammalian ODC gene. The structure of ODC gene is remarkably well conserved among mammalian species. In rodents and human the gene comprises 12 almost identical exons and 11 intervening sequences[2—4]. The actively expressed human ODC sequences segregate with the short arm of the chromosome 2[5] and those of the mouse ODC with the chromosome 12[6] that is homologous to the short arm of the human chromosome 2. Rodent genome harbors a number of pseudogenes, the human genome apparently harbors only one located at the chromosome 7[4].

Amplification and methylation of the human ODC gene. The ODC genes are readily amplified under appropriate selection pressure (such as an exposure to specific inhibitors of the enzyme) both in rodents[7, 8] and in human[9]. The exact mechanisms of ODC gene amplification are not known, as they are obscure for any mammalian genes, yet distinct methylation changes appear to accompany the human ODC gene amplification[10]. Upon amplification of the human ODC gene, a particular cell clone with a specific ODC gene methylation pattern seems to be selected for the amplification process[10].

The expression of the ODC gene is influenced by DNA methylation as the increased expression rate is associated with hypomethylation[11] and, more directly, a methylation of the human ODC gene *in vitro* prior to transfection abolishes its transient expression in the recipient cell[12].

Expression of the ODC gene in transfected cells. When the human ODC gene containing all the exons and introns together with some 800 nucleotides of the 5′ and 1000 nucleotides of the 3′ flank was transfected into Chinese hamster ovary cells devoid of endogenous ODC activity and hence auxotropic for putrescine, the transfected cells became able to grow without putrescine supplementation[13, 14]. The gene also appeared to be properly regulated as indicated by serum stimulation, short half-life and sensitivity to the polyamines of the human gene-derived ODC[13]. Among the transfected cell clones with different number of integrated gene copies, no correlation, whatsoever, was found between the rate of expression and the gene dosage indicating a strong chromosomal position effect[13, 14].

II. Transgenic Mice Harboring the Human ODC Gene

1. *Gene Constructs Used*

We initially used two different human ODC gene constructs to generate transgenic mice: (i) a full length gene shown to be actively expressed in transfection experiments[13] and (ii) a 5′ truncated gene lacking the 5′ flanking region and the first (noncoding) exon[15]. A further heterologous gene construct consisting of the mouse ODC promoter fused with the bacterial chloramphenicol acetyltransferase (CAT) gene was used for comparative purposes[16].

2. *Transgene Expression*

We have generated altogether 9 transgenic mouse lines (or founder animals) carrying the full length or truncated human ODC in their genome. Although the role of ODC promoter governing the expression of the gene may not be very critical, the 5′ flanking region and the first noncoding exon are required for the expression of the gene, as transgenic mice harboring the 5′ truncated gene construct did not produce human-specific ODC mRNA in any of their tissues studied[15]. Human-specific ODC mRNA, however, was readily detectable in all tissues of the transgenic mice carrying the full length human ODC transgene[15]. It subsequently became evident that the human ODC transgene was expressed in a strikingly aberrant fashion. The human ODC transgene-derived enzyme activity was practically in all tissues much higher than the endogenous mouse ODC activity[15]. Not only was the transgene overexpressed, but the expression pattern also was highly distorted,

i. e. strikingly elevated (up to 100-fold) ODC activity in tissues, such as brain and muscle, which normally display barely detectable ODC activity[15]. A further puzzling feature was the finding indicating that the transgene expression apparently occurred in a gene copy number-dependent fashion with no indications of a chromosomal position effect[16]. Interestingly, mouse ODC promoter-driven CAT displayed almost identical ectopic reporter gene expression pattern as did the human ODC gene in the transgenic animals[16]. Although the reasons leading to this position-independent expression, which is highly unusual in transgenic animals created with the microinjection techniques, of the ODC transgene constructs are not known, the probably simpliest explanation would imply that ODC gene expression is normally governed by remotely located strong genetic silencer elements that were not included in our gene constructs. However, at the moment of writing this hypothesis remains to be experimentally tested.

3. *Phenotypic Changes Associated With the Transgene Expression*

A subsequent determination of the polyamine concentrations in the tissues of the transgenic animals produced a surprise. In spite of the grossly elevated transgene-derived ODC activity, the tissue polyamine pools were only marginally influenced[17]. There were, however, two distinct exceptions, namely testis and brain. In these particular tissues, the enhanced transgene-derived ODC activity led to a massive (20 to 100-fold) tissue putrescine accumulation[17]. The mechanism of the clearing of the polyamines from rest of the tissues displaying high ODC activity is a total mystery. Enzyme analyses of the tissues of the transgenic animals clearly showed that the catabolic pathway of the polyamines was not activated to any appreciable extent[17] nor was the urinary excretion increased in the transgenic animals [unpublished results].

The striking accumulation of putrescine in the testes of the transgenic males appeared to result in morphological abnormalities in the testicular tissue. Depending on the testicular transgene-derived ODC activity, the spermatogenesis of the transgenic animals was slowed down to varying extent ultimately leading to a complete male sterility in the case of very high ODC activity[15]. According to our *in situ* hybridization analyses[16] both the endogenous and the transgene-derived ODC expression took place exclusively in the testicular Sertoli cells. Sertoli cells are the nursing cells of the germinal epithelium providing nutrients to the developing cells of the spermatogenic lineage. It is thus possible that high concentrations of putrescine formed in and released from the Sertoli cells are toxic to the spermatogenic cells leading to a maturation arrest. Even though the polyamines are generally believed to function as growth supporting compounds that are required for animal cell proliferation to occur, some recently expressed views[18] imply that these substances may also be involved in the process called programmed cell death. The mechanism of the polyamine-mediated cell death would probably involve the generation of cytotoxic radicals upon their oxidation[18].

In addition to the testicular tissue, a massive putrescine accumulation likewise occurred in the brain of the transgenic animals[17]. Histological examination of the brain tissue did not reveal any overt morphological abnormalities[15]. However, our nuclear magnetic resonance spectroscopy studies indicated that the dramatic accumulation of putrescine in the brain of the transgenic mice was associated with a marked (about 40%) decrease in the concentration of free magnesium ions[19]. Whether this change together with the elevated brain putrescine levels render the transgenic animals prone to epileptic seizures or postischemic brain damage[20] remains to be tested.

4. *Potential Uses of the Transgenic Animals Overexpressing the ODC Gene*

ODC definitely is a growth-related enzyme, an inhibition of which renders animal cells incapable of cellular proliferation[1]. There likewise exists some circumvential experimental evidence indicating that an overexpression of ODC, such as resulted from gene amplification, would confer certain growth advantage at least on cultured tumor cells manifested as an ability to grow on semisolid media[21]. The transgenic animals overexpressing the human ODC transgene may thus offer a valuable model for studies aimed to elucidate the initiation and progression of tumorigenesis in a number of tissues. Most obvious examples are the two-stage skin carcinogenesis (in which ODC plays a critical role), liver carcinogenesis and gastrointestinal carcinogenesis. Moreover, supposing that the polyamines are involved in the process of programmed cell death, these animals may also serve as models for postischemic brain damage or for necrotizing damage of any tissue. The exact mechanisms involved in the position-independent expression of a transgene could be of critical importance for our understanding of the regulation of the gene expression. In any event, either mouse or human ODC promoter can be used to direct a high-level expression of heterologous gene constructs into various tissues of transgenic animals in a gene dosage-dependent fashion.

References

1 Jänne, J. Alhonen, L. and Leinonen, P., *Ann. Med.*, **23**(1991), 241.
2 Coffino, P. and Chen, E. L., *Nucleic Acids Res.*, **16**(1988), 2731.
3 van Steeg, H., van Oestrom, T. M., Hodemaekers, H. M. *et al.*, *Gene*, **93**(1990), 249.
4 Hickok, N. J., Wahlfors, J., Crozat, A. *et al.*, *Gene*, **93**(1990), 257.
5 Winqvist, R., Mäkelä, T. P., Seppänen, P. *et al.*, *Cytogenet Cell Genet*, **42**(1986), 133.
6 Cox, D. R., Trouillo, T., Ashley, P. L. *et al.*, *Cytogenet Cell Genet*, **48**(1988), 92.
7 McConlogue L., Gupta, M., Wu, L. *et al.*, *Proc. Acad. Natl. Sci. USA*, **81**(1984), 540.
8 Kahana, C. and Nathans, D., *Proc. Natl. Acad. Sci. USA*, **81**(1984), 3645.
9 Leinonen, P., Alhonen-Hongisto, L., Laine, R. *et al.*, *Biochem. J.*, **242**(1987), 199.
10 Wahlfors, J., *Biochem. J.*, **279**(1991), 435.
11 Leinonen, P., Alhonen-Hongisto, L., Laine, R. *et al.*, *FEBS Lett.*, **215**(1987), 68.
12 Halmekytö, M., Hirvonen, A., Wahlfors, J. *et al.*, *Biochem. Biophys. Res. Commun.*, **162**(1989), 528.
13 Hälttä, E., Hirvonen, A., Wahlfors, J. *et al.*, *Gene*, **83**(1989), 125.

14 Jänne, J., Alhonen, L., Hirvonen, A. *et al.*, *Adv. Enz. Regul.*, **28**(1989), 81.
15 Halmekytö, M., Hyttinen, J-M., Sinervirta, R. *et al.*, *J. Biol. Chem.*, **266**(1991), 19746.
16 Halmekytö, M., Alhonen, L., Wahlfors, J. *et al.*, *Biochem. Biophys. Res. Commun.*, **180**(1991), 262.
17 Halmekytö, M., Alhonen, iL., Wahlfors, J. *et al.*, *B ochem. J.*, **278**(1991), 895.
18 Coffino, P. and Poznanski, A., *J. Cell. Biochem.*, **45**(1991), 54.
19 Kauppinen, R., Halmekytö, M., Alhonen, L. *et al.*, *J. Neurochem.*, (in press).
20 Paschen, W., Schmidt-Kastner, R., Djuricic, B. *et al.*, *J. Neurochem.*, **49**(1987), 35.
21 Polvinen, K., Sinervirta, R., Alhonen, L. *et al.*, *Biochem. Biophys. Res. Commun.*, **155**(1988), 373.

Section A

Biochemistry and Molecular Biology of Cancer

Pleiotypic Changes in Expression of the N-*myc* Gene in Neuroblastoma Cell Lines Treated With Anti-cancer Drugs

Hikoji Shindo[1, 2], Chizuru Nakagawa[1], Hiromichi Hemmi[1], Sachio Otsuka[2] and Hiroyuki Shimatake[1]

([1]*Department of Molecular Biology and* [2]*1st Department of Internal Medicine, School of Medicine, Thho University, Tokyo, Japan*)

Abstract The relationship between N-*myc* protein expression and cell cycle progression induced by antitumor agents in the human neuroblastoma cell line IMR 32 was studied. Expression of N-*myc* was observed at any phase of cell cycle, when cells were forced to a particular phase by antitumor agents. These results suggest that the N-*myc* expression occurs independently of the cell cycle.

The N-*myc* gene, a member of the *myc* oncogene family, is activated with gene amplification in neuroblastomas[1] and in other childhood malignanacies[2]. An examination of the degree of the N-*myc* gene amplification has offered an excellent test system to evaluate a prognosis of neuroblastoma cases[3, 4]. Roughly 30% of neuroblastoma cases show a sign of N-*myc* gene amplification and are highly maligant in prognosis[3]. The N-*myc* gene is not necessarily amplified in many cases of neuroblastomas and retinoblastomas. Most of retinoblastoma cases and approximately 70% of neuroblastoma cases carry only single copy of the N-*myc* gene, and some of these tumors are highly malignant[3, 5]. Conventional examination of gene amplification[3], however, failed to examine a possible over-expression of the N-*myc* gene[5]. Detection of the gene product is important to understanding the relationships between the malignancy and either the gene amplification or the over-expression. Recently, we prepared a series of antibodies against N-*myc* gene product engineered genetically[6—9]. By using these antibodies, immunohistochemical studies revealed that the N-*myc* protein was not uniformly expressed among the neuroblastoma cells of both cell lines and primary specimens[6, 7, 10]. Heterogeneous contents of N-*myc* protein in each cell could not be explained by an unequal distribution to daughter cells, because cells with a single copy of the N-*myc* gene showed the heterogeneity[4, 11]. One possibility to explain this heterogeneous expression depends on cell cycle, because c-*myc* gene expression is known to depend on the cell cycle[12]. Thus, we study here the relationship between N-*myc* gene expression including mRNA and protein and cell cycle progression induced by antitumor agents. We demonstrate that the N-*myc* expression occurs independently of the cell cycle.

I. Materials and Methods

1. *Cell Culture and Treatment*

The human neuroblastoma cell line IMR 32[13] was grown in Eagle's minimum essential medium (MEM) supplemented with 10% fetal bovine serum (FBS) and maintained at 37°C in a humidified atmosphere of 5% CO_2 in air.

IMR 32 at an initial cell density of 5×10^6 cells/75 cm^2 flask was in ubated for 2 — 3 days, growing exponentially. The culture medium was then replaced with the growth medium without or with 10 μmol/L cisplatin, 54 nmol/L vincristine, 50 nmol/L demecolcine, 100 μmol/L hydroxyurea or 10 μmol/L retinoic acid. Cell culture was continued further for 48 h. For the low serum experiments, 2% FBS-containing MEM was used. The viability of cells was more than 85% in any culture condition.

2. *Antibody*

Antibody to the human N-*myc* gene product was prepared as described previously[9]. High titer serum of a rabbit immunized with the purified N-*myc* fusion protein was purified to IgG fraction. Diluted antibody (10^{-4}) could detect 243 pg of the antigen molecule.

3. *Cell Cycle Analysis and Detection of N-myc Protein*

To analyze cell cycle and the N-*myc* protein content per cell, FACS (fluorescence-activated cell sorting) analysis with a FACStar (Becton-Dickinson) was performed. Cells prepared by the protocol mentioned above were digested with 0.1% trypsin and 25 mmol/L ethylenediaminetetraacetate to obtain a single cell suspension and washed 3—4 times with phosphate buffered saline (PBS, pH 7.2) by centrifugation. Then, cells were fixed with BOUIN's solution. Prior to addition of the antibody, samples were incubated with blocking solution consisting of 3% bovine serum albumin (BSA) in PBS for 30 min at 20°C and then with anti-N-*myc* antibody (3×10^{-2} dilution with 1% BSA) for 18 h at 4°C. After being washed with PBS, samples were incubated for 18 h at 4°C with fluorescein isothiocyanate (FITC)-labeled anti-rabbit IgG antibody diluted 5-fold. Then, 50 μg/ml propidium iodide was added to each sample to stain nuclear DNA, and 1×10^4 cells were applied to an FACStar.

4. *Preparation of RNA and Northern Blot Analysis*

Total RNA of IMR/32 was prepared by the method using the ethanol precipitation as described[14]. The prepared RNA was used for Northern blot analysis as described[14]. As probes, AluI/AluI (1849-2350) DNA fragment of human N-*myc* gene exon-1 and XhoI/RsaI (3430-4133) DNA fragment of exon-2 were used.

II. Results

The cell cycle analysis by an FACStar was designed to quantitate the amount of the N-*myc* protein and to determine the stage of cell cycle simultaneously. IMR 32 in untreated control culture was 60% of G_0/G_1 phases, 22% of S phase and 18% of G_2/M phase and showed different amounts of the N-*myc* protein (Fig.1). Although G_2/M phase cells showed approximately twice the amount of the N-*myc* protein as the G_0/G_1 phase, major heterogeneity was observed even within any one of the same phases of the cell cycle.

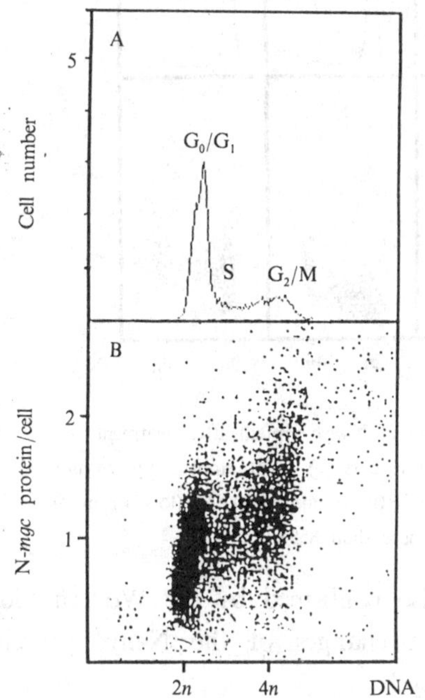

Fig.1 FACS analysis of IMR 32 cells for cell cycle (A) and quantitation of the N-*myc* protein (B). Horizontal line denotes DNA content. Vertical line denotes the relative cell number (A) and relative amount of N-*myc* protein per cell (B).

The effects of agents such as cisplatin, vincristine, demecolcine, retinoic acid, and hydroxyurea, which are known to perturb the cell cycle events, on the cell cycle and the amount of the N-*myc* protein were next examined. The treatment with cisplatin was increased in the population of S phase cells and decreased in other phase cells, compared to the untreated control (Fig. 2a). A higher amount of the N-*myc* protein in all phases was found (Fig.2a). Thus, the increase in the N-*myc* protein by cisplatin may not be due to an increase in the population of S to G_2/M phase cells that contain more N-*myc* protein than cells in G_0/G_1 phase. Vincristine and demecolcine interfered further with the proficiency in the G_2/M phase and increased it in the N-*myc* protein as well as cisplatin did (Fig.2a — c). In contrast to the above, hydroxyurea was caused a decrease in the amount of the protein at any phase of cell cycle without changing the profile at the concentration used (Fig.2d). Retinoic acid also decreased in the ratio of the G_2/M phase cells and the amount of the N-*myc* protein was decreased in all phases (Fig. 2e). Low serum treatment (2% as opposed to 10% in the control experiments) did not significantly affect the amount of the N-*myc* protein, although the ratio of the S to G_2/M phase cells was decreased (Fig. 2f). Longer treatment of IMR 32 with the agents for 72 h substantiated the increase more clearly (data not shown). The heterogeneity of the N-*myc* protein content was consistently observed in all treatments tested. Further, the changes of the N-*myc* protein content were observed throughout the whole period of the cell cycle. The changes of the N-*myc* protein

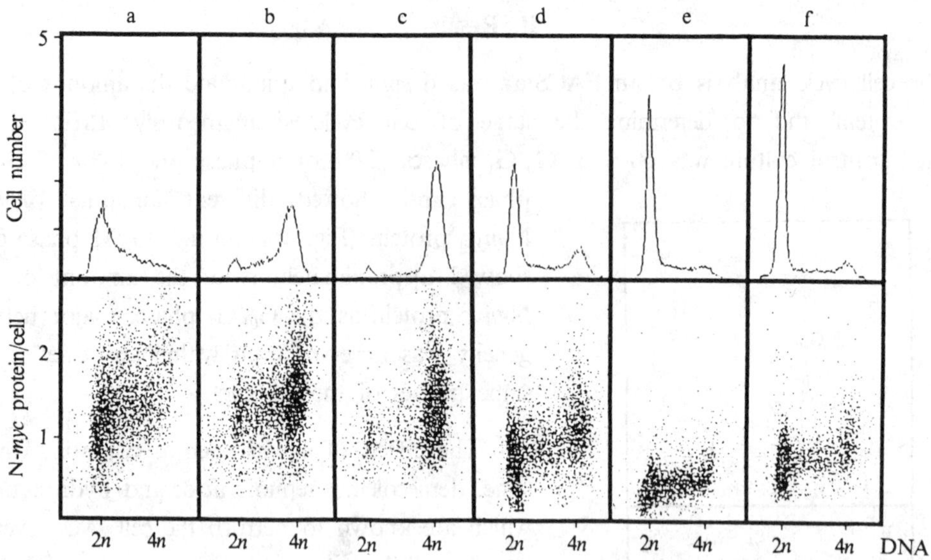

Fig.2 FACS analysis of IMR 32 for cell cycle and the quantitation of N-*myc* protein after treatment with 10 μmol/L cisplatin (a), 54 nmol/L vincristine (b), 50 nmol/L demecolcine (c), 100 μmol/L hydroxyurea (d), and 10 μmol/L retinoic acid (e) and after the cultivation in 2% FBS-containing MEM (low serum: f). The cells were treated or cultivated for 48 h and the viability was more than 85%.

contents in IMR 32 cultured with these agents were also confirmed by the Western blot analysis (data not shown). These results indicate that changes of the N-*myc* protein content of IMR 32 are not specific to a stage of cell cycle.

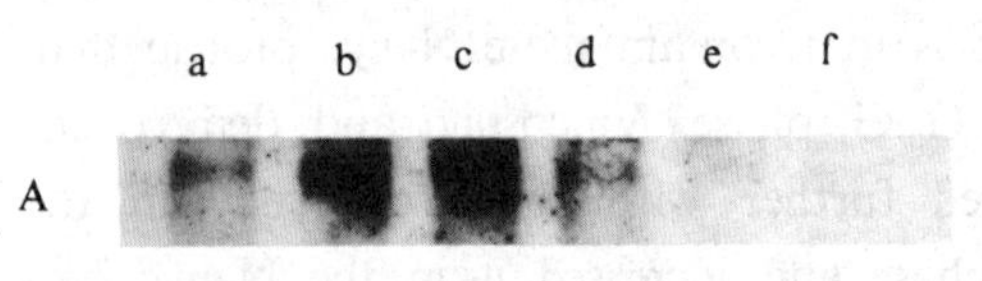

Fig. 3 Northern blot analysis of N-*myc* mRNA in IMR 32 cells. Human N-*myc* gene exon-1 (A) and exson-2 (B) were used as DNA probes. Cells were treated for 48 h with control medium (a), 10 μmol/L cisplatin (b), 54 nmol/L vincristine (c), 50 nmol/L demecolcine (d), 10 μmol/L retinoic acid (e), and 100 μmol/L hydroxyurea (f). For each lane, 10 μg total RNA was loaded.

Northern blot analysis was carried out to clarify whether the change of the N-*myc* protein content by the carcino-static agents was transcriptionally controlled or was affected by post-transcriptional events such as translational efficiency or regulation of protein turn over. N-*myc* mRNA was detected as a 3.3 kilobase (kb) band, and the intensity of the band was increased by the treatment with cisplatin, vincristine, and demecolcine and decreased by retinoic acid and hydroxyurea (Fig.3). These changes were parallel to the changes of the N-*myc* protein as detected by the cell cycle analysis with FACStar and by Western blot analysis. Thus, it was confirmed that the changes of the N-*myc* protein content were either through transcriptional control or through regulation of mRNA stability. The results of the studies on the cell cycle analysis, N-*myc* protein contents, and N-*myc* mRNA expression mentioned above are summarized in Table 1.

Table 1 Summary of the Effect of Antitumor Agents and Low Serum on Cell Cycle, N-*myc* Protein Contents, and N-*myc* mRNA in IMR 32 Shown in Figs.1 and 2

Culture Condition	Cell Cycle*[a)]	N-*myc* Protein[a)]	N-*myc* mRNA[b)]
Cisplatin	S	↑	↑
Vincristine	G_2/M	↑	↑
Demecolcine	G_2/M	↑	↑
Retinoic acid	G_0/G_1	↓	↓
Hydroxyurea	~	↓	↓
Low serum	G_0/G_1	~	n.d.

*The phase increased after the treatment.

a) The phase of cell cycle and the amount of N-*myc* protein were determined by FACS analysis.

b) N-*myc* mRNA was determined by the Northern blot analysis.

↑, increased; ↓, decreased; ~, no change; n.d., not done.

III. Discussion

We have demonstrated that the expression of N-*myc* protein by a human neuroblastoma IMR 32 cell line is an event independent of a particular phase of the cell cycle. The heterogenous expression seems to be dependent on the individual cell characteristics expressed in microenvironment, rather than dependent on a phase of the cell cycle, though some proteins are known to increase at a specific phase of cell cycle[15−18]. This heterogeneity was reported to be not only in clinical specimens of neuroblastoma and other tumors including retinoblastoma[4, 10] but also in human embryos[19]. Therefore, the heterogeneity of N-*myc* protein expression seems to be a universal phenomenon in N-*myc*-expressing cells. In the C-*myc* protein, another *myc* gene family, the heterogeneity has been also reported in breast carcinoma[20], though it was not clear whether the cell cycle played a major role in the heterogeneity. A retinoblastoma protein is reported to be phosphorylated during S and G_2/M phases without changing the protein level through the cell cycle[16]. It is possible that the N-*myc* protein might be modified during specific phases of the cell cycle. The amount of the N-*myc* protein as detected with FACS analysis reflects the rate of the N-*myc* protein synthesis in individual cells, since the N-*myc* protein turns over very rapidly ($t_{1/2}=30-40$ min)[7, 8]. The modified form of the N-*myc* protein may play an important role, physiologically.

Unexpectedly, cisplatin and vincristine, used for the clinical treatment of neuroblastomas increased in the amount of the N-*myc* oncoprotein which occurred through the increase in mRNA levels. Moreover, this increase was observed throughout all phases of cell cycle. Thus, the increase was independent of the cell cycle shift by the drug treatment. A possibility that the increase in cellular content of N-*myc* protein was caused by cell volume enlargement after treatment of drugs was excluded, because no change in the cell volume was found (unpublished results). Although cisplatin and vincristine are known to interfere with cell cycle progression with different mechanisms, these chemicals shared the same effect on increased N-*myc* mRNA level and N-*myc* protein level in IMR 32 neuroblastoma cells. It would be interesting to inquire further into their mode of action to see if they share the same mechanism to increase the N-*myc* mRNA.

We thank Dr. Y. Shidoji for his useful discussion and to H. Fujii and N. Kohyama for their excellent assistance in preparing the manuscript.

References

1 Brodeur, G. M., Seeger, R. C., Schwab, M. *et al.*, *Science*, **224**(1984), 1121.
2 Lee, W. H., Murphree, A. L. and Benedict, W. F., *Nature*, **309**(1984), 458.
3 Seeger, R. C., Brodeur, G. M., Sather, H. *et al.*, *N. Engl. J. Med.*, **313**(1985), 1111.
4 Yokoyama, T., Thukahara, T., Nakagawa, C. *et al.*, *Cancer*, **63**(1989), 2134.
5 Thuchida, Y., Kanda, N., Shimatake, H. *et al.*, *Exp. Cell. Biol.*, **56**(1988), 277.
6 Slamon, D. J., Boone, T. C., Seeger, R. C. *et al.*, *Science*, **232**(1986), 768.
7 Ikegaki, N., Bokovskv, J. and Kennett, R. H., *Proc. Natl. Acad. Sci. USA*, **83**(1986), 5929.
8 Ramsy, G., Stanton, L., Schwab, M. *et al.*, *Mol. Cell. Biol.*, **6**(1986), 4450.
9 Nakagawa, C., Thukahara, T. and Shimatake, H., *J. Med. Soc. Toho*, **36**(1989), 207.
10 Nakagawa, C., Thukahara, T. Kikuchi, T. *et al.*, *Biomedica*, **2**(1987), 1036.
11 Shimatake, H., Nakagawa, C., Kikuchi, T. *et al.*, *Saishin-igaku*, **42**(1987), 1491.
12 Rabbitts, P. H., Watson, J. V., Lamond, A. *et al.*, *EMBO J.*, **4**(1985), 2009.
13 Tumilowicz, J. J., Nichols, W. W., Cholon, J. J. *et al.*, *Cancer Res.*, **30**(1970), 2110.
14 Ausubel, F. M., Brent, R., Kingston, R. E. *et al.*, *Current Protocols in Molecular Biology*, 1988, John Wiley & Sons, New York.
15 Draetta, G., Piwnica-Worms, H., Mobrison, D. *et al.*, *Nature*, **336**(1988), 738.
16 Buchkovich, K., Duffy, L. A. and Harlow, E. D., *Cell*, **58**(1989), 1097.
17 Kikuchi, Y., Shimatake, H. and Kikuchi, A., *EMBO J.*, **7**(1989), 1175.
18 Kipreos, E. T. and Wang, J. Y. J., *Science*, **13**(1990), 217.
19 Shimatake, H., Nakagawa, C., Thukahara, T. *et al.*, *Clin. Chem. Enzym. Comms.*, **2**(1990), 227.
20 Walker, R. A., Senior, P. V., Jones, J. L. *et al.*, *J. Pathol.*, **158**(1989), 97.

Modes of Binding and Internalization of Monoclonal Antibodies Against Human Gastric Cancer*

CHEN Xitao, CAI Xuejun, HU Jialu, ZHANG Xueyong and FAN Daiming

(*Department of Gastroenterology, Xijing Hospital, Xi'an* 710032, *China*)

Abstract The processes of binding and release of monoclonal antibodies(McAb) are greatly influenced by the biology of the respective antigen. We studied the kinetic characteristics of iodine-125-labelled McAbs (MGb2, MGc1, MGd1, MGg1, MG7) using cellular radioimmunoassays. Radiolabeled McAbs were allowed to bind to live or aldehyde-fixed human gastric cancer cell lines (SGC-7901, KATOIII) at 4°C and 37°C. MGb2 was found to bind at the highest level at 4°C with live cells and this was reversed by the treatment with isoosmolar acid buffer, together with rapid release upon 37°C, suggesting the corresponding antigen shedded from cell surface and MGb2 could not internalize well into SGC-7901 cells. Glutaraldehyde-fixed cells showed lower uptake at both temperatures. Concordant results were observed with MGg1. The binding of MGc1 to its glycoprotein antigen was higher at 37°C than at 4°C. The surplus in binding corresponded to a steadily increasing portion nondesorbable by pH 2.8 buffer treatment, pointing to the temperature-dependent internalization; while the fixed cells showed almost the same amount of uptake at both temperatures. In this situation the release of MGc1 was particularly slow at 37°C. The same finding was obtained with MGd1 and MG7. We concluded that McAbs (MGc1, MG7, MGd1) could internalized into specific cells and might be stored over the a term *in vivo*. These McAbs may have some advantages for targeting immunoconjugates to tumors for imaging or therapy.

The processes of binding and release of monoclonal antibodies (McAb), which are of great concern with respect to tumor targeting therapy, are greatly influenced by the biology of the respective antigen and the structure of the antibody.

A series of monoclonal antibodies against human gastric cancer with high specificity and sensitivity have been established in our laboratory[1, 2]. In the present study, their kinetic characteristics of binding, releasc and internalization were investigated.

I. Materials and Methods

1. *Monoclonal Antibodies and Labelling of McAbs With* ^{125}I

The McAbs used and the characteristics of the corresponding antigens are listed in Table 1[3]. McAbs were labelled with ^{125}I by the chloramine-T method. The immunoreactive fraction of labelled McAbs was determined by a “double inverse plot” as described by Lindmo[4].

* Project supported by the National Natural Science Foundation of China.

Table 1 List of Anti-gastric Cancer Cell McAbs and Characteristics of the Respective Antigens

McAbs	Antigen Detected		
	S Designation	Density	Cell line
MGb_2	NI	NI	SGC-7901
MGc_1	Glycoprotein		KATO III
MGd_1	Neutral glycolipid	20 kd	KATO III
MG_7	Neutral glycolipid	30 kd	KATO III
MG_9	Glycoprotein	110—120 kd	KATO III
MGg_1	NI	NI	KATO III

2. *Gastric Cancer Cell Lines*

SGC-7901 was grown a a monolayer in RPMI 1640 (GIBCO) supplemented with 10% heat-inactivated fetal calf serum. Near-confluent cultures were detached by incubation at 37°C for 10 min in trypsin-EDTA. The cells were then washed twice with D-Hank's fluid and resuspended in D-Hank's fluid. In some experiments where fixed cells were used, the procedure was similar to that described, but, after resuspending in D-Hank's fluid, the cells were fixed by incubation with 0.05 glutaraldehyde for 5 min at 37°C, then washed twice again. KATO III cells were grown as floating aggregates in the same complete medium. Single cell suspensions were obtained by gentle pipetting and treated as described.

3. *Uptake of Labelled McAbs*

The uptake McAbs were measured on living cells and glutaraldehyde fixed cells (2×10^6) by incubating them at 4°C or 37°C with 20,000 cpm of labelled McAb (11-13 ng/ml) in a RPMI 1640 medium containing 10% FCS. After various periods of incubation, unbound labelled McAbs were removed by washing three times with cold D-Hank's fluid. The radioactivity associated with the cells was measured in a gamma counter. Nonspecific binding was determined in the presence of a 10-fold excess of unlabelled McAb. Cell pellets were then resuspended in 1 ml of 0.05 mol/L glycine-HCl buffer and were kept for 20 min at room temperature. Thereafter, radioactivity of the samples was counted to determine the radioactivity of the acid-resistant cell precipitate fraction.

4. *Release of Bound Radioactivity*

Live cells (2×10^6/ml) were incubated for 2 h at 4°C or 37°C in a complete medium containing 20, 000 cpm of radiolabelled McAbs. Loaded cells were washed twice and counted to measure the initial uptake. Thereafter, the cells were suspended in a fresh complete medium and incubated for various periods at 4°C or 37°C. At each time point, cells were washed and treated with Glycine-HCl buffer and the acid-resistant cell precipitate fraction was counted.

II. Results

The basic assumption of the experiment was that the McAbs bound to targeted cells by simple diffusion should reach steady-state levels at 4°C and 37°C and should be completely reversible upon treatment with pH 2.8 buffer. Any difference from this behaviour would indicate interference by temperature dependent functions of putatively cellular origin.

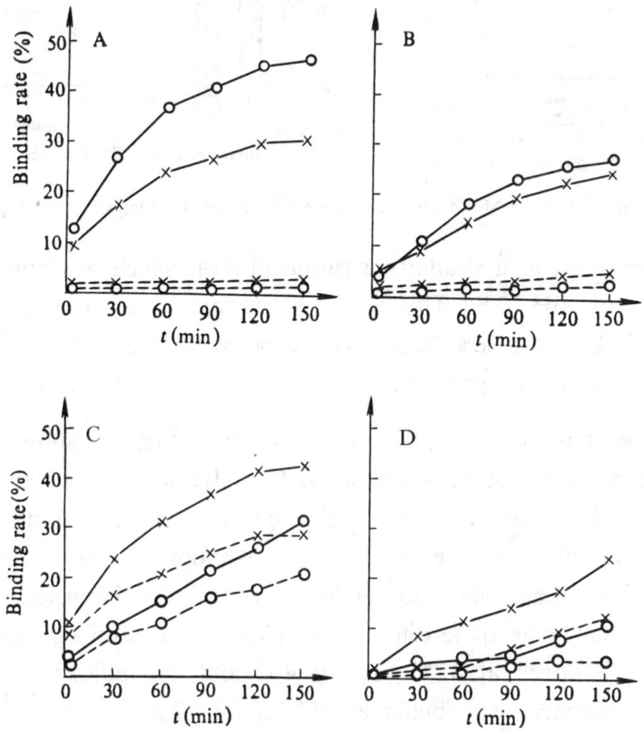

Fig.1 Uptake of ^{125}I-labelled monoclonal antibodies by gastric cancer cells.
A, B, MGb_2 binding to SGC-7901 cells; C, D, MGc_1 binding to KATO III, ○, binding at 4°C, ×, binding at 37°C, ——, total uptake, – – –, residual uptake after pH 2.8 treatment of cell; B, D, glutaraldehyde fixed cell.

Fig. 1 shows two major kinds of binding behaviour. Plots A and B indicate that MGb_2 binds with live cells at a higher level at 4°C, while the uptake by glutaraldehyde-fixed cells was found to be roughly the same at both temperatures. However, bound antibodies were totally desorbed by pH 2.8 buffer. Absolutely a similar result was obtained with McAb MGg_1.

Plots C and D show another characteristic of the binding. Here, the binding of MGc_1 to its glycoprotein antigen was greater at 37°C than that at 4°C. The excess of

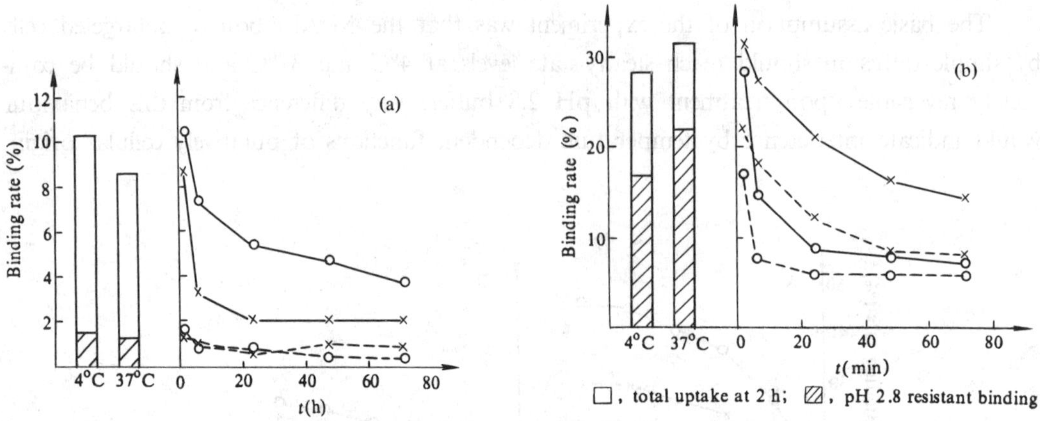

Fig.2 Release of ^{125}I-labelled McAb MGg_1 (a) and McAb MGc_1 (b). Symbols as in Fig.1.

bound antibody corresponded to a steadily increasing portion which was nondesorbable by treatment with buffer of pH 2.8. This type of uptake was also present in the glutaraldehyde-fixed cells but to a less degree. The same results were obtained with MGd_1 and MG_7 which, according to the preliminary evidence, can recognize a glycolipid antigen.

There were also two types of desorption of the McAbs which are shown in Fig.2. After an initial phase of rapid release of MGg_1 at 37°C, stable retention of radioactivity followed. But cells kept at 4°C showed a slow and progressive release of radioactivity. After treatment with buffer at pH 2.8, the acid-resistant component was almost negligible at both temperatures. The release behaviour of MGb_2 was similar. However, the release dynamics observed with MGc_1 were quite different. In these antigen-antibody systems, the release of MGc_1 was much slower at 37°C than at 4°C and the radioactivity remained at a high level even after treatment with buffer at pH 2.8 for 72 h.

III. Discussion

Antitumour McAbs have been used in imaging and therapy. The rationale of using McAb is to obtain a high target: nontarget ratio. The ratio can be influenced by many factors, e.g. the antigen density on the target cell, the antigen cross-expressed on normal tissues, the presence of circulating antigen in the blood, and the fate of McAbs subsequent to binding (stable localization outside the cell membrane or internalization or shedding). In the present communication, the modes of binding to, and the release of McAb to human gastric cancer cell lines were analyzed.

The data obtained from these studies are interpreted as follows. With McAb MGb_2, it was demonstrated that MGb_2 binding with live cells occurs at the highest level at 4°C, and this could be reversed by treatment with pH 2.8 buffer. It was also observed that there was rapid release of the antibody at 37°C, suggesting that its corresponding antigen was being shed from the cell surface. The same results were observed with MGg_1, but the uptake was minimal under all conditions.

McAb MGc_1 was another monoclonal antibody whose binding was higher at 37°C than that at 4°C. The excess bound antibody corresponded to a steadily increasing portion which was nondesorbable by pH 2.8 buffer treatment. In this situation, MGc_1 release was particularly slow at 37°C, suggesting temperature-dependent internalization. Furthermore, the increase in uptake with time could be clearly attributed to entry of radioactivity into the pH 2.8 resistant component. Similar results were obtained with MGd_1 and MG_7. It can be concluded that MGc_1, MG_7 and MGd_1 could be internalized into specific cells and might be stored over the long term *in vitro*. These McAbs may have some use for targeting immunoconjugates to tumors for imaging or therapy. A study of effect of internalization of monoclonal antibodies on McAb-directed cell-killing by immunoconjugates is under way.

References

1 Fan, D. M. *et al.*, *Chin. Med. J.*, **101**(1988), 188.
2 Deng, J. L. *et al.*, *Chin. J. Dig.* (in press).
3 Zhang, J. R. *et al.*, *J. Med. Coll. PLA*, **5**(1990), 63.
4 Lindmo, T. *et al.*, *Cancer Res.*, **46**(1986), 3848.
5 Matzku, S. *et al.*, *Cancer Immunol. Immunother.*, **24**(1987), 151.

A Method to Determine the Affinity Constant of an Antibody and Antigen Density on Cell Surfaces*

GUO Xuegang, CHEN Xitao, HU Jialu and ZHANG Xueyong

(*Institute of Gastroenterology, Xijing Hospital, Fourth Military Medical University, Xi'an, China*)

Abstract A binding assay was employed to assess the affinity constant of monoclonal antibody MGb_2 against gastric cancer and the density of MGb_2-Ag at the cellular surfaces of several live cell lines (SGC-7901, KATO III, BGC-823, MGC-803). Labelling of the antibody, MGb_2, with ^{125}I was performed according to the chloramine-T method[1]. The immunoreactive fraction of the antibody was determined by linear extrapolation to conditions representing infinite antigen excess. This ensures that the true value of the immunoreactive fraction is obtained, at about 92.3%. Two aliquots of the live cell lines were made up at a predetermined concentration in 1% BSA Hank's fluid. To one of the aliquots, unlabelled MGb_2 antibody was added in order to saturate the binding sites for subsequent determination of nonspecific binding. Eight serial 1:2 dilutions of ^{125}I-labelled MGb_2 antibody were made up in 1% BSA. After incubation, the paralleled samples were washed twice and the cpm values were measured. By Scatchard analysis, the affinity constant of MGb_2 was obtained, at about $2 \times 10^9\ M^{-1}$. The result shows that the density of the MGb_2-Ag at the cell surface is different in different cell lines, KATO III: 2×10^5/cell, SGC-7901: 4×10^6/cell, BGC-823: 5×10^5/cell, MGC-803: 2.5×10^6/cell.

Monoclonal antibodies against tumors have been successfully used in diagnostic localization of tumor tissue by external imaging[1]. Experimental approaches to cancer therapy by means of monoclonal antibody conjugates have also been reported[2]. In selecting an antibody for use in these studies, it is important to know the affinity constant of the antibody and the associated antigen density on the surfaces of the target cells. In this report, we use a binding assay for radiolabelled monoclonal antibody in which the immunoreactive fraction of the antibody was determined by linear extrapolation to conditions representing infinite antigen excess[3]. Further, by Scatchard analysis the affinity constant of the antibody and the associated binding site per cell were obtained.

I. Materials and Methods

1. *Cell Cultures*

Four cell lines of gastric cancer were used in our studies: Kato III, SGC 7901, BGC

* This study was funded in part by the National Natural Science Foundation of China.

823, and MGC 803. The Kato III cells were grown as floating aggregates and the others were grown as monolayers in cultures in RPMI 1640 medium supplemented with 10% FBS. Single cell suspensions were made by first rinsing the cell monolayer with PBS, then detecting the cells by incubation at 37°C for 5 min in 0.025% trypsin-0.02% EDTA in PBS. The cells were then washed twice with PBS and resuspended in PBS with 1% BSA or fixed by 0.25% glutaraldehyde. Care was taken to use cells in their logarithmic phase of growth, and the cultures routinely received fresh medium 1 or 2 days prior to the experiment.

In addition, Sl_7 (normal human embryogenic lung cell) was used as a control.

2. *Antibody and* ^{125}*I-labelling*

The monoclonal antibody against gastric cancer, MGb_2 (made by our laboratory) was purified from the ascites fluid of hybridoma-inoculated BALB/c mice. The purified antibody was examined by sodium dodecul sulfate polyacrylamide gel electrophoresis (SDS-PAGE). Labelling of the MGb_2 antibody with ^{125}I was performed according to the chloramine-T method (Ch-T)[4], using 0.5 mCi (1.85 MBq) of ^{125}I for 100 μg of the antibody. The labelling reaction was initiated by adding 10 μg chloramine-T and it was stopped by adding 20 μg sodium metabisulfate in equal volume. The total reaction volume was less than 100 μl, A Sephadex G-50 column was used for the separation of protein-bound and free ^{125}I and the protein concentrations were determined by Lowry's method.

3. *Time Course*

A time-course of the association of ^{125}I-MGb_2 with SGC 7901 was determined at 37°C using radiolabelled MGb_2 at a saturable dose in the absence (total binding, B) and presence (non-specific binding, NB) of unlabelled MGb_2. At various times, cold Hank's fluid was added to stop the reaction separately and the reactants were centrifuged, washed and counted to give CPM values. The specific binding (SB) was equal to B-NB.

4. *Confirmation of antibody specificity*

^{125}I-MHb_2 1.8 ng/10 μl, unlabelled MGb_2 10 μg/10 μl, irrelevant monoclonal antibody C_4 30 μg/10 μl (against epidemic haemorrhage fever virus, donated by Lab 403 of the University). SGC-7901 1.6×10^5/100 μl, untargeted cells Sl_7 4×10^6/100 μl. The binding sites of SGC 7901 or Sl_7 cells were either blocked or unblocked with unlabelled MGb_2 or C_4 while reacting with ^{125}I-MGb_2 at 37°C. The reaction was terminated 30 min later and the cells were centrifuged and washed twice for gamma counting.

5. *Determination of immunoreactive fraction of labelled antibody*

The equilibrium amount of antibody bound to antigen in an ideal binding reaction is determined by the law of mass action[3], i. e.

$$[B]=Ka[F][T\text{-}B]$$

where Ka is the association constant, [B] is the concentration of bound antibody, [F] is the concentration of free antigen, and [T-B] the concentration of unbound amount of antibody, i.e. the total micus the bound. If not all but only a fraction (r) of the total amount of antibody is immunologically reactive, the law of mass reaction applies only to the reactive amount of antibody, thus the concentration of reactive, free antibody is [rT-B], and

$$[B]=Ka[F][rT\text{-}B]$$

i.e.

$$\frac{[T]}{[B]}=\frac{1}{r}+\frac{1}{r\text{Ka}[F]}$$

According to the equation, five serial 1:2 dilutions of SGC 7901 were then made up in 1% BSA and reacted with ^{125}I-MGb$_2$ (final concentration 9 ng/mL) at 37°C for 30 min.

6. *Determination of antigen density and antibody affinity*

Eight serial 1:2 dilutions of ^{125}I-MGb$_2$ were made up in 1% BSA (final concentration 9-1150 ng/mL) and reacted with 4 gastric cancer cell lines at predetermined concentrations, respectively (Kato III: 1×10^6/ml, SGC 7901: 5×10^5/ml, BGC 823: 1.5×10^6/ml, MGC 803: 5×10^5/ml) at 37°C for 30 min. The data were analyzed as described by Scatchard[5].

II. Results

1. *Antibody purity determined by SDS-PAGE*

The test showed that there were only two bands, one light chain and the other, heavy chain, which indicated that the MGb$_2$ possessed high purity (Fig.1).

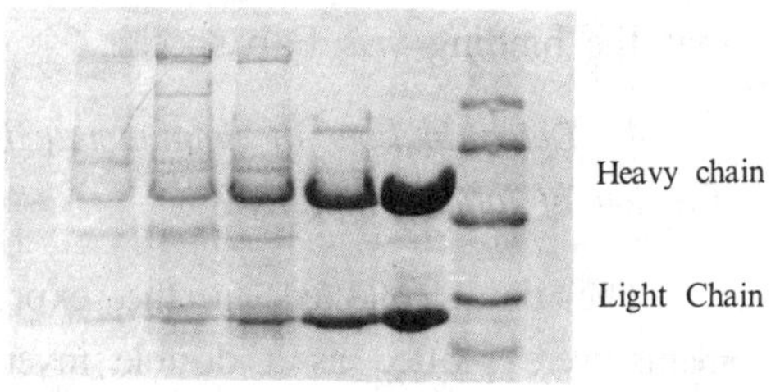

Fig. 1 SDS-PAGE photograph.

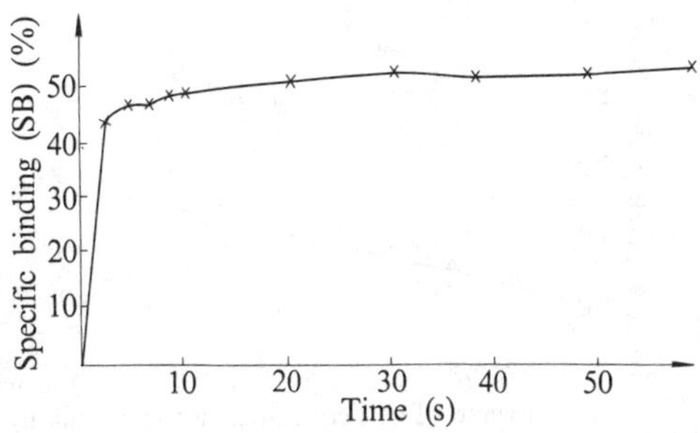

Fig. 2 Time course.

2. *Time-course*

The binding of monoclonal antibody to target cells varies with time (Fig. 2). The binding was approximate to saturation after 2 min and reached saturation at 10 min. The findings showed that MGb_2 and MGb_2-Ag reacted rapidly. Subsequent experiments were conducted for 30 min so that full equilibrium was attained.

3. *Antibody specificity*

As indicated in Fig.3a and b, the binding rate of ^{125}I-MGb_2 to target cells was as high as 74.2%, and, when blocked by irrelevant antibody C_4, the binding rate was 70.9% at highest, the two results showing no significant difference. When blocked by unlabelled MGb_2, the highest binding rate was only 5.2%, which was significantly lower than that of the former two results. When ^{125}I-MGb_2 reacted with Sl_7, the binding rates of the antibody unblocked or blocked to MGb_2 or C_4 were 2.8%, 3.5% and 3.6%, respectively, i.e. there was no significant difference between them. The findings indicated that MGb_2 can only react with its own target cells and cannot react with non-targeted cells and that the binding was Fab specific.

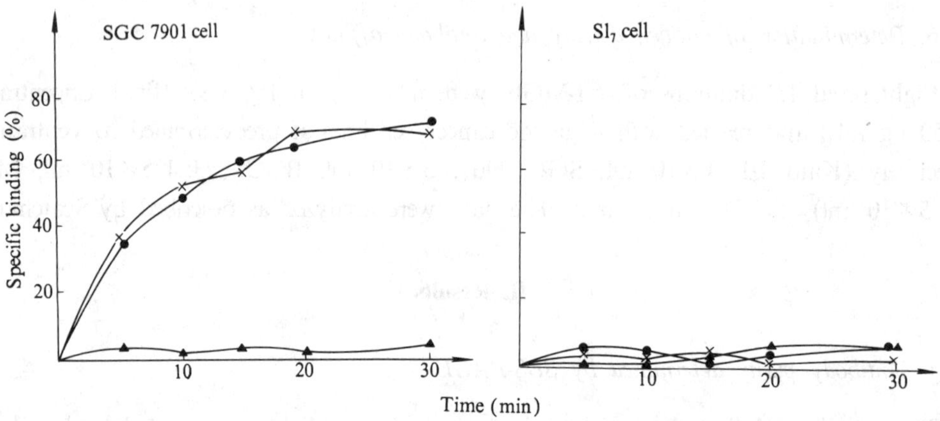

Fig. 3 Confirmation of specificity of antibody. ●, Reacted with ^{125}I-MGb_2; ×, block with MGb_2; ▲, block with C_4.

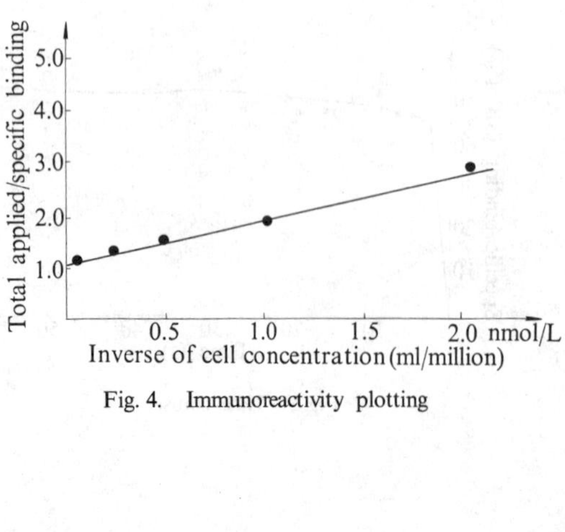

Fig. 4. Immunoreactivity plotting

4. *Determination of immunoreactive fraction of labelled antibody*

The data collected in the experiments were plotted as a double inverse plot of the applied radiolabelled antibody over the specific binding as a function of the inverse cell concentration (r=0.9998) (Fig. 4). The intercept value at the ordinate was $1/r$(=1.084) and so the immunoreactive fraction (r) was 0.9227, which was similar to Lindmo's results (93%). These findings demonstrated that the monoclonal antibody against gastric cancer prepared in our laboratory was of high immunoreactivity and the labelling process using the Ch-T method had virtually no effect on the immunoreactivity of the antibody.

5. *Antigen density and antibody affinity constant*

The experimental data were plotted with antibody concentration as abscissa and specific binding (SB) as ordinate (Fig. 5). As indicated in the figure, as the concentration of added antibody increased, the amount of specifically bound antibody rose and reached a maximum when the concentration of antibody added reached a certain level. Thus, the binding of the antibody with its target cell was saturable.

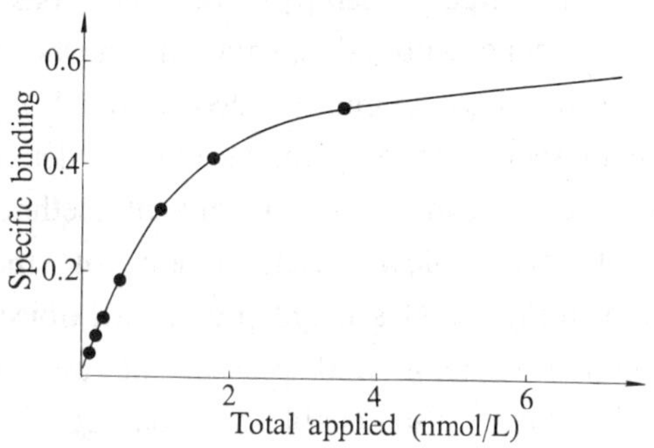

Fig. 5 Saturation curve.

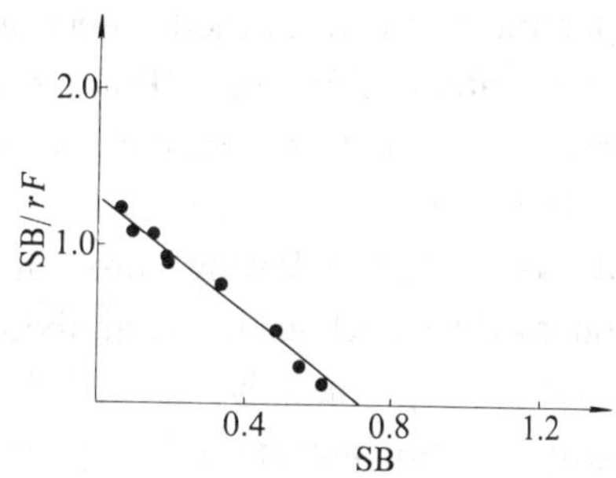

Fig. 6 Scatchard plotting.

The same data were plotted as described by Scatchard (Fig. 6). The reaction of MGb_2 against gastric cancer with four gastric cancer cell lines gave a straight line on the plot (r=0.99). Antigen density on the surface of single cell of the four cell lines and the affinity constant of the monoclonal antibody MGb_2 could be calculated using the Scatchard analysis (Table 1).

Table 1 Density of MGb_2-Ag and Affinity Constant of MGb_2

Cancer Cell Lines	MGb_2-Ag (Sites/cell)	Affinity Constant (M^{-1})
Kato III	$(2.24\pm0.20)\times10^5$	$(2.32\pm0.34)\times10^9$
SGC 7901	$(3.97\pm0.27)\times10^6$	$(1.89\pm0.20)\times10^9$
BGC 823	$(5.13\pm0.30)\times10^5$	$(2.07\pm0.13)\times10^9$
MGC 803	$(2.55\pm0.02)\times10^6$	$(2.15\pm0.16)\times10^9$

(n=3)

As indicated in the table, though MGb_2 might react with each of the four cell lines, antigen density on each cell line was different. The antigen density of Kato III and BGC

823 was 10^5, which was very similar to Lindmo's result while that of SGC 7901 and MGC 803 was 10^6. The reaction of the monoclonal antibody with target cells was actually that of MGb_2 with MGb_2-Ag, and, though the cell lines were different, the affinity between antibody and antigen was identical, as proved by the present experiment. The ffinity constants of MGb_2 with the four cell lines were very similar, and, therefore, the affinity constant of MGb_2 was $(2.1 \pm 0.25) \times 10^9$ ($n = 12$).

III. Discussion

There have been many reports of its successes in the preliminary clinical use of monoclonal antibodies against tumors. Many problems still exist before full application of monoclonal antibody can be made. For example, when radioimmunoimaging gave negative results, it was not known whether the negative results were due to the low immunoreactivity of the antibody or to the absence of the tumor. Also, it had to be determined which antibodies were more effective in serological diagnosis and selecting antibodies of high affinity was the key to success in target therapy. In the past, immunohistochemical methods were adopted for selecting antibodies, but the methods lacked quantitative accuracy. For instance, the four cell lines immunostained with MGb_2 showed positive but no distinguishing results. The present method might be able to detect the difference in antigen density of the four cell lines. In conclusion, the present method might solve the following problems: Firstly, it may allow determination of the immunoreactive fraction of the antibody or immunoconjugate. This might provide an objective evaluation of negative results obtained by immunoimaging and prevent the use of antibody of no immunoreactivity in patients. It would also enable the damage to immunoreactivity by the conjugation of drugs and antibody to be accurately assessed. Secondly it may allow determination of the turmor-associated antigen density on the cell surface. This might distinguish tumor cells giving identical immunohistochemical results of different origins and further the investigation of the effect of various biochemical factors on the expression of antigen on the cell surface. Thirdly, it may allow the determination and comparison of the affinity constants of the various monoclonal antibodies, which would be of use in selecting an antibody of high affinity in target therapy. This might also enable the affinity of the conjugates to be assessed so that an ideal conjugating method or conjugate might be obtained.

References

1 Goldenberg D. W. *et al.*, *J. Cancer Res. Clin. Oncol.*, **113**(1987), 3: 203.

2 Badger C. C. *et al.*, *Cancer Res.*, **46**(1986), 6223.

3 Lindmo T. *et al.*, *J. Immumo. Mech.*, **72**(1984), 77.

4 Mcconahey P. J. *et al.*, *Int. Arch. Aller.*, **29**(1986), 185.

5 Scatchard G., *Ann. N. Y. Acad. Sci.*, **51**(1949), 660.

Effect of 6-Thioguanine and Interferons on c-*myc* Protooncogene Expression in HL-60 Cells*

TAN Yuying, SUN Xinghua, TAN Huiying, ZHOU Hong,

(*Cancer Research Institute, Harbin Medical University, Harbin 150040, China*)

TAN Xuezhong and SUN Rei

(*The First Hospital of Harbin, Harbin 150040, China*)

Abstract A synergistic effect produced by combination of the anti-metabolite 6-thioguanine (6-TG) and the cytokines IFN-α, IFN-γ has been reported previously. In order to study the molecular biological basis of those agents and the relationship between c-*myc* protooncogene expression, the cell proliferation and cell differentiation we have evaluated the effect of 6-TG, IFN-α and IFN-γ on HL-60 human leukemia cell growth, cell differentiation and the expression of c-*myc* mRNA and an interferon inducible gene, PIFN-IND-2 gene, RNA(56 k mRNA).

The results show that 6-TG has a strong inhibition effect and IFNs have only a minimal inhibition effect on HL-60 cell growth. However, both of them produce similar induction of functional terminal differentiation of HL-60 cells in an NBT assay. Northern blot autoradiagraphy analysis showed that 6-TG and IFNs produce a similar effect on the expression of mRNA related genes. 6-TG has a very rapid effect on c-*myc* mRNA with a biphasic response. After the first 3h c-*myc* mRNA increases rapidly; after 6h it decreases; by 48h less than 10% remains. IFNs produce a similar effect although slowly and weakly. The effect on 56kDa mRNA is obvious: IFNs induce a marked and rapid increase in 56kDa mRNA. Unexpectedly, 6-TG produces a similar effect. It is of interest that the concentrations of the IFNs used in all of the experiments did not have any cytotoxic effect on the cells, but a marked effect was produced on cell differentiation and cmyc mRNA expression.

The results suggest that the expression of the c-*myc* oncogene is closely related to cell differentiation. The rapid increase in c-*myc* mRNA soon after drug treatment can be identified with the differentiation process. The subsequent decrease is related to the terminal differentiation. The PIFN-IND-2 gene may also be involved in the cell differentiation. The results also suggest that 6-TG and the IFNs may produce a similar regulation in the expression of some related genes. This may be the molecular biological basis of their synergistic effect.

The expression of the c-*myc* protooncogene has been proposed to be related to a variety of conditions in malignant cells including the growth rate of the cells and the level of development or differentiation. The ability to affect c-*myc* expression may therefore be a useful target in attempting to control or eradicate a particular malignancy. It remains unclear however whether c-*myc* expression is linked to growth or to differentiation. The

* Project supported by the National Natural Science Foundation of China.

ability of currently available therapeutic agents to produce this action has been of particular interest. The purine antimetabolite 6-thioguanine (6-TG) is one of the most effective agents in the treatment of human acute myelogenous leukemia, and is used in other anticancer regimens as well. 6-TG is quite clearly a potent cytotoxic agent that incorporates into both DNA and RNA. In addition to its cytotoxic activity, it has been shown recently that 6-TG can stimulate myeloid differentiation, and that it can alter the physiology of cells very rapidly.

Considerable attention has been afforded the cytokines such as α and γ interferon (IFN). These agents, although not generally having tumorocidal activity themselves, appear to enhance the host's immune activity against tumor cells. In addition, it is now recognized that these agents can be potent differentiation agents. Several genes, such as 2-5a synthetase, have been identified as being regulated by IFN. One recently characterized gene code for a 56 kDa cytoplasmic protein in hematopoeitic cells.

A synergistic effect produced by a combination of the anti-metabolite 6-thioguanine (6-TG) and the cytokines IFN-α, IFN-γ has been reported previously[1]. In order to study the molecular biological basis of these agents and the relationship between c-*myc* protooncogene expression, cell proliferation and cell differentiation, we evaluated the effect of 6-TG, IFN-α, and IFN-γ on HL-60 human leukemia cell growth, cell differentiation and the expression of c-*myc* mRNA and an interferon inducible gene, PIFN-IND-2 gene, mRNA(56 k mRNA).

I. Materials and Methods

1. *Cell Culture and Clonogenic Survival*

HL-60 human promyelocytic leukemia cells were maintained as a suspension culture in RPMI-1640 medium supplemented with 15% FCS at 37°C and with 5% CO_2. The cell density used for experimentation was 1×10^5 to 8×10^5 cells/ml, which was at the logarithmic growth stage. Cells at a density of 1 to 2×10^5 cells/ml were treated with either 6-TG or IFN. Drug toxicity was determined by using a soft-agar cloning procedure as described previously[2], with each set of conditions being run in triplicate. The plating efficiency of the control was about 60%. Percent growth was calculated as the ratio of the clones under each conditions divided by the control.

2. *NBT Assay for Measuring Differentiation*

Cells were exposed continously to the drugs for 5 days, with the cell density maintained at 2 to 4×10^5 cells/ml by diluting the cells twice during this period. Differentiation of HL-60 leukemia cells was measured by using a standard NBT reduction assay, which has been described previously[3]. After being washed once,

2×10^5 cells were resuspended in 0.2 ml of NBT solution (2 mg/ml NBT and 2×10^{-4} mg TPA in 1 × PBS), mixed well and incubated at 37°C for 20 min. NBT positive cells containing cytoplasmic blue-black precipitate were quantitated using a hemacytometer. A minimum of 200 cells were counted and the percent of NBT positive cells was calculated.

3. *RNA Extraction and Analysis*

Following drug treatment for a certain period, HL-60 cells were centrifuged at 1000 rpm at 4°C for 10 min, washed once with ice cold 1 × PBS, suspended in 10 volumes of lysis buffer A (0.14 mol/L NaCl, 0.0015 mol/L $MgCl_2$, 0.01 mol/ L Tris-Cl pH8.6, 0.2% Triton x-100, and freshly added 0.01 mol/ L VRC), and vortexed for 8 seconds. Immediately, to the cell suspension was added the same volume of lysis buffer B (lysis buffer A containing sucrose 24% w/v) and the mixture was centrifuged at 10,000 × g for 20 min at 4°C. The upper layer, which contained cytoplasmic RNA, was incubated with proteinase K (200 μg/ml). At 37°C for 30 min, and then the protein was extracted with phenol/chloroform/isoamyl alcohol (25/24/1, v/v/v) twice and then chloroform/isoamly alcohol (24/1, v/v) twice. The RNA was precipitated with 2.5 volumes of ethanol at −20°C for 12 hours. Extraction of the nuclear RNA was completed by adding GIT buffer (4mol/L guanidine isothiocyanate, 0.025 mol/L sodium acetate pH6, 0.1 mol/L β-mercaptoethanol) 6ml per 0.5 ml of nuclei which was carefully layered on the top of 4 ml CsCl Buffer (5.7 mol/L cesium chloride, 0.025 mol/L sodium acetate pH 6). This mixture was then centrifuged at 174,000 × g at 20°C for 21 h. The supernatant was carefully removed without disrupting the pellets which were then suspended in 0.5 ml of 0.3 mol/L sodium acetate (pH 6). The RNA remaining in the solution was precipitated with ethanol. The combined RNA was extracted by the guanidinium/cesium chloride method as described previously[4]. Then the RNA was measured using a Beckman spectrophotometer at 260 nm. A sample of the RNA (5 μg) was dot blotted with a 60-hole aspiration dot blot apparatus onto a piece of Zeta-probe membrane apper, then the paper was baked at 80°C in vacuum.

A second sample of the RNA (5 μg or 10 μg) was fractionated on a vertical 1.6% agarose slab gel which contained 6 mol/L urea and 0.015 mol/L iodoacetate, with a TPE running buffer at 40 V for 4 to 5 h. RNA bands were visualized under UV light after staining with ethidium bromide for photography. The RNA was then transferred to Zeta-probe paper (Biorad Laboratories) by electroblotting at 1.3 amps for 2h at 4°C, then baked in vacuum at 80°C for 1 h. After pre-hybridization the paper was hybridized at 42°C for 48 h with either *c-myc*-cDNA-plasmid or pIFN-IND-2 cDNA plasmid which had been previously labeled by nick-translation with [α-^{32}P] dCTP, (3×10^7 cpm/ml). The papers were then autoradiographed at −70°C for 1—5 days.

II. Results

1. *Effect of 6-TG and Interferon on Cell Viability*

The effect of a 24 h exposure to different concentrations of 6 - TG, or to a continuous exposure of IFN, on the viability of HL - 60 cells was determined by measuring their clonogenic survival in semi-soft agar. The results are shown in Fig. 1. The LD50 of 6-TG was observed to be 0.55 μmol/L with greater than 99% of cells killed at concentrations exceeding 10 μmol/L. It is of interest that even when the concentration of 6 - TG was increased to 100 μmol/L, the toxicity of 6 - TG never exceeded 99.95% (in these instances, 5,000 cells per cloning experiment were evaluated rather than the 100 cells per experiment used for the results in Fig. 1). An increase in the exposure time to 72 h did not alter this result, so it was not aparently related to cell cycle/exposure time.

Neither IFN-α nor IFN-γ exhibited significant reductions of cell viability even under conditions of continuous exposure at 1000 IU/ml.

2. *Differentiation of HL-60 Cells*

In addition to the cytotoxic activity exhibited by 6-TG, it has been also shown to be able to stimulate HL-60 myeloid differentiation. Similarly, although not potent cytotoxic agents, as was illustrated in Fig. 1, the interferons have been shown to be potent differentiation agents. The results are shown in Table 1. As a differentiation control,

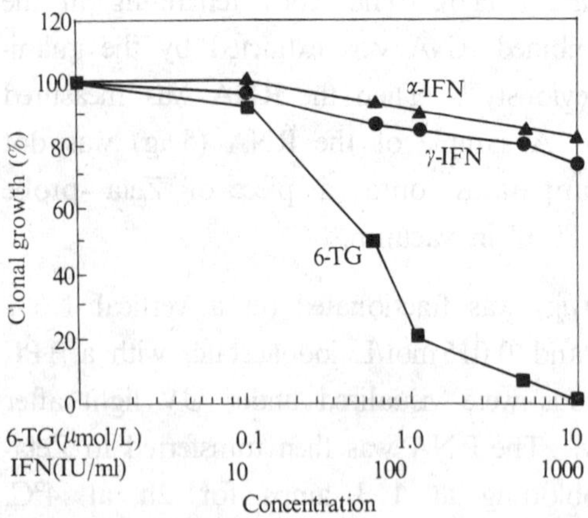

Fig. 1 Clonal growth of 6-TG and IFN-treated HL-60 cells. Cells were treated with either 6-TG (24 hours), α-IFN or γ-IFN (2 weeks), and then cloned as deseribed under Materials and Methods. Values represent the mean ($n=3$).

Table 1 Effect of 6-TG and Interferon on HL-60 Differentiation

HL-60 cells were exposed to each agent for five days, and the differentiation was examined by NBT reduction assay as described in Materials and Methods

Treatment	%NBT$_+$ [a]	Fold increase[b]
Control	13±4	–
0.1 mol/L DMSO	30±7	1.3
0.5 μmol/L 6-TG	26±9	1.0
1 μmol/L 6-TG	32±5	1.5
100 IU/ml α-IFN	31±7	1.3
1000 IU/ml α-IFN	35±2	1.6
10 IU/ml γ-IFN	30±3	1.3
100 IU/ml γ-IFN	36±4	1.7

a) % NBT$_+$ = percent of cells containing the black-blue deposits as noted in the Materials and Methods.
b) Fold increase = [%NBT$_+$ of sample/%NBT$_+$ of control] − 1.

we also evaluated the effect of DMSO. Using a standard NBT reduction assay, 0.5 μmol/L 6-TG, 100 IU/ml IFN− and 10 IU/ml IFN− were each found to induce HL-60 cell differentiation to a similar, or greater level than that produced by DMSO (dimethyl sulfoxide). Among these agents, IFN-α and IFN-γ were found to be the most potent, with 6-TG also exhibiting significant activity. In contrast to the cytotoxicity results presented above, all three agents have strong differentiating activity.

3. *Effect on c-myc and 56K mRNA*

We measured the expression of c-*myc* mRNA in cells exposed to 1 μmol/L 6-TG, 100 IU/ml IFN-α or 10 IU/ml IFN-γ. Figs. 2— 5 illustrate the relative level of c-*myc* mRNA in HL-60 cells following exposure to 1μmol/L 6-TG from 30min to 48h. Fig. 2 is a photograph of the ethidium bromide stained gel showing that relatively constant amounts (10 μg) of RNA were electrophoresed in each lane. An autoradiograph of the northern blot of the RNA which was hybridized with [α-^{32}P] dCTP labeled c-*myc* cDNA is also shown. The total cellular RNA, illustrated in the picture with the rRNA, did not change during the treatment period, although the level of cMyc mRNA was markedly changed over this period. These results are more clearly illustrated in Fig. 3. 6-TG had a rapid effect on c-*myc* mRNA as both nuclear and cytoplasmic mRNA levels initially increased after exposure to the drug for 30 min and were found to be increased by almost 3-fold after 3 h. The levels of c-*myc* mRNA were then observed to markedly decrease with time, and c-*myc* mRNA was almost undetectable after 48 h treatment.

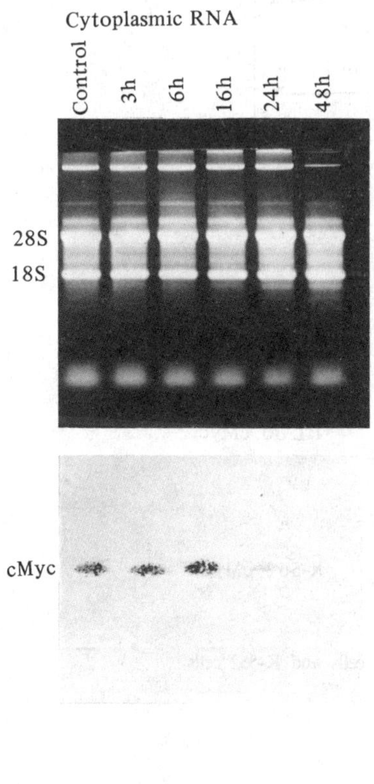

Fig. 2. Agarose/urea gel electrophoresis and autoradiography of HL-60 cytoplasmic and nuclear RNA. Following 1 μmol/L 6-TG treatment, nuclear and cytoplasmic RNA were isolated from HL-60 cells, and 10 μg of RNA was electrophoresed at 40V for 7 hours at described in Materials and Methods. Illustrated is a photograph of the ethidium bromide stained gel prior to transfer, and the autoradiograph of the transferred RNA following hydridization with a [^{32}P]-labelled human c-*myc* cDNA.

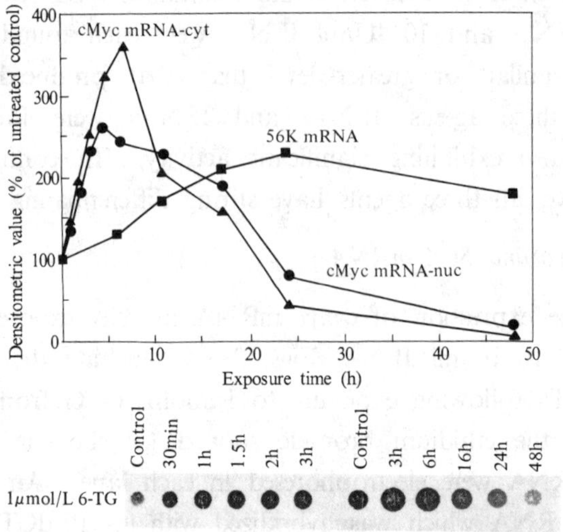

Fig. 3. Effect of 6-TG on c-*myc* mRNA and 56K mRNA in HL-60 cells.

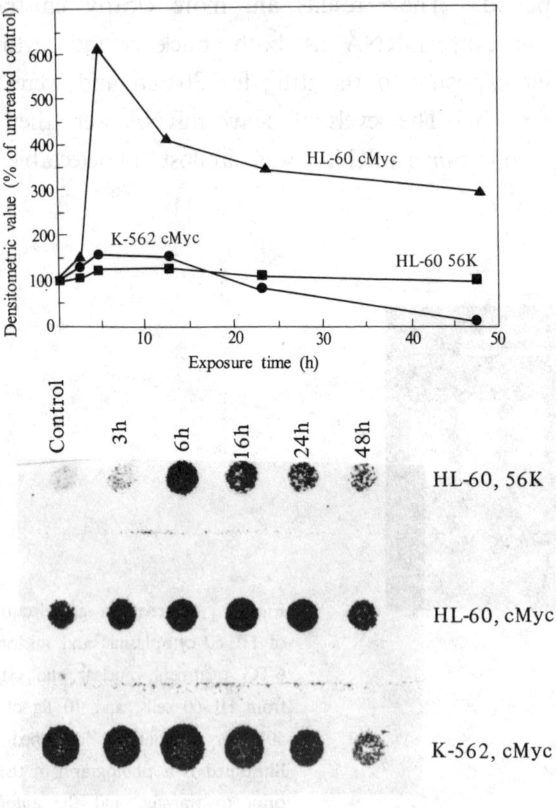

Fig. 4. Effect of α-IFN on mRNA in HL-60 cells and K-562 cells.

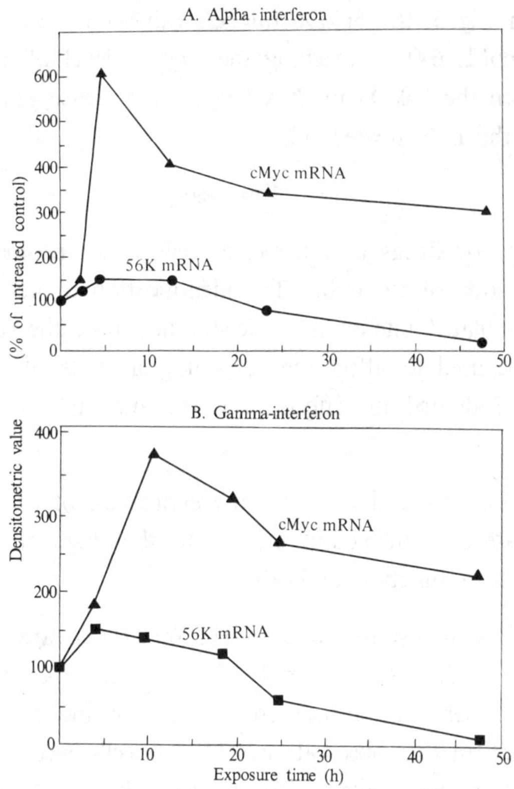

Fig. 5. Effect of IFNs on c-*myc* mRNA and 56kDa mRNA in HL-60 cells.

The effect of IFN on c-*myc* mRNA was similar, as is shown in Fig. 5 A, B. Both IFN-α and IFN-γ produced an initial increase of c-*myc* mRNA after treatment for 3 h, although the level of increase was considerably less than that observed with 6-TG. However, with time the level of c-*myc* mRNA declined markedly so that again after 48 h, the level was very low.

Evaluation of 56kDa mRNA was also completed. Following exposure of the HL-60 cells to 100 IU/mL of IFN-α, the level of 56kDa mRNA was found to be rapidly increased (Fig. 5) reaching values 5-fold greater than those in untreated control cells within 6 h following treatment with IFN-α, and 3-fold in cells treated with IFN-γ. The rate of increase in 56kDa mRNA however was slown at approximately 6 h, and then the level of 56kDa mRNA began to decrease with time, although the level remained elevated compared to the control at all times examined. The 56kDa mRNA began to decline at the same time as the c-*myc* mRNA in the cells was also declining (Fig. 4), although it remained 3 and 2.5 fold greater than the control, during the period when the c-*myc* mRNA levels were negligible.

The effect of 6-TG on this supposedly IFN-specific mRNA was evaluated as well.

As can be observed in Fig. 3, the 56kDa mRNA exhibited a slow but steady increase in cells treated with 1 μmol/L 6-TG, reaching the highest level of almost twice that of the control after 24 h. Then the 56kDa mRNA began to decrease, showing behaviou similar to that observed with the IFN treated cells.

IV. Discussion

The use of anti-tumor drugs to kill cancer cells or to promote differentiation of the cells remains an active area of research. The identification of key genes in the malignant growth process has stimulated interest in understanding how the control of the expression of these genes might be used to affect the physiological state of the malignant cell. The studies presented here evaluated the effects of 6-TG and IFN in the expression of some important genes.

Previous investigations have shown that the expression of c-*myc* appears to be related to either the growth rate of a malignant cell, or to the stage of functional differentiation of the cell, or it may be a function of both.

Filmus and Buick[5] demonstrated that in HL-60 cells treated with DMSO or grown under serum depleted conditions, the level of c-*myc* mRNA appeared related to the differentiation process rather than to the growth rate of the cells. Our studies, using a different approach, confirm this observation. HL-60 cells were examined under optimal conditions of growth, but were treated with an agent that was both cytotoxic and able to promote differentiation (6-TG), and compared with the results of an agent that was able to produce differentiation but which was not cytotoxic (IFN). The results show that 6-TG has a very rapid effect on c-*myc* mRNA, with a biphasic response. The rapid and large induction of c-*myc* mRNA in the first 3 h of exposure to 6-TG concurs with other reports that this type of response is important as a "precommitment phase" to the differentiation process. The differentiation activity of 6-TG has only recently become recognized as possibly being an important factor in its clinical activity. The loss of cMyc mRNA in the cells treated with either of the IFNs under conditions which did not alter the apparent proliferation of the cells, supports the view that the expression of this gene is strongly related to the level of cell differentiation. The activity of 6-TG as an immunosuppressant may also relate to the rapid changes in mRNA expression that occur in response to it .

The functional role of the interferon regulated genes in cells is also an area of great interest, as exemplified by the IFN inducible 56kDa protein[6]. Considering the potent differentiating activity of IFN, we felt that this 56kDa protein might be involved in differentiation. Our results demonstrate that this gene is rapidly induced in HL-60 cells by IFN under conditions that result in both cytodifferentiation as well as modulation of the c-*myc* mRNA. Similar stimulation by the 6-TG would have supported this theory. However, these results do not rule out that the normal expression of the 56k gene is either a function of differentiated hematopoetic cells, or may be involved in promoting the normal activity of these cells.

In conclusion, these studies demonstrate that both 6-TG and the interferons can promote HL-60 differentiation which is accompanied by an initial stimulation of c-*myc* mRNA and is followed by a large suppression of its expression. Only 6-TG was able to reduce the proliferation of these cells, adding support to the concept that c-*myc* expression is a function of the stage of cell development rather than the proliferative capacity of the cell. These results also add evidence for there being a large increase in the expression of c-*myc* as a part, or indeed as the signal, of a precommitment phase for the differentiation process. The 56kDa mRNA in HL-60 cells was shown to be induced by both IFN-α and IFN-γ, as well as 6-TG (on a delayed basis), and may be necessary for the differentiated function of the cells. Our results also suggest that 6-TG and the IFNs produce a similar regulation of the expression of some related genes and this might be the molecular biological basis of their synergistic combination.

References

1 Tan, Y.Y. et al., *Cancer Res.*, **49**(1989), 4431.

2 Armstrong, R.D. et al., *Biochem. Biophys. Res. Comn.*, **109**(1982), 2: 595.

3 Yen, A. and Guerrey, D.L. *Cancer Res.*, **46**(1986), 4156.

4 Tan Y.Y. et al., *Chinese Journal of Oncology* (in press).

5 Filmus, J. and Buick, R.N., *Cnacer Res.*, **45**(1985), 822.

6 Moutichen, S. et al., *Molecular and Chemical Aspects of the Interferon-Regulated Pathway,* 1985, p. 183.

The Purification and Characterization of a Carbohydrate Recognized by Concanavalin A in Gastric Cancer Tissue and Its Significance in the Diagnosis of Patients With Malignancies

ZHANG Jiren[1] and ZHANG Xueyong[2]

1. *Department of Oncology, Zhu Jiang Hospital, Guangzhou 510282, China*
2. *Laboratory of Gastroenterology, Xi Jing Hospital, Xi'an 710032, China*

Abstract A neutral glycolipid and a glycoprotein defined by Concanavlin A (Con A), were purified from gastric cancer tissue and used in the serological diagnosis of tumours.

Fresh gastric cancer tissue was obtained from the surgical department, and proved to be reactive with Con A by ABC method, minced up, homogenized and centrifuged according to the routine method. The supernatant, containing the receptors recognized by Con A, was collected and incubated with sepharose 4B coupled with Concanavalin A at 4°C for 6 h. By means of affinity chromatography, the substances defined by Con A were isolated from the extract of gastric cancer tissue.

Analysis of the substances defined by Con A was performed on an HPTIC plate and SDS-PAGE gel according to the procedures of Hakomori and Towbin. It was confirmed that the receptors of Con A in gastric cancer tissue contain two components, a neutral glycolipid and a glycoprotien with a molecular weight of 35—80 kDa.

The glycoprotein purified from tumor tissue was conjugated with HRP and used to investigate the levels of the receptors defined by Con A in the serum of patients with malignancies, using the ELISA inhibiting method. The results suggest that there is a high expresson of these receptors in the serum of patients with tumors. The positive rates were found to be 51.3% in gastric cancer, 60.7% in liver cancer, 57.4% in lung cancer and 52.9% in ovarian tumors.

Recently, many carbohydrates in the serum of patients with tumors have been shown to be associated with carcinoma. They can be carried by both the glycolipids and glycoproteins of a malignant cell. Examples include sialyl Lewis a, CA50, Tn, Cal, MGd1-Ag and MG7-Ag[1—3]. Most of these tumor-associated carbohydrate antigens can be recognized, not only by a specific antibody, but also by some lectins[3, 4]. The results of an earlier study demontrated that the oligosaccharide specific agglutinin can be used as a tool in the analysis of the tumor-associated antigen and in the immunopathological diagnosis of carcinoma. During the last decade, much attention has been focused on the possibility that cellular recognition is mediated by carbohydrates on the surface of the cell membrane.

There are strong indications that in many cases carbohydrates modify the activities of the proteins to which they are attached and also serve as markers for cell differentiation, development and pathological states[5]. Concanavalin A (Con A), a mannose-linked oligosaccharide sepecific agglutinin has been used in the detection of an oligosaccharide chain on gastrointestinal cancer tissues and in the isolation of tumor-associated antigens, such as CEA, AFP and MG-Ags[1, 3, 5]. In this study Con A was used to purify and characterize carbohydrates in gastric cancer tissue, and its possible use in the serological diagnosis of patients with malignant tumors was investigated.

I. Materials and Methods

1. *Preparation of carbohydrate Extract*

In order to prepare a large amount of carbohydrate extract, fresh gastric cancer tissue of a patient who had been diagnosed with gastric adenocarcinoma was obtained from the surgical department in our hospital. After removal of normal and necrosis tissue, the stomach neoplasm tissue, which was shown to be active with Con A by the ABC method, was minced up, homogenized in phosphate-buffered saline solution containing 0. 25% ninedet p40 (pH 7.4), and centrifuged at 100000×g for 1 h. The supernatant was collected and stored at 20°C[6].

2. *Purification of carbohydrate defined by Con A*

The carbohydrate extract from gastric cancer tissue was dialysed against PBS buffer solution containing 0.15 mol/L sodium chloride, and 1 mmol/L each of magnesium chloride, manganese chloride, and calcium chloride (all from Sigma Chemical Co.) overnight, and then centrifuged at 20000×g for 10 min. The supernatant was collected and passed through a sepharose 4B column (2.5 cm×25 cm) to remove materials absorbed by sepharose 4B. The fraction collected was applied onto a Concanavalin A-sepharose 4B (Pharmacia) column (1.5 cm×15 cm) and allowed to equilibrate for 4 h at 4°C. The solution was chromatographed using a flow rate of 10—15 ml/h. The unbound proteins were eluted from this column with phosphate-buffered saline solution (pH 7.4). The carbohydrate bound by the Con A on the column was subsequently eluted with PBS buffer containing 500 mmol/L α-methylmannopyranoside (Sigma)[7]. The purified carbohydrate was collected and dialysed against water solution.

Analysis of the carbohydrate defined by Con A: To isolate the glycolipid and glycoprotein from the carbohydrate purified from gastric cancer tissue, the carbohydrate fraction was extracted with chloroform/methanol and partitioned according to the method described elsewhere. The glycolipid-containing layers were collected and evaporated to dryness, and then dissolved in a suitable quantity of chloroform/methanol (1:1 v/v). The glycolipid component from gastric cancer tissue was chromatographied on a high performance thin layer chromatography plate (E. mark) according to the published method[3]. The solvent system for TLC was chloroform/methanol/0.5% $CaCl_2$ in H_2O (55/40/10; v/v/v). The ganglioside mixture prepared from a calf brain served as the TLC control. After chromatography the TLC plate was treated with Orcinol H_2SO_4 and Resorcinol-HCl respectively[3].

Analysis of glycoprotein. The glycoprotein component purified from gastric cancer tissue was analyzed by sodium dodecyl sulfate polyacrylamide gel electrophoresis (SDS-PAGE) according to the previously published procedure[6]. The carbohydrate extract from the gastric cancer tissue was used as a control in this experiment.

3. *Preparation of the conjugate of glycoprotein and horseradish peroxidase*

25 mg of the glycoprotein purified from gastric cancer tissue, with Con A affinity chromatography, was dialysed against $NaHCO_3$ buffer (pH 8.5) and conjugated with 5 mg of horseradish peroxidase[8].

4. *Specimen*

Serum samples from 100 individuals were collected at the blood bank in our hospital. Samples were also collected from 104 patients with benign diseases of the digestive system. These included 29 gastric, 12 colorectal, 30 liver, 14 lung and 18 other diseases. A total of 218 sera specimens were collected from cancer patients, including those with gastric (110), liver (23), lung (37) and ovarian (34) tumors.

5. *Determination of carbohydrate in serum*

Serum levels of the carbohydrate defined by Con A were measured by a competitive binding method[9]. In brief, 50 μl samples were reacted with Concanavalin A coated on the bottom of 96-well plates, for 4 h at 4°C. The excess serum was removed by washing, and then glycoprotein labelled with peroxidase was added to this system and allowed to react for 4 h at room temperature. The excess glycoprotein labelled with peroxidase was removed by washing with PBS buffer solution. The peroxidase activity associated with Con A was measured according to the published method[8]. Carbohydrate purified from gastric cancer tissue in a concentration range of 5—70 μ/mL was used instead of serum as a standard. In this assay carbohydrate activity is expressed in arbitrary units and is not related to protein concentration.

II. Results

1. *Purification of the carbohydrate defined by Con A from gastric cancer tissue*

Carbohydrate extract solution (60 ml) was prepared using 15 mg of stomach neoplasm tissue. It was determined that the carbohydrate recognized by Con A was present in this extract. By means of Con A affinity chromatography, the carbohydrate associated with Con A in gastric cancer tissue was eluted from a Con A column using 500 mmol/L α-methylmannopyranoside. The results of the assay suggested that in the fraction containing carbohydrate purified from gastric cancer tissue there are both glycolipid and glycoprotein components. They can both be recognized by Con A. The results of thin layer chromatography demonstrated that the glycolipid components of the carbohydrate recognized by Con A were not made visible by resorcinol-HCl reagent, since they are not gangliosides. However a band was visible on treatment with orcinol-H_2SO_4 reagent indicating that neutral glycolipids were present (Fig.1).

On SDS-PAGE gel, the glycoprotein components of the carbohydrate purified by Con A affinity chromatography showed five subunits with molecular weight of 80, 70, 60, 35 and 20 kDa, under reducing conditions when stained with Coomassie blue.

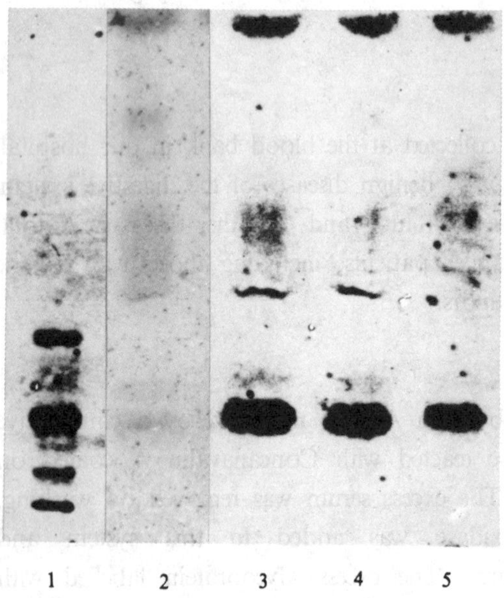

Fig. 1 Analysis of the glycolipids defined by Con A on TLC plate. Result of resorcinol-HCl reaction of the TLC plate: band 1, standard ganglioside from calf brain; band 2, glycolipid recognized by Con A. Result of orcinol-H_2SO_4 reaction of the TLC plate: bands 3, 4 and 5, glycolipid recognized by Con A.

Detection of the carbohydrate defined by Con A in serum. In this experiment, the amount of Concanavalin A coated on the bottom of the 96-well plates was known, that is 0.3 mg/ml and 50 μl in each well. When there was a greater amount of carbohydrate in the serm samples which could combine with Con A, there would be less of the glycoprotein labelled with peroxidase. The results of the determination of carbohydrate in the serum are summarized using a reference level, 51 U/ml (i.e. the value of the normal group times 2.5), in Table 1. Altogether, 218 patients with various malignant diseases were tested for carbohydrate levels associated with Con A. Its sensitivity is 53.7%.

Values greater than 51 U/l were seen in only 3.0% of 100 normal individuals tested. However, the specificity of the carbohydrate-associated Con A is reduced by such benign diseases as chronic gastritis, cirrhosis and pulmonary emphysema.

Table 1 Incidence of Elevation of Carbohydrate-Associated Con A in Serum

Patients	Number of cases	Positive Number	Positive rates
Gastric carcinoma	119	61	51.3[a)]
Hepatonoma	28	17	60.7[a)]
Lung carcinoma	37	21	56.7[a)]
Ovarian tumors	34	18	52.9[a)]
Benign diseases	104	12	11.5

a) vs benign diseases $P<0.01$

III. Discussion

To date, tumor markers are becoming ever more important in the diagnosis of malignant diseases. But, there have been few studies of the significance of the detection of oligosaccharides recognized by lectins serological detection or of the nature of the carbohydrate defined by lectin in tumor tissue. Concanavalin A is a mannose-linked oligosaccharide-specific agglutinin. One of the essential core structures in glycopeptides which interact with this agglutinin is shown below[10].

R 1— Man 1, 3 ↓

R 2— Man 1— 4 GlcNAc 1— 4GlcNAC 1— Asn

R 3— Man 1, 6 ↑

Con A has a great affinity for a trimannosidic core structure substituted by two GlcNAc residues (R1) at the nonreducing end; the affinity is not affected when this structure is modified by the addition of a 1—4 linked GlcNAc on the linked mannose (R2). Previous studies demonstrated that Concanavalin A can be used to isolate the tumor-associated antigen containing this core structure, and that detection of its receptor on gastrointestinal tract tumor tissues is significant in the analysis of carcinoma[11]. However, the question remains of how the carbohydrates are recognized by Con A in gastric cancer tissue whether in the form of a glycoprotein or a glycolipid? The answer is not clear. The results of this study confirmed that the carbohydrate defined by Con A in gastric cancer tissue exists in the form of neutral glycolipid and glycoprotein. They can secrete into the serum and their expression in the serum of patients with tumors bears a relationship to mutagenesis and oncogenesis. In the serum of patients with malignant diseases there is a high expression of the oligosaccharide molecules. Approximately 51. 3% of 119 patients with gastric malignancies showed a level greater than 51 U/ml. In patients with advanced disease, this number rose to about 60% of the cases. It is suggested that in addition to CEA AFP MG-Ags[1, 3, 4], other tumor-associated antigen containing mannose-linked oligosacharides may exist. Analysis of the oligosaccharide recognized by Con A in serum can provide useful information for cancer research and for the clinical diagnosis of malignant diseases.

References

1 Hakomori, S. and Kannagi, R., in *Handbook of Experimental Immunology* (eds. Weir, D. M. & Herzenberg, L.) Blackwell Scientific Publishing Inc., Boston, 1986, Vol. 1, pp.9.1—9.39.

2 Mangnani, J.1L., *et al., J. Biol. Chem.*, **257**(1982), 4365.

3 Zhang, J. R. *et al., Chin. Med. J.*, **104**(1991), 3: 212.

4 Zhang, J. R. *et al., J. Med. PLA.* (in Chinese), **15**(1990), 5: 246.

5 Hakomori, S. and Kannagi, R., *J. Natl. Cancer Inst.*, **71**(1983), 231.

6 Zhang, J. R. *et al., J. Med. Coll. PLA,* **5**(1990), 1: 63.

7 Zhang, J. R., Zhang, X. Y. and Chen, X. T. *Chin. J. Immunol.* (in Chinese), **5**(1989), 6: 359.

8 Zhang, J. R. *et al.*, Chin. Med. J., **104**(1991), 4: 300.

9 Zhang, J. R., Zhang, X. Y. and Chen, X. T. *Chin. Inter. Med. J.* (in Chinese), **39**(1991), 4: 204.

10 Leeb Krogerus, MD and Leifc Andersson, MD., *Cancer*, **66**(1990), 15: 1802.

11 Kellokumpu, *Cancer Res.*, **46**(1986), 4620.

Quantum Biological Studies of DNA Methylation and PAH Carcinogenic Activity*

WANG Ying, LIU Ciquan and HUANG Jingfei

(*Laboratory of Cellular and Molecular Evolution, Kunming Institute of Zoology, Academia Sinica, Kunming* 650223, *Yunnan, China*)

Abstract Methylation clearly affects the molecular electrostatic potential of DNA and enhances the reaction of methylated B-DNA with carcinogenic PAH. Using quantum mechanical calculations, we have systematically studied the relationship between DNA methylation and the attack of electrophilic PAH. We have examined the molecular electrostatic potentials (MEP) of a segment (10 bp) of the B-DNA double helix containing both methylated and unmethylated DNA, using the *ab initio* SCF method and a computer molecular graphic technique. The results indicate that introduction of a methyl group into the C5 position of cytosine, an exposed site in the major groove of DNA, markedly affects the MEP. DNA methylation reduces the minimum value range of the MEP in the methylated helix compared to the unmethylated helix. The minimun value range of the MEP for the unmethylated helix -G-C-G-C-G-C-G-C-G-C, -C-G-C-G-C-G-C-G-C-G was found to be from −452.22 to −406.90 kcal/mol, while that for the methylated helix -G-C-G-m^{5}C-G-m^{5}C-G–C-G-C-, -C-G-C-G-m^{5}C-G-m^{5}C-G-C-G was found to be from −498.45 to −445.90 kcal/mol. The range of the minimum value of the MEP of the latter is wider than that of the former[2]. Further, the reactivity of the segment of methylated B-DNA helix with the ultimate carcinogenic form of the PAH is greater than that of the unmethylated segment. These results seem to explain why methylation of DNA enhances the electrophilic attack of the active carcinogenic PAH on the methylated DNA.

For a long time, researchers of chemical carcinogenesis and molecular biologists have been studying the interaction of PAH with DNA. A number of experimental studies have indicated that the active electrophilic matter which is formed by the metabolic activation of PAH *in vivo* could produce carcinogenesis only by interaction with biological macromolecules in the cell, such as, DNA, i.e. abnormal DNA in the cell is the internal cause of the growth of cancer. What factors do actually affect the electrophilic reaction of PAH with DNA? Answers have been provided by quantum biological calculations using the method of molecular electrostatic potentials (MEP)[1].

In recent years, we have systematically pursued quantum biological research on DNA methylation and gene function and DNA methylation and PAH carcinogenesis. In the area of DNA methylation and PAH carcinogenesis, some of our research results were reported in an International Workshop-Symposium on the Basic Mechanisms of Chemical

* Project supported by the National Natural Science Foundation of China.

Carcinogenesis which was held in Shanghai (1982)[2]. Reported in this paper are new results concerning the relationship between methylated DNA and PAH carcinogenesis, which were obtained by quantum biological computations using the method of MEP.

I. Computing Methods and Results

1. *PAH Methyl Substituted Derivates*

Many studies have indicated that methylation of PAH can either activate or inhibit the carcinogenesis of PAH[3]. When the methyl group is substituted into some sites, the carcinogenicity of PAH can be increased, but when the group is substituted into other sites, its carcinogenicity is decreased.

In investigating the relationship of the structural carcinogenic activity between PAH and its methyl substituted derivates, we have used the superdelocalizability index in quantum chemistry[4] to calculate the values of $\Sigma S_r^E - \Sigma S_r^N$ in 63 different methyl-substituted derivatives of PAH, e.g. BaA and BaP, etc. The results show a good correspondence with the experimental carcinogenicity[5, 6]. In addition, we have compared our results from computing the values of $\Sigma S_r^E - \Sigma S_r^N$ with those of Memory[7] from computing the S_r^E values of the K region (Table 1).

Table 1 A Comparison of the Computed Values of $\Sigma S_r^E - \Sigma S_r^N$ With the S_r^E Values Computed by Memory[a)]

BaA Methyl Substitutive Derivatives	The Computed Values of $\Sigma S_r^E - \Sigma S_r^N$	S_r^E Values in K Region From Memory	Carcinogenicity
Monomethyl derivates			
7-methyl	0.6436	2.126	++++
12-methyl	0.5830	2.090	+++
8-methyl	0.4757	2.091	++
6-methyl	0.4610	2.180	++
5-methyl	0.4607	2.180	++
11-methyl	0.4606	2.082	++
4-methyl	0.3948	2.106	0
10-methyl	0.3693	2.091	+
2-mehtyl	0.3592	2.107	0
9-methyl	0.3541	2.082	+
1-methyl	0.3540	2.082	0
3-methyl	0.3185	2.083	0
Dimethyl derivates			
7,12-dimethyl	1.284	2.141	++++
6,7-dimethyl	1.004	2.230	++
8,9-dimethyl	0.867	2.094	+++
9,10-dimethyl	0.729	2.094	+
2,9-dimethyl	0.713	2.110	0
3,10-dimethyl	0.688	2.102	0

a) S_r^E : the electrophilic superdelocalizability, S_r^N : the nucleophilic superdelocalizability.

From Table 1, it can be seen that our computed values are more in accordance with the experimental carcinogenicity than Memory's computed values.

2. *The methylated Segment of B-DNA Double Helix*

Firstly, we computed the electronic wave functions of some of the constituent units of the nucleic acid, that is, the bases, the phosphodiester and the ribose, and then proceeded to calculate the MEP of a segment of B-DNA with 5-methylcytosine (m^5C)/as a comparison. We also computed the MEP of an unmethylated segment of the B-DNA double helix. The base constituents are

(a)		(b)
-G-C-G-C-G-C-G-C-G-C-		-G-C-G-m⁵C-G-m⁵C-G-C-G-C-
. . . .	and	. . . .
-C-G-C-G-C-G-C-G-C-G-		-C-G-C-G-m⁵C-G-m⁵C-G-C-G- .

The calculated minimum values of the MEP of various nucleic acid positions on some bases in different molecules are listed in Table 2.

Table 2 The MEP Minimum Values of Some Nucleophilic Positions on Guanine (G) and Cytosine (C) in Different Molecules (kcal/mol)

Position	Single Base	Nucleoside	Nucleotide	Single Helix
N7 (G)	−88.2	−88.0	−146.8	−220.6
N3 (G)	−55.6	−58.9	−100.9	−168.5
06 (G)	−75.0	−74.4	−115.2	−152.7
02 (C)	−82.3	−84.7	−122.6	−209.1
N3 (C)	−85.7	−85.2	−126.7	−202.4

The minimum values of unmethylated B-DNA (a), from this computation, are −452.22— −406.90 kcal/mol, and the minimum values of methylated B-DNA (b) are −498.45— −445.45 kcal/mol. In order to obtain a more objective picture, we also used a computer drawing technique to draw MEP models (Fig. 1) for the methylated and unmethylated B-DNA double helix.

II. Discussion

Firstly, it can be seen from Table 1, that the calculated values of $\Sigma S_r^E - \Sigma S_r^N$ correspond more closely to the experimental carcinogenicity than the S_r^E values of the K region calculated by Memory.

Secondly, it is agreed by researchers in the field of chemical carcinogens that the ultimate carcinogenic forms of PAH are epoxides. They also stress the importance of the reaction between carboncations and biological macromolecules. Research has indicated that a

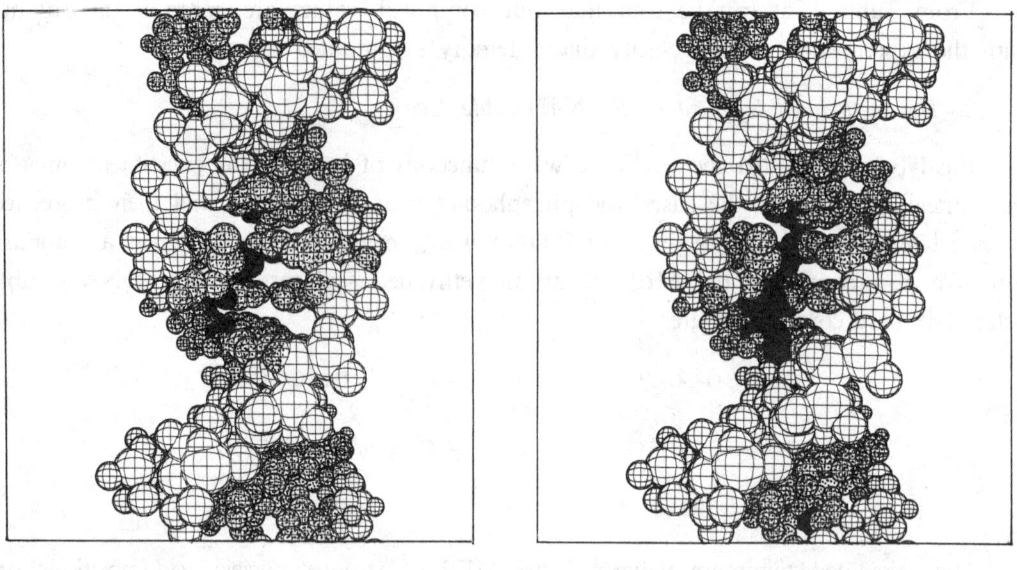

Fig. 1 The MEP in a segment of B-DNA double helix. (a) The unmethylated B-DNA double helix; (b) the methylated B-DNA double helix.

methyl group can stabilize carboncations by the electronic effect, and that hydroxylation of the methylated carbon atoms plays an important role in the mechanism of activation. The methyl group can also be metabolized by organisms to form an electrophilic methylcation which can take part in many biochemical reactions.

Because MEP can reflect the electrostatic character of the total molecule, thus indicating the effect of the whole structure on the reactive sites and activity, we chose a segment of the B-DNA double helix as the main object of study, and therefore did not only consider MEP calculations of the isolated bases, base pairs, nucleosides and nucleotides. However, to allow comparisons, we also computed the MEP minimum values of some nucleophilic positions on guanine (G) and cytosine (C) for different cases (Table 2). From the results (see Fig.1), we can see that the depth of the MEP potential well in bases, nucleosides, nucleotides, single helices and double helices gradually increases.

From this analysis, it can be seen that the effect of a methyl group on the MEP in a segment of the B-DNA double helix is localized and the MEP minimum values are distributed along the relative positions of the major groove. In the methylated helix (b), the distribution of the MEP minimum values is relatively concentrated in the regions between the 4th and 7th base pairs. The most conspicuous feature is that the methylated helix has the strongest MEP. Thus, the minimum values are between −452.22 and −406.90 (kcal/mol) for the unmethylated helix and between −498.45 and −445.44 (kcal/mol) for the methylated helix. The spread of the minimum values of the latter is also extended. Since methylation causes the MEP to change in localized region, it could change the affinity of the DNA with a specific protein. Therefore, on the one hand, it could affect the interaction between the DNA and the regulatory proteins, protecting the DNA from being degraded or inhibiting its transcription etc. On the other hand, it could favor the combination with the final carcinogenic form of the electrophilic PAH. Moreover, the methyl cations which are produced by the metabolized PAH could form methylated G, adenine (A) and C. However, the action of PAH substituted by a methyl group which has a higher delocalization energy (thus behaving almost like a methyl cation) in the methylation reaction, is still a problem to be explored further. The data in Table 3 indicate that the finding energy of the alkylation of the nucleophilic position of cytosine is strongly related to the polarization energy, charge transfer energy and exchange repulsion energy[8]. Therefore, the effects of these factors need to be considered in detail.

Table 3 The Binding Energy and Its Constituents in the Methylation of the Nucleophilic Position on Cytosine (kcal/mol)[a)]

Position	ΔE	E_e	E_{del}	E_{ex}
N3	−201.7	−136.6	−199.3	134.3
O8	−202.0	−105.5	−201.9	105.4

a) E_e = electrostatic energy, E_{del} = delocalized energy = polarization energy + charge transfer energy, E_{ex} = exchange repulsion energy.

In the methylated reaction, whenever the methylation is catalyzed by methylase or S-adenosylmethionine or by methyl cations produced by PAH metabolism, the methyl group will cause a change in the conformation of DNA and its charge distribution by both steric and electronic effects.

As has been described, our theoretical studies show that PAH carcinogenic activity is also affected by substitution of the methyl group into certain positions. Details of the relationship of these effects to PAH carcinogenic activity need to be studied further. In the same way, more experimental data needs to be accumulated on the relationship of the methylation of DNA with the carcinogens which, when metabolized, give rise to methyl cations. This would allow further discussion.

Some EP values have been listed in Table 2 and Fig. 1, and the regularity of the changes has also been analyzed in a preliminary fashion. It is well known that a negative MEP indicates attraction to electropositive groups, and that the active forms of many PAH are carbocations. The bases of nucleic acids are one of the most important targets of these carcinogenic forms of the PAH. Our calculations indicate that the depth of the MEP potential well in bases, nucleosides, nucleotides, single helices and double helices gradually increases. Experiments show that this increase in MEP parallels the increase in reactivity of DNA with the electrophilic carcinogenic materials. Therefore, our calculations can provide an explanation for the interaction of electrophilic carcinogens with nucleic acids and their constituents. It is worth reporting that the calculated values of the MEP seem to explain why DNA methylation enhances the reaction of the methylated DNA with active forms of PAH.

References

1 Wen, Y. and Shao, J., *Exploration of Nature,* **3**(1984), 85.
2 Liu, C. *et al.*. *An International Workshop-Symposium,* Shanghai, 1982, p.56.
3 Arcos, J. C. and Argus, M. F., *Chemical Introduction of Cancer,* Academic Press, New York and London, 1974.
4 Fukui, K., Yonezawa, T. and Nagata, C., *Bull. Chem. Soc. Jpan.* (Jpn.), **27**(1954), 423.
5 Liu, C. *et al.*, *J. Mol. Sci.*, **2**(1981), 19.
6 Liu, C. *et al.*, *An Introduction to Quantum Biology,* Science Press, Beijing, 1989.
7 Memory, J. D., *Int. J. Quant. Chem.*, **15**(1979), 363.
8 Liu, C. *et al.*, *J. Theor. Biol.*, **148**(1991), 145.

Changes of Immunological Properties of Serum Copper-Zinc Superoxide Dismutase in Cancer Patients and Their Clinical Application*

SHEN Wenmei, TIAN Yaping, JIANG Chaoguang,
ZHOU Dong, FANG Yunzhong** and HUANG Xiaomei

(*Great Wall Hospital, Beijing* 100853, *China*)

Abstract A very sensitive and more specific chemiluminescent immunoassay for estimating CuZn-SOD has been successfully established. This method has been used to study the change in the immunological properties of CuZn-SOD in the serum of cancer patients. To date, no reports on this topic have been published. A series of subsequent studies definitely showed an antigen-antibody reaction between antibovine CuZn-SOD antisera and CuZn-SOD in cancer patients which was very useful clinically.

1. *Chemiluminescent immunoassay*[1, 2]

In order to observe the change in the immunological properties of CuZn-SOD in the serum of the cancer patients in terms of antigen-antibody reaction between antibovine CuZn-SOD antisera and CuZn-SOD, a chemiluminescent immunoassay was thoroughly studied and finally established. This method is based on the combined detection of a crossimmunity reaction and a luminescent immunoassay, since bovine CuZn-SOD labelled with a luminescent substance can react with antibovine CuZn-SOD antisera to form an immunological complex. By measuring the luminescent intensity of the complex which was formed by thc cross reaction of antibovine CuZn-SOD antisera and CuZn-SOD in the sample, the level of immunologically changed CuZn-SOD (CuZn-SOD-I) in human serum could be measured.

2. *Detection of CuZn-SOD-I in the serum of cancer patients*[3]

By using the luminescent immunoassay established by us, the level of CuZn-SOD-I in the serum of healthy adults (105 males and 105 females, 20—45 years of age) was determined to be 0.43±0.07 μg/L ($\overline{X}$±SE). In the group, 70% did not have CuZn-SOD-I, whereas less than 30% showed only a very mild cross reaction with antibovine CuZn-SOD antisera.

---

* Project supported by the National Natural Science Foundation of China.

** Institute of Radiation Medicine, Beijing 100850, P. R. China.

Forty one of the cancer patients admitted to the ward of internal medicine were definitely diagnosed by the doctors in the Department of Pulmonary Medicine, being 12 cases of squamous cell carcinoma, 13 of adenocarcinoma, 12 of small cell cancer, 2 of mucoepidermoid carcinoma, 1 of carcinoid, and 1 of pulmonary metastasis of endometrium carcinoma. Eleven cases of noncancer patients {pneumonia (2), pulmonary tuberculoma (3), chronic bronchitis (4) and asthma (2)} were also diagnosed. Their sera were collected for detection of CuZn-SOD-I and the results showed that the level of CuZn-SOD-I in the serum of the cancer patients was significantly higher than that in the healthy adults as well as in the noncancer patients ($P<0.001$) as shown in Table 1.

Table 1 Serum CuZn-SOD-I Levels in Pulmonary Carcinoma Patients and Pulmonary Noncancer Patients

Patients	No. of Cases	CuZn-SOD-I (μg/l)
Pulmonary carcinoma	41	$8.98 \pm 0.84^{a)}$
Pulmonary noncancer disease	11	2.10 ± 0.90

a) Comparison between two groups, $P<0.001$.

Patients suffering from lung cancer of different cell types have different levels of CuZn-SOD-I in their sera and among the patients the order of the appearance of the carcinoma is as follows: squamous cell carcinoma>adenocarinoma>small cel carcinonma.

To further study the relationship between cancer and the CuZn-SOD-I level in the serum of cancer patients, two observations were made to allow differential diagnosis between malignant and benign tumors by detection of the cross reaction between serum CuZn-SOD and antibovine CuZn-SOD antisera. In the first observation, three groups of patients were selected as experimental subjects. The first group included 36 cases of primary hepatic carcinoma (31 males and 5 females, 27—73 years of age) and 19 cases of hepatitis hepatocirrhosis (15 males and 4 females, 38—73 years of age). The second group consisted of 18 cases of breast carcinoma (all females, 29—72 years of age) and 9 cases of mammary noncancer diseases (all females, 21—59 years of age). The third group had 11 cases of cancerous obstructive jaundice (7 males and 4 females, 32—67 years of age), diagnosed as pancreas cancer (5), choledochous carcinoma (4), ampullary carcinoma (2) and 8 cases of benign obstructive jaundice (4 males and 4 females, 34—73 years of age) including 6 cases of cholelithiasis and 2 of the choledochous cyst. As shown in Table 2, the levels of CuZn-SOD-I in the serum of the malignant tumor patients in all three groups were significantly higher than those in the benign tumor and noncancer patients.

In the second observation, two groups of patients were selected from the Department of Thoracic Surgery for comparative studies. The patients suffering from those diseases were carefully diagnosed by histopathological examinations. In the first group there were 18 cases of lung cancer (13 males and 5 females, 44—65 years of age) including 12 cases

Table 2 The Levels of CuZn-SOD-I in the Serum of the Patients With Malignant and Benign Tumors or Noncancer Diseases

Group	Units for Obtaining Serum Sample	Disease Suffered by Patients	No. of Cases	CuZn-SOD-I (μg/1)
1st	Department of Digestive Medicine	Primary hepatic carcinoma	36	$5.71 \pm 0.90^{a)}$
		Hepatocirrhosis	19	2.72 ± 1.01
2nd	Department of	Breast carcinoma	18	$6.00 \pm 1.24^{a)}$
	General Surgery	Mammary noncancer diseases	9	1.46 ± 1.04
3rd	Department of General Surgery	Canceroms obstructive jaundice	11	$7.68 \pm 2.10^{a)}$
		Obstructive jaundice	8	0.95 ± 0.80

a) Compared with corresponding benign tumor patients or noncancer patients, $P < 0.05$.

of squamous cell carcinoma, 3 of low differentiate adenocarcinoma, 1 of mucoid adenocarcinoma, 1 of adenoid squamous cell carcinoma and 1 of carcinoid, and 10 cases of the thoracic noncancer (5 males and 5 females, 29—55 years of age) including 2 cases of pulmonary tuberculoma, 1 of pseudo-tumor, 1 of pulmonary hamartoma, 1 of teratoma, 1 of thyrophyma, 1 of pyothorax, 1 of thoracic tuberculosis, 1 of spontaneous pneumothorax and 1 of bronchopleural fistula. In the second group 12 cases of esophageal carcinoma or carcinoma of the cardiac end of the stomach (11 males and 1 female, 44—66 years of age) were observed. They included 6 cases of squamous cell carcinoma, 4 of adenocarcinoma and 2 of signetring cell carcinoma. On the other hand, 8 cases of the thoracic noncancerous disease (4 males and 4 females, 19—55 years of age) were also observed. They served as a control group. As indicated in Table 3 both in the first group and in the second group, the levels of CuZn-SOD-I in the serum of cancer patients were very significantly higher than those in the noncancerous patients.

Table 3 The Levels of CuZn-SOD-I in the Serum of Patients With Cancer or Noncancer

Patients	No. of Cases	CuZn-SOD-I (μg/1)
Pulmonary carcinoma	18	$7.66 \pm 1.92^{a)}$
Thoracic noncancer disease	10	1.57 ± 0.75
Esophageal carcinoma or Carcinoma of the cardiac end of the stomach	12	$10.59 \pm 2.25^{a)}$
Thoracic noncancer disease	8	1.51 ± 0.68

a) Compared with corresponding noncancer patients, $P < 0.01$.

The results from the two observations confirmed our preliminary experiments in which the levels of CuZn-SOD-I in the serum of cancer patients reflected the changed immunological properties of CuZn-SOD. This is a most important finding in the study of the relationship between free radicals and cancer. The results are detailed in Table 4 and

Table 4 Overall Comparison of the Concentration of Serum CuZn-SOD-I Between Cancer Patients and Patients With Noncancer Diseases

Patients	Total Cases	Serum CuZn-SOD-I (μg/1)
Cancer	158	7.77±1.83[a)]
Noncancer	79	1.71±0.61

a) Compared with noncancer diseases, $P<0.001$.

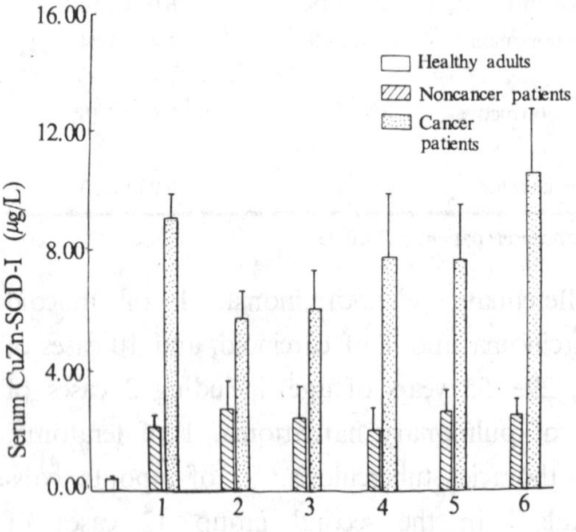

Fig.1 Comparison of CuZn-SOD-I among the sera of cancer patients, noncancer patients and healthy adults.

Fig.1.

By using the chemiluminescent immunoassay, it was found that the immunological cross reaction of CuZn-SOD in the serum of cancer patients was more significant than that in patients with noncancer diseases or healthy adults. This indicated the definite existence of CuZn-SOD-I in cancer patients. This is the first finding in cancer research that might be an important criterion for the relationship between oxygen free radicals and cancer, giving bright prospects in this field.

3. *Serum CuZn-SOD-I levels in cancer patients before and after an operation*[4, 5]

In order to further verify our findings, a comparative study of serum CuZn-SOD-I levels in cancer patients before and after an operation was made. As shown in Table 5, the results showed that the serum CuZn-SOD-I levels in cancer patients were significantly decreased after an operation as compared with those before the operation.

Table 5 Serum CuZn-SOD-I Levels in Cancer Patients Before and After an Operation

Patients	No. of Cases	CuZn-SOD-I (μg/l)	
		Pre-operation	Post-operation
Pulmonary carcinoma	11	8.46±1.32	3.52±0.71[a)]
Esophageal carcinoma or carcinoma of the cardiac end of the stomach	12	10.59±2.25	3.83±1.36[a)]

a) Compared with pre-operation, $P<0.01$.

Since the patients selected had not had irradiation treatment or chemical drug therapy, the higher levels of CuZn-SOD-I in their serum before the operation were very likely to result from their cancer. Moreover the strikingly increased level of the serum CuZn-SOD-I must reflect the CuZn-SOD-I produced by the cancer, therefore after the operation, no CuZn-SOD-I was transferred into the serum, resulting in a decrease in the immunologically changed CuZn-SOD.

4. *Differential diagnosis of malignant and benign tumors by cross reaction between antibovine CuZn-SOD antisera and CuZn-SOD in the serum of the patients with undetermi ed pulmonary carcinoma.*

Before operation, five patients suffering from pulmonary diseases were diagnosed as having malignant tumors. However no CuZn-SOD-I was detected in their sera, and in fact the tumors removed from these patients after the operation were definitely diagnosed by pathological examination to be benign (one case of tuberculoma, 2 cases of post-inflammatory pseudo-tumor of the lungs, one case of hamartoma and one case of multiple foci abscesses). After the examination, two cases were described as follow:

case III Clinical diagnosis: Pulmonary carcinoma (Fig. 2); Histopathological diagnosis: Post inflammatory pseudo-tumor of the lungs (Fig. 3). No existence of CuZn-SOD-I in serum.

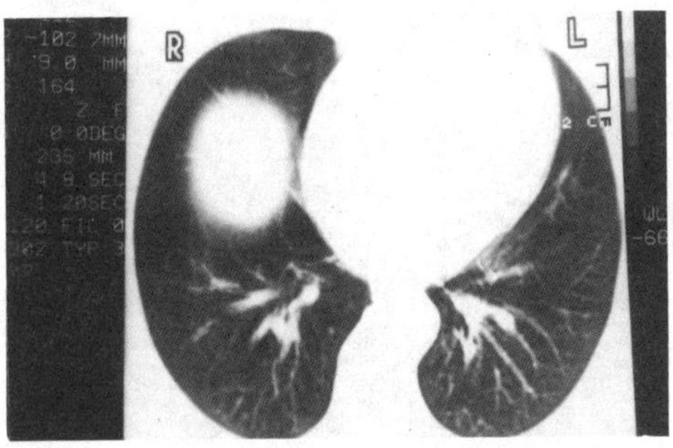

Fig. 2 CT scanning of lungs (Liu Yuqin).

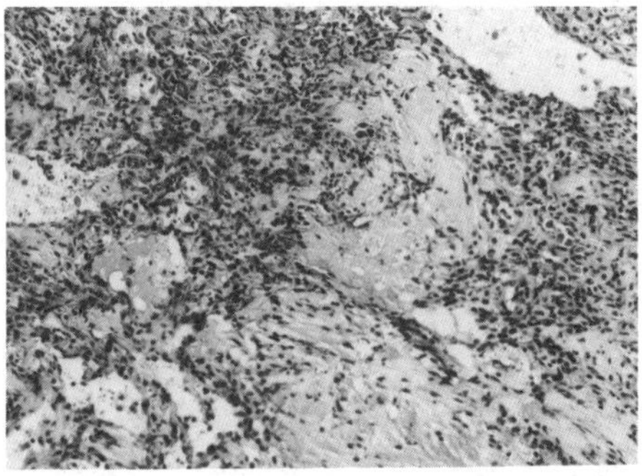

Fig. 3 Histopathological observation of a lung slice (Liu Yugin).

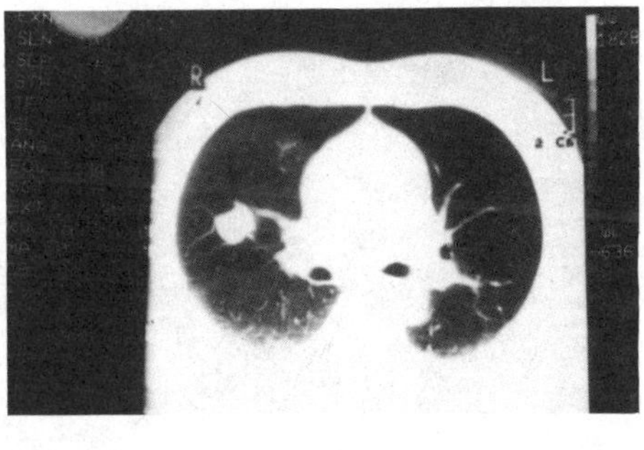

Fig. 4 CT scanning of the lung (Liu Guxin).

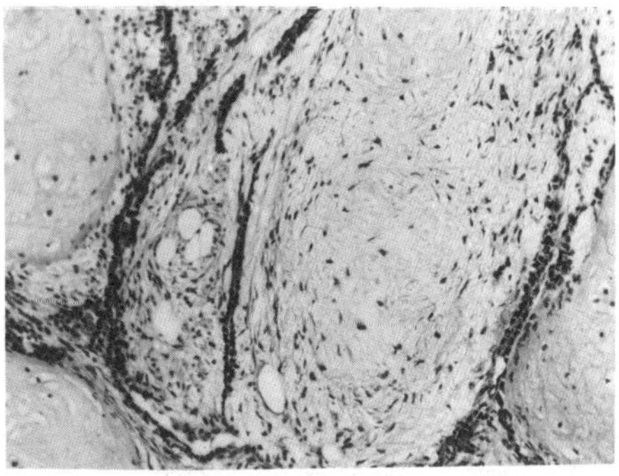

Fig. 5 Histopathological observation of a lung slice (Liu Guxin).

case IV Clinical diagnosis: Pulmonary carcinoma (Fig. 4); Histopathological diagnosis: hamartoma (Fig. 5).

The results reported here definitely indicate that the detection of immunologically changed properties of serum CuZn-SOD not only has valuable clinical application in the differential diagnosis between malignant and benign tumors, but also is theoretically significant. The results are therefore of importance. Further investigations will be carried out and the results will be reported later.

References

1 Tian Yaping, Shen Wenmei *et al.*, *Progress in Biochemistry and Biophysics* (in Chinese), **16**(1989), 4: 310.

2 Tian Yaping, Shen Wenmei *et al.*, *Bullentlin of the Academy of Military Medical Sciences*, 1989, 1: 80.

3 Shen Wenmei, Tian Yaping *et al.*, *National Medical Journal of China*, **69**(1989), 5: 286.

4 Jiang Chao-guang, Huang Xiao-mai *et al.*, *Chinese Journal of Thoracic and Cardiovascular Surgery*, **6**(1990), 1: 62.

5 Jinag Chao-guang, Huang Xiao-mai *et al.*, *Cancer* (in Chinese), **10**(1989), 2: 89.

Studies on Antibody-IgY Against Stomach Cancer*

LIU L. R., WANG H. P., YONG T. L. and FENG S.

(*Institute of Genetics, Academia Sinica, Beijing* 100101, *China*)

Abstract An antibody IgY against human stomach mucoid adenocarcinoma was prepared from the yolk of hens' eggs. The antibody can specifically recognize the human stomach mucoid adenocarcinoma cell line, MGC-80-3. The IgY also recognized stomach cancer cells that were from a patient. Further, it does not react with normal human cells. A type of immunotoxin was made from conjugation of the antibody IgY with ricin A. The immunotoxin can kill MGC-80-3 cells, but it did not react with normal human cells. The therapeutic effects of the immunotoxin have been studied. Thus TA2 mice were transplanted with S-78-4 cancer. One week after transplantation the tumor had grown to 0.5 cm in diameter, the immunotoxin was injected into the mice carrying the tumor. In 80% of the treated mice the cancer disappeared. Different methods of treatment gave different therapeutic effects. When the immunotoxin was injected into the tumor intramuscularly, the effects were 84%, better than in untreated mice. However, when it was given intravenously, the effects were 63%. The effects also differ in different sexes, being 91.5% in female and 80% in male.

When we studied gene expression of eukaryotic cells we found that the yolks of the eggs of immunized hens contained an antibody[1, 5]. This antibody was transferred into progeny. An egg yolk from an immunized hen yielded 15—25 mg of antibody. From studies of IgY against RNA polymerase, it was found that the serial subunits of the polymerase can be recognized by the antibody IgY. The antibody IgY was suitable for the immunoanalysis of high conservation antigens in animals.

Ricin is a toxin which is composed of A and B polypeptide chains. The antibody was coupled with the chain of ricin A to form the immunotoxin. The immunotoxin recognized specific cells and killed the cells[4, 6, 8, 12].

The stomach mucoid adenocarcinoma cell line was originally from a human cancer (it was named MGC-80-3 cell line)[2]. A cancer specific protrein was isolated from the cell line. To make this protein an antigen a laying hen was immunized, and the antibody IgY, effective against MGC-80-3 cells, was obtained from egg yolk. This antibody IgY is specific in its recognition of a conservative antigen. The immunotoxin, formed by coupling IgY with the chain of Ricin A was synthesized. It is reported in this paper that the immunotoxin recognized and killed cancer cells *in vitro* and had therapeutic effects against the tumor S-78-4 in TA2 mice.

* Project supported by the National Natural Science Foundation of China.

I. Materials and Methods

1. *Protein extraction*

MGC-80-3 cells were cultured in RPMI 1640 medium with 10% calf serum. After harvesting, the cells were resuspended in a buffer (10 mmol/L NaCl, 1. 5 mmol/L $MgCl_2$, 10 mmol/L Tris-HCl, pH 8.0, 0.1 mmol/L PMSF, 0.1 mmol/L EDTA). The suspension of cells was sonicated and ammonium sulfate was added and stirred for 30 min. The pellet was redissolved in a buffer (20 mmol/L Tris-HCl, pH 8.0, 2% SDS, 10 mmol/L EDTA, 0.1% 2-mercaptoethanol). The solution was extracted three times with phenol. The phenol phase was dialyzed against a buffer (0.25 mmol/L sucrose, 0.01 mmol/L phosphate, 0.1% SDS, 0.01% 2-mercaptoethanol pH 8.0) until all of phenol was removed. The protein was used as the antigen to immunize a hen.

2. *Antibody IgY purification*

A one year old laying hen was immunized with 200 μg of the oncoprotein of MGC-80-3 cells in a complete Freund adjuvant[3]. After the first immunization, it was further immunized every 10 days with same amount of protein but in an incomplete Freund adjuvant. About 3—4 immunizations, the antibody appeared and the eggs were collected. The antibody IgY was isolated from the egg yolks according to Carroll and Stollar' s method[5].

3. *Immuno-fluorescence reaction*

The antibody IgG against IgY was obtained from immunized rabbit serum. 5 mg IgG was dissolved in 5 ml phosphate buffer (pH 9. 5). The IgG solution and fluorescein isothiocytonate (1 mg/ml) was mixed. The mixture was dialyzed against PBS (pH 8.0) for 9 h at 20°C. After dialysis it was chromotographed on Sephadex G25. The eluate was FITC-TgG.

Culture cells were grown on slices in a 5% CO_2 atmosphere in an incubator at 37°C for 24 h. The slices were put into 50% acetone for 10 min and dried in the air. One drop of antibody IgY (1 mg/ml) was applied to a slice and left for one hour at 37°C. The slices were washed twice with PBS (pH 7.6) and sterilized water respectively. One drop of FITC-IgG was applied to a slice and the slice was washed again. The slices were stained by Evan's blue for 2 min and then sealed with 5% glycerol.

4. *Therapeutic effects of IgY-ricin A*

According to Domigo and Trowbridge' s method[7], the antibody IgY against MGC-80-3 cells was conjugated with ricin protein A chain. The cancer cells were cultured to subconfluence. The medium containing 0— 20 μg/ml IgY-ricin A was added to the culture. After 4 h the IgY-ricin A medium was removed and fresh medium was added to the culture. It was continuously cultured for 24 h. Finally the surviving cells were counted. The IgY-ricin A was injected into mice by I. V. and I. M. The mice had been transplanted with S-78-4 tumors.

II. Results

Antibody IgY against NGC-80-3 cells can specifically recognize stomach tumor cells.

The IgY was isolated from the egg yolk of a laying hen which had been immunized with MGC-80-3 cell oncoprotein. 15—25 mg antibody per egg was obtained. The antibody IgY was present in the eggs laid during the six months after immunization.

An indirect immunization test was performed. In the indirect immnoreaction the IgY was found to specifically recognize MGC-80-3 cells. The IgY was also found to recognize human stomach adencarcinoma cells from a patient. The IgY cross-reacted with HeLa cells, but not with 2BS cells, Nal cells, 3T3 cells, human embryo cells or normal human stomach cells.

1. *IgY-ricin A reacted with cancer cells*

The antibody IgY was conjugated with ricin A to yield an immunotoxin. The immunotoxin can kill some types of cells. The results are shown in Table 1. The MGC-80-3 cells were sensitive to the immunotoxin. When the concentration of the immunotoxin in the medium was 0.1 μg/ml, 0.13% of the MGC-80-3 cells survived. Other types of cells had survival levels of 16—75% at the same immunotoxin concentration.

Table 1 The Ability of IgY-ricin A to Kill Cells

Cells	IgY-ricin A Doses Affected Cells (survivor rate %)					
	0	0.1	1.0	5.0	10.0	20.0 μg/ml
MGC	96.4	0.13	0.08	0.03	0.0	0.0
HeLa	87.5	29.0	7.0	1.8	2.4	0.0
Nal	90.0	16.0	8.0	7.0	8.0	8.0
HE	74.2	67.4	47.0	23.4	26.0	20.0
Re	100	75.0	52.0	38.0	26.6	20.0

Nal: lymphocytoma cell HE: human embryo cell, Rc: rat sarcoma cell.

2. *Toxicity of IgY-ricin A*

To test the toxicity of IgY-ricin A, IgY, and ricin A were injected into normal TA2 mice. The results showed that the IgY antibody is not toxic to the mouse. When 0.02 mg of ricin A was injected into a mouse, the mouse died after 5 min. When 0.5 mg of IgY-ricin A was injected into a mouse, the mouse died after 48 h. (Table 2). The LD50 of IgY-ricin A was found to be 18.4±3.5 mg/kg.

Table 2 The Toxicity of IgY-ricin A and Ricin A

Agent	Dosage/Mouse	Treated Mice	Number of Mice That Died	Time Until Death
IgY	0.5 mg	5	0	—
IgY-ricin A	0.5 mg	5	5	48 h
Ricin A	0.02 mg	5	5	5 min

3. *Therapeutic effects of IgY-ricin A*

The S-78-4 strain of cancer was transplanted into TA2 mice. When the tumor grew to 1 cm in diameter, the IgY-ricin A was injected into cancer-carrying mice. As controls, mice were also injected with IgY and a protein from a normal egg. The experimental results showed that the tumors disappeared in the IgY-ricin A-treated mice and they became healthy. The antibody IgY was found to partially inhibit the cancer growth while the egg protein did not have any therapeutic effect (Table 3).

Table 3 The Therapeutic Effects of IgY-ricin A, IgY and Protein

Agent	Dosage (mg/ml)	Treated Mice	Time to death (days)
Protein	0.4	5	15
IgY	0.4	5	53
IgY-ricin A	0.1	15	cancer disappeared

The IgY-ricin A was injected into the cancer-carrying mice both at the seat of the tumor and by I. V. When 15—30 μg was injected into the tumor, the cancer disappeared in 24 days. When the IgY-ricin A was injected by I. V. into the cancer-carrying mice, three days after injection the cancer became dark from the centre and 30 days later the cancer disappeared. Therefore, different therapeutic methods give different therapeutic effects. Injection at the seat of the tumor gives better results; 84% of the animals became healthy. When the IgY-ricin A was injected by I. V., 63% of the animals recovered (Table 4).

Table 4 Therapeutic Effects of IgY-ricin A to Cancer-carrying Mice

Method	Treated Mice	Heal Mice	Heal Rates %
Injection at cancer	56	47	84
Injection I. V.	17	12	63
Total	75	59	80

To find the most effective dose of IgY-ricin A, the effects of different dosages and number of injections were analyzed. 15 μg IgY-ricin A was injected once every three days into mice, a total of three times. The rate of recovery from cancer of the mice was 83.3%. When 30 μg was used each times, after three injections the recovery rate was 71.4%. This dosage had effects on the health of the mice, so it did not give good results. If treatment was only once with 30 μg IgY-ricin A, the tumor disappeared slowly, but the rate of recovery rose to 86.5% (Table 5).

Table 5 Treatment Effects of Different Dosages and Different Numbers of Injections of IgY-ricin A

Dosage (μg/mouse)	Number of Injections	Total Dosage (μg/mouse)	Number of Mice Treated	Number of Mice that Recoveved	Rate of Recovery (%)
15	3	45	24	20	83.3
30	3	90	28	20	71.4
30	1	30	37	32	86.5

To determine whether the IgY caused animal sensitization, 0.4 mg of antibody IgY was injected subcutaneously into mice weighing 20 g. One week after the first injection the same dosage was injected into the same mice intravenously. Results were observed after the injections had been repeated four times. They showed that 50% of the mice had light sensitization. There were no deaths and no mice were strongly sensitized.

III. Discussion

The antibody IgY against human stomach mucoid adenocarcinoma cells MGC-80-3 was obtained from the yolks of the eggs of an immunized hen. The antibody IgY was easily obtained. A large amount of purified IgY was prepared from the immunized hen eggs. The antibody is suitable for conservative mammalian antigen analysis. The IgY was found to be much better than the monoclone for the structural analysis of RNA polymerase.

It was demonstrated that the human stomach mucoid adenocarnoma MGC-80-3 cells expressed v-myc oncogene in our hybridization experiments. There is a 110 kDa protein in the cells which we have purified. The laying hen was immunized with this protein. The antibody IgY which was isolated from the immunized hen eggs was found to specifically recognize MGC-80-3 cells. The antibody cross reacted with HeLa cells, but did not react with other tumor cells or normal cells. Using indirect immuno-fluorescence reaction experiments, it was demonstrated that the IgY can specifically bind to human stomach cancer cells. However it did not bind to normal stomach cells. It may be that HeLa cells and MGC-80-3 cells have some similar antigens.

The IgY-ricin A has the ability to kill cancer cells. In our experiment it was demonstrated that 0.1 μg/ml IgY-ricin A can kill most of the cultured cancer cells MGC-80-3; a high concentration of IgY-ricin A also kills HeLa and Nal cells. The IgY-ricin A can kill cancer cells so that tumors disappear. It was found that a dosage of 30 μg per mouse is optimal. Higher concentrations of the immunotoxin had adverse side effects on the health of the mice.

References

1 Wang, B., *Hereditas,* **4**(1982), 5.

2 Wang, K. H., *Acta Biologiae Experimentalis Sinica,* **16**(1983), 3: 256.

3 Liu, L. R., *Annual Report of Inst. Genet. Acad. Sinica,* 1985, p.12.
4 Bast, R. C., *Cancer Res.,* **45**(1985), 499.
5 Carroll, S. and Stollar, B. D., *J. Biol. Chem.,* **258**(1982), 24.
6 Cushly, W. *et al., Toxicon,* **22**(1985), 265.
7 Domigo, D. L. and Trowbridge, I. S., *Meth. in Enzymology,* **112**(1985), 238.
8 Lappi, D. A. *et al., Proc. Natl. Acad. Sci. USA,* **75**(1978), 1069.
9 Merrian, J. M. *et al., Cancer Res.,* **44**(1984), 3178.
10 Olsens, S. *et al., J. Biol. Chem.,* **257**(1980), 13263.
11 Ueda, R. *et al., Cancer Res.,* **45**(1985), 1314.
12 Vessella, R. L. *et al., Cancer Res.,* **45**(1985), 6131.

Observations on Manganese-Containing Superoxide Dismutase Activity in Human Lung Cancer

JIANG Chaoguang, HU Zhongyang, JIN Yuquan,

(*Department of Thoracic Surgery Chinese PLA General Hospital, Beijing* 100853, *China*)

SHEN Wenmei, ZHAO Houan and FANG Yunzhong

(*Depatment of Biochemistry, Chinese PLA General Hospital, Beijing* 100853, *China*)

Manganese-containing superoxide dismutase (Mn SOD) activities in lung cancer tissues from 5 patients with pulmonary carcinoma were measured by the nitrite formation method, lipid peroxide (LPO) values were measured spectrophotometrically using the thiobarbituric acid reaction. The results obtained show that Mn SOD activity is higher in lung cancer tissues, and lower in normal peripheral lung tissues. This trend was verified by statistical treatment ($P<0.01$). In addition, LPO values were found to be lower in lung cancer tissues than in normal peripheral tissues. The fact that lung cancer tissues possess a higher Mn SOD activity than peripheral pulmonary tissues may conceivably be of importance both for molecular biology and physiological pathology.

Superoxide dismutase (SOD) protecting against the superoxide radical has recently received much attention in connection with malignant tumors. Much has been written about the manganese-containing superoxide dismutase (Mn SOD) in malignant cells and tumors during the last few years. However, different conclusions were obtained, and those mainly on animal tumors[1—5]. To make a more comprehensive study of the Mn SOD in malignant tumors we measured Mn SOD activities and lipid peroxide (LPO) values in lung cancer tissues from 5 patients with pulmonary carcinoma. For comparison, we also analyzed the enzymes in peripheral tissues around the lung cancer and normal peripheral lung tissues. In the present survey, Mn SOD activities in lung cancer tissues was found to be much more than in normal peripheral lung tissues.

I. Materials and Methods

Patients. Of the 5 patients with primary pulmonary carcinoma aged from 44 to 65 years, 3 were male and 2 female. According to the histological classification of WHO, the pathohistogenetic diagnosis of the surgically dissected specimens included 2 cases of squamous cell carcinoma, 2 cases of low-differentiated adenocarcinoma and 1 case of carcinoid.

Tissue specimens. Specimens were taken from the main part of the cancer tissue, peripheral tissues around the lung cancer and normal peripheral pulmonary tissues. These were correspondingly numbered I, II, III. The volume of each specimen was about 0.5—0.7 cm^3. All samples were immediately placed in a refrigerator at −25°C until tested for enzyme activity and LPO value.

Enzyme activity and LPO value. The tissues were homogenized using a glass homogenizer with glass pestle. The total SOD activity was measured by the nitrite formation method. Mn SOD activity was assayed at pH 8.2 and then 2 mmol/L cyanide was used to inhibit the copper- and zinc-containing superoxide dismutase (CuZn SOD) activity[6]. LPO values were measured spectrophotometrically using the thiobarbituric acid reaction[7].

A statistical comparison of the mean concentrations was done using the Student's t-test.

II. Results

Table 1 lists the results of the total SOD activity, Mn SOD activity and LPO value in cancer tissues, peripheral tissues around the cancer and normal peripheral lung tissues. The mean total SOD and Mn SOD activities in lung cancer tissues were found to be 11.4±5.31 and 5.19±1.76 U/mg protein, while the correspounding activities in normal peripheral lung tissues were 3.89±2.20 and 1.52±0.75 U/mg protein. The assay indicated a lower value from cancer tissues compared to normal peripheral tissues and this was confirmed statistically ($P<0.01$). On the other hand, LPO values were found to be lower in lung cancer tissues than in normal peripheral tissues. This result was consistent with the previous investigation[8].

Table 1 Total SOD and Mn SOD Activities and LPO Values in Cancer Tissues (I), Peripheral Tissues Around the Cancer (II) and Peripheral Normal Tissues (III)

Sample	No. of Determinations	Units/mg Protein		
		Total SOD	Mn SOD	LPO
I	5	11.45±5.31	5.19±1.76	0.96±0.36
II	5	5.85±3.10	3.36±1.78	1.10±0.19
III	5	3.89±2.20	1.62±0.75	1.13±0.18

The differences in the values between cancer tissues and normal peripheral tissues (i.e. I/III) are compared in Table 2. They varied between 1.8 and 6.0. The average value was exceeded in 2 patients with hilus lymph node metastasis.

Case 1. A 60-year-old woman had a lobectomy for primary pulmonary carcinoma in the right upper lobe. The mass of cancer was 3×2×2 cm in diameter and pathological diagnosis was poorly differentiated adenocarcinoma. Lymph node metastasis in the hilus was 2/2. The difference in the values of the Mn SOD activities (I/III) was 43 greater than the mean value.

Case 2. A 55-year-old man underwent lobectomy for primary pulmonary carcinoma

Table 2 Difference and Ratio of Mn SOD Activities in Cancer Tissues (I) and Peripheral Normal Tissues (III)

Patients	Mn SOD Activity (Units/mg protein)			
	Cancer (I)	Noncancer (III)	(I-III)	(I/III)
1 M 44yr	5.12	1.76	3.36	2.9
2 F 60yr	5.30	1.24	4.06	4.3
3 M 53yr	7.96	2.15	5.81	3.7
4 F 65yr	4.38	2.42	1.96	1.8
5 M 55yr	3.18	0.53	2.65	6.0
X±SD	5.19±1.76	1.62±0.75	3.57±1.49	3.70±1.60

in the left lower lobe. The lump of cancer was 3×2.5×2 cm and pathological diagnosis was squamous cell carcinoma. Metastatic lymph node in the hilus was 1/5. The difference in the values of the Mn SOD activities (I/III) was 6.0. The value differences were less than the 3.7 in the other three cases where lymph node metastasis was not found (0/4—0/7). This result is worth noting.

III. Discussion

Oberley has reported that a lowered Mn SOD activity has been found in all tumors measured to date, measurements having been begun in 1979. It has been suggested that the reduction in Mn SOD activity is intimately related to cancerous phenotypes[1]. Iizuka reported that no significant difference was seen between the Mn SOD activity in normal lung cells and lung cancer cells[4]. Marklund et al.[2,3] analyzed the activity in human tissues from accident or suicide victims and also from neoplastic cell lines. They found the activity of Mn SOD in cultivated neoplastic cells to vary within wide limits, sometimes a very high level of activity being present. They also observed the Mn SOD activity in tumors removed in an opeation. Mn SOD activity was detected in all of the tumors investigated. The malignant tumors had a higher Mn SOD activity than the benign tumors. As seen from their results, the Mn SOD activity in mammary low-differentiated ductal carcinoma was higher than that in mammary fibroadenosis. Marklund believed that the difference in the Mn SOD may be due to the fact that Mn SOD is present in both the cytoplasm and the mitochondrial matrix in primates, whereas in other animals, Mn SOD is found only in the mitochondrial matrix.

Because of the different investigations reported in literature, we made an effort to ensure that the identities of enzymes in the specimens were comparable. The enzymes present on both the cancer and noncancer tissues came from the same pulmonary lobe which had been surgically dissected. This may reduce differences among individuals. This method of collecting samples was more reasonable than that of Marklund *et al.*[3].

The fact that lung cancer tissues possess a higher Mn SOD activity than peripheral pulmonary tissues may conceivably be of importance both for molecular biology and pathophysiology.

References

1 Oberley, L. W. *et al., Cancer Research,* 1979; **39**: 1141.

2 Westman, N. G. *et al., Cancer Research,* 1981; **41**: 2962.

3 Marklund, S. L. *et al., Cancer Research,* 1982; **42**: 1955.

4 Iizuka, S., *The Hokkaido J. Med. Sci.* (in Japanese), 1984; **59**: 739.

5 Hoffman, C. E. *et al., Br J Cancer,* 1985; **51**: 127.

6 Zhao, H. A. *et al., J. Biochem.* (in Chinese), 1988; **4**: 29.

7 Ohkawa, H., *Analytical Biochemistry,* 1979, **95**: 351.

8 Lesko, S. A. *et al.*, in *Free Radical, Lipid Peroxidation and Cancer* (eds. Mc Brien, D. C. *et al.*), Academic Press, London, 1982, p. 401.

Section B

Molecular Mechanism of Carcinogenesis by Chemical, Virus or Physical Factors

Antitumor Activity of Diazoketones in Terms of Physical and Quantum Chemistry

L. I. Kirkovsky

(*Institute of Chemical Physics in Chernogolovka, Russia Academy of Sciences Chernogolovka Moscow Region, 142432 Russia*)

Abstract On the basis of analysis of the kinetic scheme of nucleophilic substitution reactions of the diazoketones (DKs) R-COCHN_2 the relationship between the DKs alkylating ower and their structure is established. The role of anchimeric assistance in the enhancement of the DKs alkylating power is shown. The relationship between the DKs antitumor effect and their hydrolysis rate is described (preliminary publication[1]).

The concept of the optimal stabilization of the cyclic onium intermediate (COI) of anchimeric assistance is analyzed. The method of quantum-chemical calculation of the COI stabilization energy is proposed and developed for prediction of the DKs antitumor activity.

I. Introduction

In the middle of 1950s the first antitumor compound in diazoketones (DKs) was found[2]. And then the active search of new antitumor drugs in this chemical class began. Compounds such as o-acetyl-1-serine (Azaserine)[3], 6-diazo-5-oxonorleucine (DON)[4] and 1, 2-bisdiazoacetylethane (Diazane)[5] were subjected to extensive clinical tests[6 – 11], (Diazane was developed at the Institute of Chemical Physics of the USSR Academy of Sciences). These drugs have demonstrated high efficiency and despite certain limitations (high chronic toxicity) they are used in clinical practice. These preparations are a result of screening rather than directed synthesis.

Therefore, the the aim of the present study has been to work out effective methods for the development of antitumor preparations (including DK-based), using quantitative and qualitative correlations "structure-physicochemical properties-biological effects".

1. *Relationship Between the Structure and Alkylating Power of Diazoketones*

The DKs biological activity is believed to stem from their ability to alkylate nucleophilic centers of biomacromolecules (e.g. sulphhydryl, carboxyl, hydroxyl protein groups)[12, 13]. From the chemical viewpoint, the reaction of alkylation is the nucleophilic substitution.

2. *The Kinetic Description of the DKs Alkylating Reactions*

The kinetic scheme of the nucleophilic substitution reactions which can proceed in aqueous DK solutions is shown in Scheme 1, where S_0 is DK initial concentration,

$$k_{obs} = \{k_1 k_2/(k_{-1}+k_2)\} \cdot [H^+] = k_{eff} \cdot [H^+], \qquad k_2 = k_M + k_{x2}[X] + k_{W2}[H_2O].$$

Scheme 1

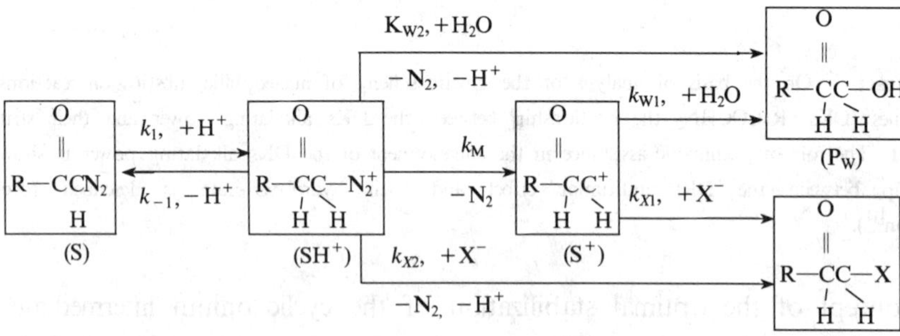

At $t \to 0$

$$\underbrace{\frac{dP_X(t)}{dt} \cdot \frac{1}{S_0[H^+]}}_{\boxed{AP}} \cong \underbrace{\frac{k_{X2}[X] + k_M\{k_{X1}[X]/(k_{X1}[X] + k_{W1}[H_2O])\}}{k_M + k_{X2}[X] + k_{W2}[H_2O]}}_{\boxed{S}} \cdot \underbrace{k_{eff}}_{\boxed{R}} \tag{1}$$

$$\boxed{AP = S \cdot R} \tag{2}$$

The reaction starts from the reversible protonation of the initial DKs and formation of the corresponding diazonium ion (SH^+). Then the diazonium ion reacts with solvent (water molecules) or external nucleophile X^- producing the corresponding products of the reaction—— the hydrolysis product P_W or the product of the nucleophilic substitution P_X. The latter is the "target" product from the viewpoint of the building-up of DKS biological effect.

Assuming that the rate of P_X accumulation can characterize the DKs alkylating power (AP), Eq. (1) is obtained (Scheme 1). Eq. (1) is formulated by using the Bodenstein principle[14] for process reactive intermediates (SH^+) and (S^+).)

The first factor (S) in Eq. (1) is the selectivity of the compound interaction with the external nucleophile X^-, the second (R) is the overall DKs reactivity. Consequently, $AP = S \times R$ (Eq. (2), Scheme 1).

3. *The Influence of the Substituent Inductive Properties on the DKs Alkylating Power*

It is known from literature that changes in the inductive properties of substituent R in the molecule R-$COCHN_2$ produce changes in the selectivity of nucleophilic substitution as well as in the reactivity of the compounds involved in the following reactions:

— *donor substituents R promote the* S_N1 *mechanism with low selectivity and simultaneously enhance the DKs reactivity by increasing the basicity of the diazocarbonyl fragment;*

— *acceptor substituents R cause the reaction to proceed via the* S_N2 *mechanism (with high selectivity) reducing thereby the basicity and, respectively, the reactivity of compounds.*

Consequently, variations in the inductive properties of the substituent R in the molecule R-$COCHN_2$ produce changes in the selectivity and overall reactivity of the nucleophilic substitution reaction. As a result, the compound alkylating power changes but insignificantly.

4. *The Influence of Anchimeric Assistance on the DKs Alkylating Power*

Simultaneous increase in the reactivity and selectivity of the substitution process can only be achieved through the S_N1 mechanism. However, in this case the resulting carbenium ion formed must be stabilized by its interaction with the intramolecular nucleophilic center (e.g. the heteroatom lone pair).

Such participation of the neighboring groups (anchimeric assistance) takes place in the cyclic onium intermediate (COI) IV (Fig. 1) and creates an energy barrier $\delta F_5^{\neq}$ to the reaction with the external nucleophiles. The existence of this barrier promotes the preferential interaction with the strong nucleophiles rather than with weak ones. It is equal to the increase in the selectivity of the nucleophilic substitution.

In accordance with Hammond postulate[15] anchimeric assistance simultaneously with COI stabilization by the value δF_i causes a decrease ($\delta F^{\neq}$) in the energy of cyclic transition state (CTS) III (Fig. 1) of such COI formation. Because this reaction step is a limiting one, the overall rate process is increased.

Thus, anchimeric assistance should enhance markedly the DKs' alkylating power, and consequently their antitumor effect.

So, the aim of the further study is to measure quantitatively the value of anchimeric assistance and to determine the relationship between the DKs' antitumor effect and the value of anchimeric assistance during their nucleophilic substitution.

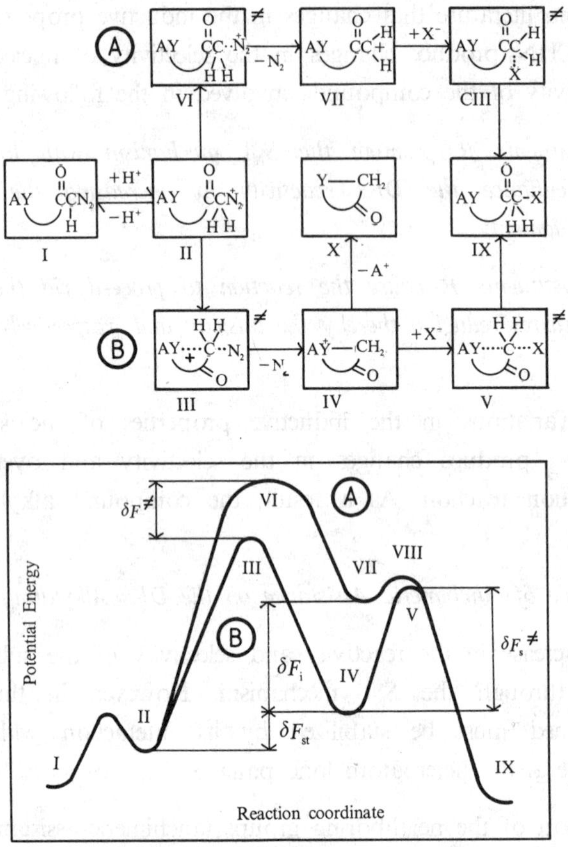

Fig. 1 Energetic diagram of the nucleophilic substitution reaction which proceeds via the S_N1 mechanism without and with stabilization of carbocation VII as a cyclic onium intermediate IV (paths A and B, respectively); the transition state VI is stabilized as a cyclic transition state III.

II. Materials and Methods

1. *Starting Materials*

The starting materials were functionally substituted DKs (formulas are shown in the legend of Fig. 2).

2. *The Kinetic Measurement*

The value of anchimeric assistance during the DKs' nucleophilic substitution is characterized quantitatively by the compound hydrolysis rate constant in aqueous $HClO_4$ solutions at 20°C. The kinetics of hydrolysis are measured spectrophotometrically according to the disappearance of the DKs characteristic bands in the UV region.

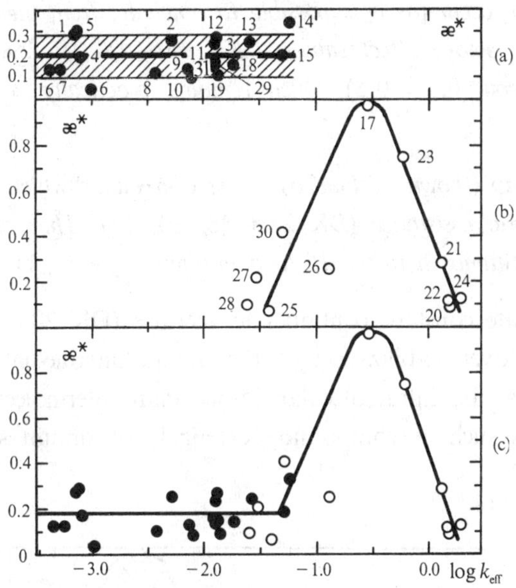

Fig. 2 Dependence of the coefficient of Sarcoma 180 growth inhibition $\mathscr{H}^*$ on $\log k_{eff}$ ($M^{-1}s^{-1}$, 20°C, $HClO_4/H_2O$) for DK 1 ÷ 31. Explanations are in the text.

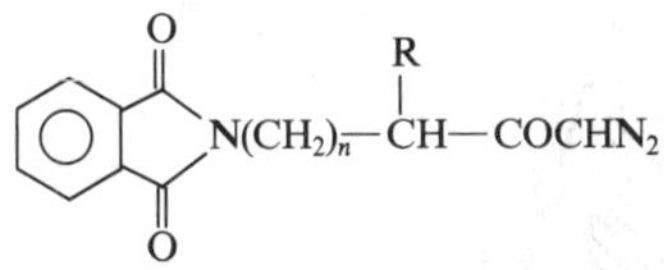

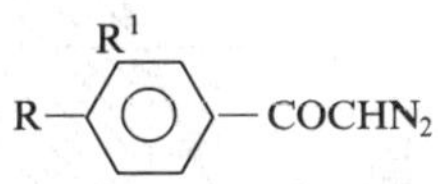

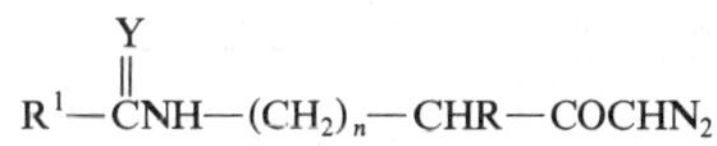

DK	R	n
1	H	0
2	H	1
3	H	2
4	Me	0
5	Et	0
6	1-Pr	0
7	CH_2Ph	0

DK	R	R^1
8	NO_2	H
9	Br	H
10	Cl	H
11	F	H
12	H	H
13	Me	H
14	MeO	H
15	MeO	MeO

DK	R^1	Y	n	R
21	PhNH	S	0	H
22	PhNH	S	1	H
23	PhNH	S	0	CH_2Ph
24	MeNH	S	1	H
25	PhNH	O	1	H
26	PhNH	O	0	CH_2Ph
27	Me	O	0	H
28	Me	O	1	H
29	Me	O	2	H
30	Me	O	0	CH_2Ph

$N_2HCOC—(CH_2)_n—COCHN_2$

DK 16: $n=0$; DK 17: $n=2$
DK 18: $n=3$; DK 19: $n=4$

DK 31: $MeCOCHN_2$

DK 20: $N_2HCOC—CHMe—COCHN_2$

3. *Relationships Between Antitumor Activity of Diazoketones and Their Hydrolysis Rate*

The dependence of the coefficient of tumor growth inhibition $\mathscr{H}^*$ on the logarithm of the hydrolysis rate constant (k_{eff}) is shown in Fig. 2.

All studied compounds are divided into two groups:

— *The first group* (*shown in Fig.* 2a) — *the compounds in which anchimeric assist-*

ance is not likely to occur (as it is possible to conclude, from their structural features, k_{eff} *and the solvent isotope effect values, DK* 1 ÷ 16, 18, 19, 29, 31). *They show a low* $\mathscr{H}$* *value (about* 0.1 ÷ 0.3) *which remains practically constant over a wide range of* $\log k_{eff}$.

— *The second group (shown in Fig.* 2b)— *the compounds which are hydrolyzed with a marked anchimeric assistance (DK* 25 ÷ 28, 30, 17). *They show a considerable enhancement in antitumor activity, up to a maximum* ($\mathscr{H}$* = 1).

If the hydrolysis rate constant continues to increase (DK 20 ÷ 24), the biological effect is reduced due to the over stabilization of the onium intermediates. Conversion of such intermediates occurs via the intramolecular rather than intermolecular interaction to give heterocyclic compounds such as compound X (Fig. 1) or onium salts but not alkylating products[16, 17].

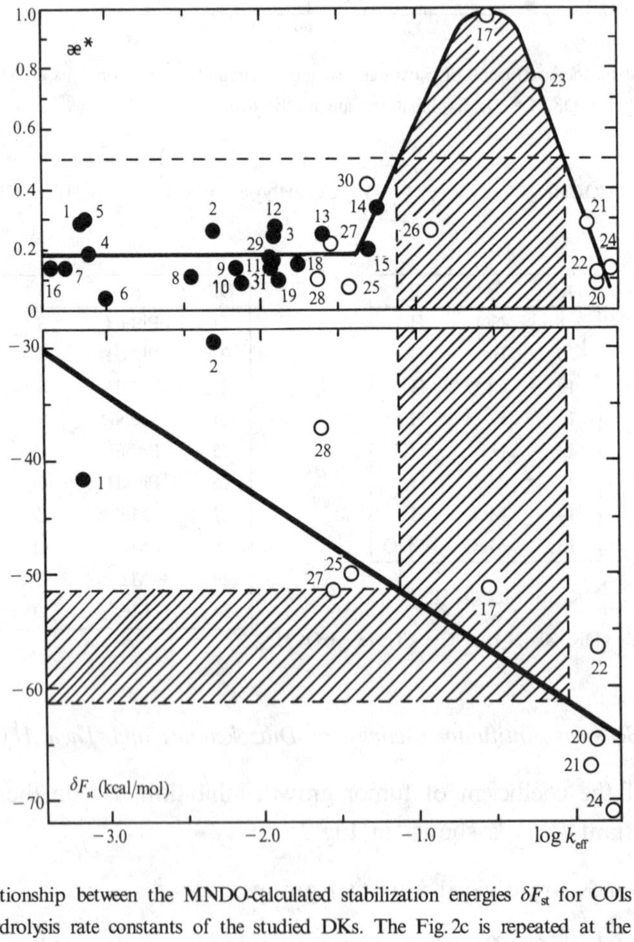

Fig. 3 The relationship between the MNDO-calculated stabilization energies δF_{st} for COIs formed during anchimeric assistance and hydrolysis rate constants of the studied DKs. The Fig. 2c is repeated at the top of this figure. Formulas of DKs are shown in the legend of Fig. 2.

The curve in Fig. 2c summarizes these two relationships. The maximum lies in the k_{eff} range from about 0.1 to 1 $M^{-1}s^{-1}$.

Summing up, for diazoketones to show the highest antitumor activity, the acidic conversion should proceed with the optimum anchimeric assistance. The highest antitumor activity is shown by compounds with the hydrolysis rate constant varying in the range about $0.1 \div 1\ M^{-1}\ s^{-1}$ (20°C, $HClO_4/H_2O$).

4. *Quantum Chemical Calculations of the Diazoketone Antitumor Properties*

Proceeding from the fact that there is an optimum of anchimeric assistance, the concept of the optimal stabilization energy (δF_{st}) of COI formed due to anchimeric assistance has been proposed.

Quantum-chemical calculations can give the value of $\delta F^{\neq}$ (Fig.1). However it is easier to calculate the energy of COI IV as compared with the energy of carbocation VII (δF_i) or compared with the energy of diazonium ion II (δF_{st}).

The latter was used in this study and it was calculated as the free energy difference of nitrogen molecule elimination from the diazonium ion and formation of COI and N_2 molecule at 20°C. The equation $\delta F_{st} = \Delta H - T(n+1)\Delta S_{ir}$ was used, where ΔH is the calculated difference of the reagent heat formations, ΔS_{ir} is the mean entropy loss due to the fixation of one rotation freedom degree initially available in CH_2 groups (n is the number of CH_2 groups frozen in COI). (The value $\Delta S_{ir} \cong -4$ e.u.[18, 19] was used.)

Figure 3 shows the relationship between the MNDO-calculated stabilization energies for the COIs which can form during anchimeric assistance to nucleophilic substitution reaction and hydrolysis rate constants of studied DKs. Calculations show that for the most active compounds the δF_{st} values are in the range of about $-50 \div -60$ kcal/mol.

III. Conclusions

Based on the result obtained it is possible to predict the antitumor activity of DK before their synthesis has actually been carried out. The experimentally found relation between the DK antitumor effect and their hydrolysis rate constant can be used to assess the anticancer properties of newly synthesized compounds prior to their biological testing.

This approach can be extended to other chemical classes of alkylating compounds (arene imines and epoxides[20], β-chloroethylamines and related compounds, cyclophosphamides, triazenes, etc.) which show the antitumor, mutagenic, carcinogenic or other types of biological activity.

The author wishes to thank V. Kartsev, A. Sipyagin, S. Chapyshev, L. Tolochko for synthesis of the most studied diazoketones, E. Nosenko for assistance in some kinetic studies and N.

Konovalova, L. Vasilieva for placing at my disposal the results of their biological studies. (All the persons are from the Institute of Chemical Physics, Russian Acad. Sci.)

References

1 Kirkovsky, L. I., *Chemistry and Biological Activity of Diazo Compounds* (Materials of 2nd All-Union Meeting, July 1988, Chernogolovka, USSR), Inst. Chem. Phys. Publ., Chernogolovka.

2 Fusari, S. A. *et al., J. Am. Chem. Soc.,* **76**(1954), 2878.

3 Duvall, L. R., *Cancer Chemotherapy Rep.,* **7**(1960), 65.

4 Duvall, L. R., *Cancer Chemotherapy Rep.,* **7**(1960), 86.

5 Emanuel, N. M. *et al., Dokl. Akad. Nauk SSSR,* **183**(1968), 724.

6 Sofiina, Z. P *et al.* (eds.), *Experimental Evaluation of Anti-tumor Drugs in the USSR and in the USA,* Meditsina Pudl., Moscow, 1980.

7 Emanuel, N. M., *The Kinetics of the Experimental Tumor Processes,* Nauka Publ., Moscow, 1977.

8 Anikin, I. V., *Thesis, Tartu State University,* Tartu State Univ. Press, 1986.

9 Catane, R. *et al., Cancer Treat. Rep.,* **63**(1979), 1033.

10 Regan, R. T. *et al., Cancer Treat. Rep.,* **66**(1982), 1665.

11 Earhart, R. H., Koeller, J. M. and Davis, H. L., *Cancer Treat. Rep.,* **66**(1982), 1215.

12 Gale, E. F. *et al., The Molecular Basis of Antibiotic Action,* Wiley-Intersci., London, New York, Sydney, Toronto, 1972.

13 Buchanan, J. M., in *Enzyme-Activated Irreversible Inhibitors* (eds. Seiler, N. *et al.,*), Elsevier, New York, 1978.

14 Bodenstein, M., *Z. Physik. Chem.,* **85**(1913), 329.

15 Hammond, G. S., *J. Am. Chem. Soc.,* **77**(1955), 334.

16 Kirkovsky, L. I. and Chapyshev, S. V., *Dokl. Akad. Nauk SSSR,* **291**(1986), 847.

17 Kartsev, V. G. *et al., Khim. -Pharm. J.* (Rus.) **7**(1985), 804.

18 Page, M. I., *Chem. Soc. Rev.,* **2**(1973), 295.

19 Winnik, M. A. *Chem. Rev.,* **81**(1981), 491.

20 Szentpaly, L. V. and Schwerdtfeger, P., in *Abstr. Int. Symp. Recent Adv. Chem, & Mol. Biol. Cancer Res.* (Beijing, July 1991), Beijing Polytech. Univ. Press, 1991.

pH-dependent Protease-inhibitory Activity of v-Ha-*ras* p21 Toward Cathepsins B and L, and Papain

Takaki Hiwasa

(*Division of Biochemistry, Chiba Cancer Center Research Institute, 666-2, Nitona-cho, Chuo-ku, Chiba 260, Japan*)

Abstract v-Ha-*ras* oncogene product (p21) produced by *Escherichia coli* inhibited cathepsins B and L, and papain effectively in MES buffer at pH values below 6.0. The inhibitory activity of p21 decreased as the pH value increased.

I. Introduction

In spite of a great deal of researches on *ras* oncogenes, the action mechanism of *ras* gene products (p21s) remains to be determined. p21s have guanine nucleotide-binding activity[1] and GTPase activity[2]. However, none of the *ras*-related guanine nucleotide binding proteins has a similar transforming activity. Interaction with GTPase activating protein (GAP) might be necessary for the biological activity of p21[3], yet it can suppress the transforming activity of c-*ras*[4]. At least at present, the only possible function of p21 found which can cause effects on other molecules[5 – 8] is its protease-inhibitory activity.

The protease-inhibitory activity of p21 may be cysteine proteinase-specific because the amino acid sequence between positions 40 and 59 of Ha-*ras* p21 is quite similar to the well-conserved regions among cysteine proteinase inhibitors called the cystatin superfamily[5]. However, most cystatins inhibit both the cathepsins B and L, and papain whereas the inhibitory activity of p21 toward cathepsin B and papain was much weaker than that toward cathepsin L using the standard assay system[7]. Thus, in the present study, I have investigated the protease-inhibitory activity of p21 under various conditions, and found that p21 inhibits not only cathepsin L but also cathepsin B and papain effectively in 20 mmol/L MES (pH 5.5—6.0).

II. Materials and methods

1. *Materials*

Bovine cathepsin B and papain were purchased from the Sigma Chemical Company

(St Louis, MO). Benzyloxycarbonyl-phenyl-alanyl-arginine 4-methyl-7-coumarylamide (Z-Phe-Arg-NMec) and Z-Arg-Arg-NMec were purchased from the Peptide Institute Inc. (Osaka).

2. *Preparation of p21s*

p21 was produced by *Escherichia coli* with plasmids bearing v-Ha-*ras* gene[9] and purified according to the method of Lacal and Aaronson[10] as described previously[11].

3. *Purification of Cathepsin L*

Cathepsin L was purified from porcine kidney as described previously[12].

4. *Assay for Proteinase Activity*

Cathepsins B and L and papain were activated by incubation at 37°C for 10 min in 20 mol/L 2-(N-morpholino)-ethanesulfonic acid (MES) (pH 5.5 — 6.8), 2.5 mol/L dithiothreitol (DTT) and 1 mol/L EDTA. p21 was diluted in 20 mmol/L MES (pH 5.5—6.8), 0.5% Brij-35 and 1 mmol/L EDTA, and then mixed with the proteinases and synthetic substrates. Z-Arg-Arg-NMec was used as a substrate for cathepsin B and Z-Phe-Arg-NMec was used for cathepsin L and papain. The reaction mixture (0.25 ml) contained 100 μU proteinase, 0 — 20 μg/ml p21, 10 μmol/L substrate, 20 mmol/L MES (pH 5.5— 6.8), 0.1% Brij-35, 2 mmol/L DTT and 1 mmol/L EDTA and was incubated at 37°C for 5 min. In some experiments, phosphate buffer (0.1 mol/L, pH 5.8) or acetate buffer (0.1 mmol/L, pH 5.0 or 4.6) was used instead of MES buffer. Reaction was terminated by the addition of 0.25 ml of 100 mmol/L sodium chloroacetate, 30 mmol/L sodium acetate and 70 nmol/L acetic acid[13].

III. Results

The effect of the pH of the assay mixture on the protease-inhibitory activity of p21 was investigated. In the presence of phosphate buffer (pH 5.8), p21 did not inhibit cathepsin B significantly even at 10 μg/ml (Fig. 1A). However, its inhibitory activity increased as the pH value decreased. The half maximal inhibition concentration (IC_{50}) of p21 at pH 4.6 was approximately 5 μg/ml (240 nmol/L). Similarly, the activity of papain was inhibited by p21 under acidic conditions. IC_{50}s of p21 toward papain at pH 5.8, 5.0 and 4.6 were >20 μg/ml, 8 μg/ml and 5 μg/ml, respectively (Figure not shown).

The protease-inhibitory activity of p21 was much higher in the presence of MES buffer. p21 partially inhibited cathepsin B even at pH 6.4 and the inhibitory activity increased as the pH value decreased (Fig. 1B). The IC_{50} of p21 at pH 5.5 was approximately 2.5 μg/ml (120 nmol/L). Similar dose-response curves were obtained when cathepsin L was used (Fig.1C). The IC_{50} of P21 toward cathepsin L at pH 5.5 was approximately 2 μg/ml (100 nmol/L).

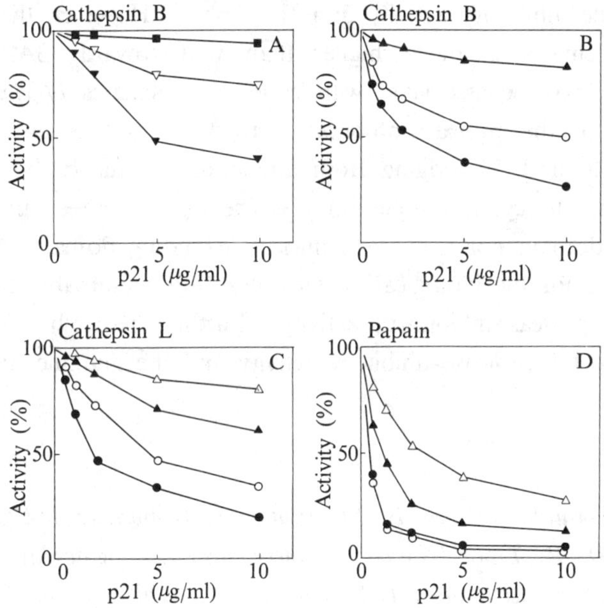

Fig. 1 Inhibition of cysteine proteinases by p21s. Relative activities of cathepsin B (A and B), cathepsin L (C), and papain (D) in the presence of varying concentrations of p21 are shown. Buffers of the reaction mixtures of A were 0.1 mol/L sodium phosphate (pH 5.8) (■), 0.1 mol/L sodium acetate (pH 5.0) (▽), and 0.1 mol/L sodium acetate (pH 4.6) (▼). MES was used as a buffer in B—D and the pH values of MES were 5.5 (●), 6.0 (○) 6.4 (▲), and 6.8 (Δ). Activities in the absence of p21s were expressed as 100%.

In the presence of MES buffer, papain activity was much more effectively inhibited by p21 than the activity of the cathepsins (Fig. 1D). Maximal inhibitory activity was observed at pH 6.0 and 5.5. The IC_{50} of p21 toward papain at pH 6.0 was approximately 0.2 μg/ml (10 nmol/L).

Addition of NaCl (100 mmol/L), $MgCl_2$ (20 mmol/L) or $CaCl_2$ (10 mmol/L) to the reaction mixture significantly decreased the inhibitory activity of p21. The presence of Nonidet P-40 or Triton X-100 instead of Brij-35 slightly decreased the inhibitory activity of p21.

IV. Discussion

The present study demonstrated that protease-inhibitory activity of *ras* p21 is inversely correlated to pH. By contrast, the protease-inhibitory activity of chicken egg white cystatin gradually decreased as the pH value decreased (data not shown). Cystatin inhibits proteases at near neutral pH (pH 6—7) while p21 works only under more acidic conditions (pH below 6). Thus, it seems that acid cysteine proteinases are inhibited by two classes of inhibitors, namely, acid inhibitors (p21s) and neutral inhibitors (cystatins).

The physiological relevance of the protease-inhibitory activity of p21 is not well understood at present. Guanine nucleotides or point mutations of p21 at positions 12 and 61 did not affect the inhibitory activity of p21s[5—8, 12, 14]. However, the affinity of p21 toward cysteine proteinases is much higher than that toward GAP[5], leading to the possibility that p21 may be associated with cysteine proteinases *in vivo*. Furthermore, the functional domain of the protease-inhibitory activity of p21 is assumed to be located between positions 40 and 59 judging from amino acid sequence homology to the conserved region among the cystatin superfamily[5]. The region between positions 40 and 60 is neither an effector domain nor a guanine nucleotide-binding domain. Nevertheless, this region is indispensable for the biological activity of p21[15] presumably because the region is required for the protease-inhibitory activity. Further research might elucidate the relationship between the protease-inhibitory activity and the guanine nucleotide-binding activity of p21.

The author is grateful to Drs. B. M. Willumsen (University Institute of Microbiology, Copenhagen) and D. R. Lowy (National Cancer Institute, Bethesda) for providing v-Ha-ras plasmid. The author also thanks T. Sawada for technical assistance.

This work was supported in part by Grants-in-Aid from the Ministry of Health and Welfare for Comprehensive 10-*Year Strategy for Cancer Control, Japan.*

References

1 Scolnick, E. M., Papageorge, A. G. and Shih, T. Y., *Proc. Natl. Acad. Sci. USA,* **76**(1979), 5355.
2 McGrath, J. P. *et al., Nature,* **310**(1984), 644.
3 Trahey, M. and McCormick, F., *Science,* **238**(1987), 542.
4 Zhang, K., DeClue, J. E., Vass, W. C. *et al., Nature,* **346**(1990), 754.
5 Hiwasa, T. *et al., FEBS Lett.,* **211**(1987), 23.
6 Hiwasa, T. *et al., Biochem. Biophys. Res. Commun.,* **146**(1987), 731.
7 Hiwasa, T. *et al., Biochem. Biophys. Res. Commun,* **151**(1988), 78.
8 Hiwasa, T. *et al., FEBS Lett.,* **233**(1988), 367.
9 Willumsen, B. M. *et al., EMBO J.,* **4**(1985), 2893.
10 Lacal, J. C. and Aaronson, S. A., *Mol. Cell Biol.,* **6**(1986), 4214.
11 Hiwasa, T., Sawada, T. and Sakiyama, S., *Carcinogenesis,* **11**(1990), 75.
12 Hiwasa, T. *et al., Biol. Chem. Hoppe-Seyler,* **370**(1989), 1215.
13 Barrett, A. J. and Kirschke, H. *Method Enzymol.,* **80**(1981), 535.
14 Hiwasa, T. *et al., Biochem. Int.,* **19**(1989), 593.
15 Zhang, K. *et al., Science,* **249**(1990), 162.

Why Are Arene Imines More Mutagenic Than Arene Oxides?

László von Szentpály[1] and Peter Schwerdtfeger[2]

([1]Dept. of Chemistry, University of the West Indies, Kingston, Jamaica
[2]Dept. of Chemistry, University of Auckland, Auckland, New Zealand)

Abstract The molecular origin of the 20-fold increase in mutagenicity of the arene imines over that of the corresponding arene oxides is investigated. Focusing on the 3 membered rings, the role of the proton affinities and the C-X bond energies of the cations is discussed.

I. Introduction

Arene oxides (epoxides) are important intermediates along the pathways leading from polycyclic aromatic hydrocarbons (PAH) to ultimate mutagens and carcinogens[1–3]. Arene imines (aziridines) are the isoelectronic nitrogen analogues of arene oxides. Glatt *et al.* have shown that the specific mutagenicity of 7 representative K-region arene imines is highly correlated ($r=0.984$) with, and ca. 20-fold higher than that of the corresponding arene oxides[4, 5]. Some arene imines belong to the most potent mutagens found so far[5]. Various *N*-substituted arene imines[5], and some aziridines derived from olefinic structures (ethylenimines) are potent mutagens and carcinogens[6]. Electron withdrawing substituents at *N* greatly reduce the mutagenicity[5], supporting an acid catalyzed mechanism via protonation at *N*, with subsequent ring opening. In the case of the epoxides, there is very little doubt that the ring opening reactions take place by an ionic mechanism[1–3]. It has been further confirmed for ethylene and haloethylene oxides that only the epoxides, not their rearrangement forms, e.g. 2-haloacetaldehydes will alkylate DNA[7].

No molecular explanation has been put forward for the increased mutagenicity of arene imines; specifically the reasons for the strikingly linear correlation and the constant factor of 20 seem to be unknown[4, 5]. In this paper, we compare the 3 membered rings (3MR) ethylene oxide (oxirane=Ox), ethylenimine (aziridine=Az) and their protonated forms (OxH^+, AzH^+), and attempt to relate their chemical properties to the mutagenicity.

The constant increase by a factor of 20 in mutagenicity seems to indicate the involvement of some energies having a nearly constant characteristic difference between corresponding pairs of oxiranes and aziridines. We will here focus on the proton affinity (PA), and the C-X bond energy of the protonated species.

II. Methods, Results and Discussion

The calculations have been performed with the GAUSSIAN 86 program developed by the Pittsburg group[8]. Several levels of approximation have been used, viz. the STO-3G and the extended 6-311+G* basis sets. The effects of valence electron correlation have been incorporated at the second (MP2) order of many body perturbation theory. The reaction coordinates leading to the transition structures (TS) along minimum energy paths have been determined using the Berny optimization method. The TSs located have been checked by the vibrational normal mode analysis.

The experimental gas phase PAs of oxirane, aziridine, and their differences to the corresponding non-cyclic molecules, dimethyl ether and dimethyl amine are well established[9, 10]. Based on most recent experiments[10], PA(AZ)=(227.8— 4.8) kcal/mol=933.3 kJ/mol, thus 139 kJ/mol larger than PA(OX)=794.3 kJ/mol[9, 10]. Table 1 contains a selection of PA values including those at the MP2/6-31G* level of theory[11]. Replacing NH by O reduces the PA by an almost constant increment ΔPA. Further examples of this near constancy are given in [11].

Table 1 Proton Affinities of 3 Membered Ring Heterocycles and Their Dimethyl Analogues

PA (kJ/mol)	Az	Ox	ΔPA	Me_2NH	Me_2O	ΔPA
Exptl	933.3	794.3	139.0	953.3	809.0	144.3
MP2/6-31G*[11]	948.3	785.5	162.8	979.3	816.1	163.2

The PAs of arene imines and oxides are larger in absolute values, this being connected to the lowering of the lone pair ionization energies. A quantitative explanation has been given in terms of sigma- and pi-conjugation[12]. These influences, however, add very similar increments to the PAs of both arene imines and oxides, and practically are canceled in calculating the differences. Therefore we assume the gas phase PA of an arene imine to be about 140—160 kJ/mol larger than that of a corresponding oxide.

Gas phase PAs may significantly differ from the solution values, and it is the latter which influences the reaction *in vivo.* We find, however, the geometries and charge distributions of the protonated AzH^+ and OxH^+ to be quite similar. According to a Mulliken population analysis at STO-3G level, $q\,(C)=0.04$, $q\,(O)=-0.16$ for OxH^+, and $q\,(C)=+0.01$, $q\,(N)=-0.31$ for AzH^+. The positive charge does not reside at the heavy atoms, but on the hydrogens. To assess solvation effects it is reasonable to compare the charges at the CH_2, NH_2 and OH groups: $q\,(CH_2)=+0.34$ for AzH^+, compared to $q\,(CH_2)=+0.39$ for OxH^+, and $q\,(NH_2)=+0.33$, vs. $q\,(OH)=+0.22$ according to STO-3G. There are small changes at the 6-311+G* level, e.g. $q(CH_2)=+0.35$ and $q(OH)=+0.29$. Similar charge distributions and geometries yield similar solvent effects. Thus solvation seems unlikely to change the picture obtained from gas phase PAs. The solution

PAs will be reduced and ΔPA probably scaled down. We believe, however, that the PA of arene imines will exceed that of the corresponding arene oxides by ca. 100 kJ/mol. This would be a rather significant amount, and it is tempted to believe that the difference in the ring opening of AzH^+ and OxH^+ cannot overcompensate the advantage gained by the imines during protonation. According to chemical intuition the C-N and C-O bond dissociation energies should be comparable; the localized bond model increments for their bond energies are $E_{C\text{-}N}=3.834$ eV and $E_{C\text{-}O}=4.149$ eV[13]. Protonation of 3MRs, however, weakens the C-X bond increments for their bond (and strenghtens the C-C bond) proportional to the electronegativity of X[11, 14]. For this reason, and because the 3MRs are known as notorious, but well understood exceptions to many rules[11, 14], we cannot use any conventional increments to the bond energy. On the other hand, it is known that STO-3G calculations overestimate the stability of cyclic isomers, and unduly favor them over acyclic ones[15, 16]. Therefore it seemed necessary to calculate the thermodynamic stability of the cyclic and open isomers of AzH^+ and OxH^+ at the 6-311+G* level of theory. Our SCF energy for OxH^+ is -153.21222 a.u. (E_h), thus 0.0304 $E_h=0.828$ eV lower than the best previous value (6-31G**) in [17]. Concentrating on the difference in C-X bond energies, we compare our calculations with earlier published data in Table 2.

Table 2 Relative Energies (kJ/mol) of the Acyclic End-on Structures of $[CH_2CH_2X]^+$ Isomers Above the Cyclic Cations

X	STO-3G	4-31G	6-31G*//4-31G*	6-311+G*	MP2/6-311+G*	exptl
NH_2	282	178[14]	192[16]	184	239	180[14]
OH	172	40[14]	38[17]	53	102	84[14]
Diff	110	138	154	131	137	96

The potential energy hypersurface of $[C_2H_4NH_2]^+$ is quite complicated. Earlier studies[14—16] have considered the 2-amino-ethyl cantion in its totally staggered conformer only, where the CH_2 and NH_2 end groups are coplanar. We find, however, that a geometry reoptimization with a $\pm 62^\circ$ rotation of the NH_2 group lowers the total energy by 38 kJ/mol at the STO-3G level. Nevertheless, the C-X bond cleavage of AzH^+ requires at least 100 kJ/mol more energy than that for OxH^+. Interestingly, this energy difference is only weekly influenced by the choice of the basis set. Two reasons seem important for this substancial difference.

a) In acyclic $[C_2H_4OH]^+$ the O-H bond points away from the CH_2 group, on the other hand, the NH_2 group in $[C_2H_4NH_2]^+$ has much less possibility to reduce the electrostatic repulsion with the CH_2 group.

b) OxH^+ is better represented as a Dewar type II-complex[14], thus the shift of the OH group into an acyclic end-on position requires less energy than that for a classical 3MR.

A plot of the potential energy vs. the C-C-X angle is shown in Fig. 1. The TSs resemble closely to the acyclic end-on structures and show very small energy barriers with respect to them: 23 kJ/mol at 98° for $[C_2H_4OH]^+$ and only 5 kJ/mol at 105° for $[C_2H_4NH_2]^+$ (STO-3G values).

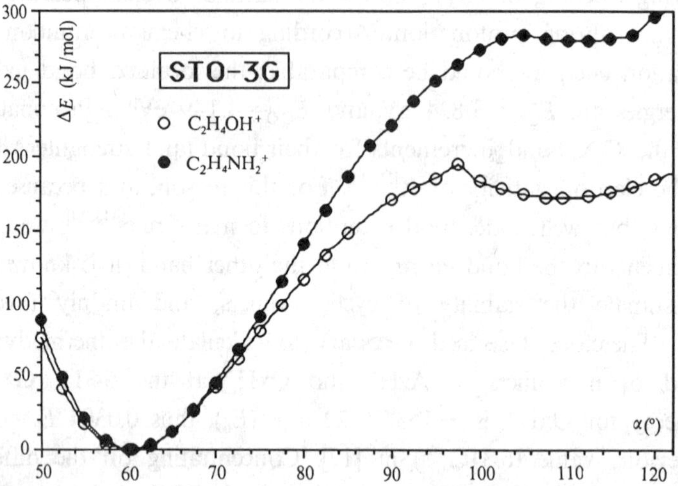

Fig. 1 Cross section of the potential energy hypersurfaces along the C-C-X angle.

At a higher level of theory, an H-shift from NH_2 can follow practically without activation. At present we are interested in a comparison of the openings of different 3MRs, therefore the follow-up H-shifts are not considered in our model. A nucleophilic attack on the positively charged end-on CH_2 group will greatly reduce the TS barrier and ease the ring cleavage. Such an interaction will particularly reduce the partial charge at the attacked CH_2, and thus scale down the electrostatic repulsion with the NH_2 and OH groups. Without nucleophile this repulsion is larger with the NH_2 group and contributes to the ca. 100 kJ/mol higher TS energy of $[C_2H_4NH_2]^+$(Fig. 1). Therefore it is reasonable to assume that this difference between imines and oxides is substancially reduced in case of a nucleophilic attack. We shall make calculations to model such reactions.

At present, the experimental evidence and theoretical results favour an acid catalyzed mechanism of the reaction of arene imines and oxides with a nucleophile. Arene imines are more easily protonated than arene oxides. The C-X bonds in their 3MRs are weakened by protonation[11]. This effect is more prominent with arene oxides, however, and counterbalances the influence of the proton affinities. The experimental fact that electron withdrawing substituents reduce the mutagenicity[5], and the electrostatic arguments just presented indicate that ΔPA is only partly compensated by the bond cleavage, leaving a nearly constant energy balance favouring the acid catalysed reaction of the imines. The role of the aromatic ring systems consists of assisting the protonation[12] and ring opening[3]. The specific assistance accounts for the wide variation in mutagenicity within the separate series of imines and oxides, on the other hand, the effects of the aromatic systems are canceled to a good approximation when comparing corresponding pairs of arene imines and oxides. Thus it is sufficient to determine the the extent of the partial compensation between PA and C-X bond cleavage, in order to rationalize the experimental observations[4, 5] concerning the mutagenicities in the series of K-region arene imines and oxides.

References

1 Sims, P. and Grover, P. L. *Adv. Cancer Res.*, **20**(1974), 165.

2 Glatt, H. R. and Oesch, F., in *Chemical Mutagens: Principles and Methods for Their Detection* (ed. De Serres, F. J.)., **Vol. 10**(1986), Plenum, New York.

3 Szentpály, L. v., *J. Am. Chem. Soc.*, **106**(1984), 6021.

4 Glatt HR, *et al.*, *Cancer Res.*, **45**(1985), 2600.

5 Glatt, H. R. *et al.*, *Envir. Mutagenesis*, **8**(1986), 829.

6 *IARC monogr eval carcino risk chem hum*, **9**(1975), 1975.

7 Bolt, H. M., Laib, R. J. and Filser, J. C., *Biochem. Pharmacol.*, **31**(1982), 1.

8 Frisch, M. J. *et al.*, *Program GAUSSIAN* 86, Canegie Mellon Quantum Chemistry Publishing Unit Pittsburg.

9 Aue, D. H. *et al.*, *J. Am. Chem. Soc.*, **102**(1980), 5151.

10 Meot-Ner, M. and Sieck, L. W., *J. Am. Chem. Sco.*, **113**(1991), 4448.

11 Cremer, D. and Kraka, E., *J. Am. Chem. Soc.*, **107**(1985), 3800.

12 Szentpály L. v., *Rev. Quim. Mex.*, **31**(1987), 186.

13 Dewar, M. J. S., Harget, A. J. and Trinajstic, N., *J. Am. Chem. Soc.*, **91**(1969), 6321.

14 Dewar, M. J. S. and Ford, G. P., *J. Am. Chem. Soc.*, **101**(1979), 783.

15 Jordan, F., *J. Phys. Chem.*, **80**(1976), 76.

16 Barone, V. *et al.*, *J. Mol. Struct.* (Theochem.), **25**(1985), 319.

17 Nobes, R. H. *et al.*, *J. Am. Chem. Soc.*, **103**(1981), 1913.

Isomerism of Active Species and Molecular Biology

Zdeněk Slanina*

(*Max-Planck-Institut für Chemie (Otto-Hahn-Institut), W-65 Mainz, FRG*)

Abstract Theoretically recognized isomerism, established as a crucial point in computation-observation comparisons, is discussed in particular relation to molecular biology. Illustrative examples are supplied with the tautomeric system of 2-pyridone and 2-hydroxypyridine and C_{50} isomeric set.

I. Potential Hypersurface and Isomers

Theoretical chemistry has been accepted[1] as a full partner to experimentation also in several areas of molecular biology. Potential energy hypersurfaces represent[2, 3] a key concept in contemporary chemical theory. Potential hypersurfaces can be employed within two different levels: (i) as a whole within molecular dynamics treatment[4], or (ii) represented by their sole (isolated) stationary points; the choice being dictated by computational demands determined by system dimensions.

Among the stationary points[5] (i.e. the hypersurface points with zero first energy derivatives with respect to nuclear coordinates), local minima and transition states (i.e. activated complexes) are particularly important for the interpretation of chemical and biological phenomena. Efficient optimization techniques are available for location of the stationary points at practically any methodological level. The energy and structural features are routinely enhanced by evaluation of the harmonic vibrational spectrum. While the location treatment is mostly based on analytical energy derivatives, the force-constant matrix is more frequently derived by numerical differentiation of the analytical gradient. This information triad (energy-structure-harmonic vibrations) has recently become standard for the quantum-chemical description of smaller chemical systems. Hence, partition functions (in the approximation[2] of rigid rotator and harmonic oscillator) can be constructed for thermodynamical evaluations.

A systematic investigation of a potential hypersurface often reveals several different local minima (i.e. several isomers), all belonging to the same species reacting in an experiment. Simple potential energy reasoning can sometimes eliminate all higher structures so

* Permanent address: The J. Heyrovský Institute of Physical Chemistry and Electrochemistry, Czechoslovak Academy of Sciences, CS-18223 Prague 8, CSFR.

that only the global minimum is really important. However, the potential energy term itself is not necessarily decisive-temperature excitation of individual motions (particularly, vibrations) within each structure also is to be taken into account. This special kind of enthalpy-entropy compensation can cause coexistence of some local minima or even overwhelming population of a local minimum other than the global one. Such situations of stability/activity interchanges can have profound consequences for molecular biology applications.

II. Computational Scheme

Let us consider a set of n isomers and let them establish an inter-isomeric thermodynamic equilibrium (characterized by the values of the mole fractions w_i of the individual isomers). We do not require the full thermodynamic equilibrium (i.e. with respect to dissociation products, etc.). The relative positions of the isomers are described by the potential energy differences ΔE_i related to the global minimum. Vibrational motions contribute to the terms through the zero-point energies, leading to the ground-state energy differences $\Delta H^o_{0,i}$. The isomeric mole fractions are given by[6]

$$w_i = \frac{q_i \exp[-\Delta H^o_{0,i}/(RT)]}{\sum_{j=1}^{n} q_j \exp[-\Delta H^o_{0,j}/(RT)]}, \tag{1}$$

where q_i stand for partition functions of the individual isomers, R is the gas constant and T is the temperature. The formula was primarily derived for gas-phase conditions, however, it can be equally well applied[7] to other environments, as long as the partition functions are adjusted accordingly. A simplified treatment is offered by means of so-called simple Boltzmann factors[8]:

$$w_i' = \frac{\exp[-\Delta E_i/(RT)]}{\sum_{j=1}^{n} \exp[-\Delta E_j/(RT)]} \tag{2}$$

based on the sole potential energy differences. However, the factors (2) do not admit a relative-stability temperature interchange.

In a thermodynamical approach[2] one can consider either the individual isomers or a pseudospecies composed of their equilibrium mixture. This creates two classes of quantities-partial and overall. Let us consider a reaction in which one component exhibits isomerism. Application of just one of the isomers leads to a partial standard term ΔX^o_i. Consideration of the pseudospecies yields the overall standard change ΔX^o_T, all the isomers contributing according to the weights w_i.

The partial and overall terms contain however some common terms. Those can be cancelled out by introduction of so-called isomerism contributions to thermodynamic terms, δX_1:

$$\delta X_1 = \Delta X_T^o - \Delta X_1^o, \tag{3}$$

which does not depend on the standard state. For convenience the most stable species (at the low temperature limit) is chosen as the reference structure labelled by $i=1$. We shall consider enthalpy ($X=H$), entropy ($X=S$), or heat capacity at constant pressure ($X=C_p$). Interesting is the heat capacity case[9] where, in addition to the full, exact (relaxation) term $\delta C_{p,1}$, its simplification neglecting the temperature dependency of w_i is considered ($\delta C_{p,w,1}$, isofractional term). The relaxation term is reduced to the isofractional part at both high- and low-temperature limits.

III. Illustrative Examples

Tautomeric equilibria are systems of great importance in organic and biological chemistry. The tautomerism of 2-pyridone (P2) and 2-hydroxypyridine (HP2) represents an interesting system studied intensively by both experimental and theoretical means. However, the P2/HP2 relative stabilities have only been evaluated in terms of the simple Boltzmann factors. Hence, our study[10] evaluated the rigorous weights w_i. It turns out that, in contrast to several other isomeric systems studied recently, the agreement of both types of weight factors is quite good (though at higher temperatures the HP2 species is significantly more stable than predicted by the simple Boltzmann factors). In other words, the contributions of rotational-vibrational motions to the partition functions are sufficiently similar for both isomers in question. This is however an exception rather than the rule[2].

Fullerenes (polyhedral, purely carbonaceous species C_n with n larger than 20) represent[11] a new system of not only chemical and physical but also biological interest. On the one hand, their possible carcinogenic effects are speculative but a fullerene-type system has served for diagnostic purposes[12]. Three minimum-energy structures were found in the MNDO study[13] each of them being built from pentagonal and hexagonal rings. The polyhedra resulted from optimization of the geometry with the D_{5h}, D_3 and C_{2v} symmetry point groups. The D_{5h} structure is the lowest in energy (the heat of formation at room temperature), the D_3 isomer being some 30 kJ/mol and the C_{2v} isomer some 1600 kJ/mol higher than an energy (Fig. 1). Fig. 2 presents the temperature evolution of the w_i and w_i' terms in a wide temperature interval. Effectively, the system behaves[14] like a two-component mixture—populations of the C_{2v} species are negligible throughout. The simple Boltzmann factors do not represent a good approximation of the exact w_i terms. The most interesting feature of the w_i temperature profile is the relative-stability interchange between the D_{5h} and D_3 structures at about 1390 K. Hence, from the thermodynamic-equilibrium point of view the D_3 species should be preferentially formed in high temperature regions. This is primarily a phenomenon of chemical importance but nevertheless one can well imagine a biological system with such a relative-stability interchange around physiological temperature optimum. Fig. 3 presents temperature evolu-

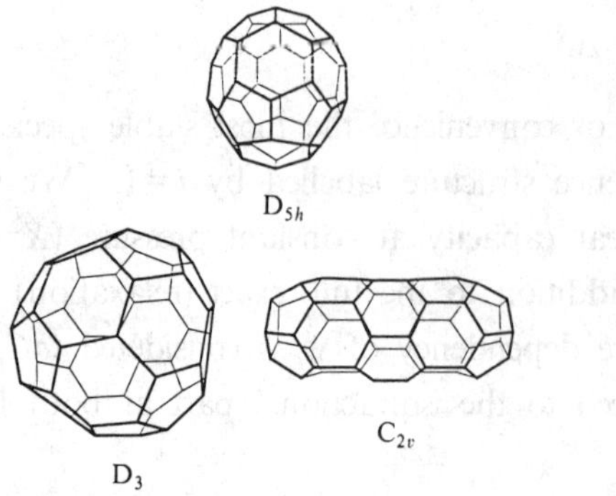

Fig. 1 Schemes of three C_{50} isomers with D_{5h}, D_3 and C_{2v} point-group symmetries[13].

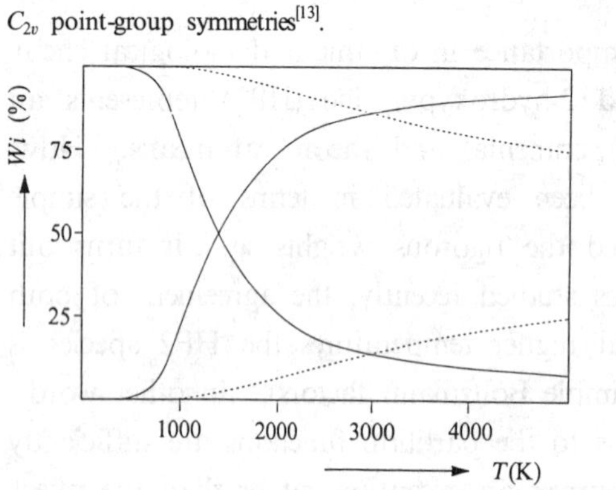

Fig. 2 Temperature dependences[14] of the weight factor w_i and simple Boltzmann factors w_i' (dashed curves) for the D_{5h} (the decreasing curves) and D_3, C_{50} isomers (C_{2v} cannot be seen).

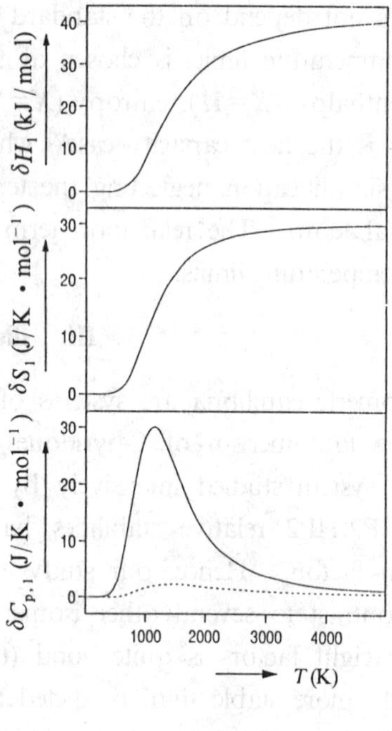

Fig. 3 Temperature evolution[14] of the the isomerism contributions (related to the D_{5h} species as the reference structure) δX_1 to thermodynamic functions of the C_{50} isomeric system ($X = H$, S or C_p; the dashed curve represents the isofractional contribution $\delta C_{p,w,1}$).

tion of the isomerism contributions to thermodynamics for the isomeric C_{50} system related to the D_{5h} species as the reference species. Features exhibited by the isomerism contributions resemble those already reported for other cluster isomeric systems[9]. Behaviour of the heat-capacity term is most interesting. The full (relaxation) term exhibits clear temperature maximum, not present in the sole isofractional term. The temperature maximum is placed closed to the relative-stability crossing. It was pointed out[9] that such a temperature maximum could serve as an experimental evidence of an isomerism discovered computationally. In conclusion, the procedure reported represents a practical method of treating conformational multiplicity (limiting in a fluxional isomeric behaviour[15]).

This paper was prepared during a research stay at the Max-Planck-Institut für Chemie (Otto-Hahn-Institut) supported by the Institute and the Alexander von Humboldt-Stiftung. The support and the valuable discussions of and with Profs. P. J. Crutzen and K. Heinzinger are greatly appreciated.

References

1 Karplus, M. *J. Phys. Chem.,* **94**(1990), 5435.

2 Slanina, Z., *Contemporary Theory of Chemical Isomerism,* Reidel, Dordrecht, 1986.

3 Mezey, P. G., *Potential Energy Hypersurfaces,* Elsevier, Amsterdam, 1987.

4 Hoover, W. G., *Molecular Dynamics,* Springer, Berlin Heidelberg New York, 1986.

5 McIver, Jr., J. W. and Komornicki, A., *J. Am. Chem. Soc.,* **94**(1972), 2625.

6 Slanina, Z., *Int. J. Quantum Chem.,* **16**(1979), 79.

7 Slanina, Z., *Comput. Chem.,* **13**(1989), 305.

8 Zimmerman, S. S. and Scheraga, H. A., *Biopolymers,* **16**(1977), 811.

9 Slanina, Z., *Int. Rev. Phys. Chem.,* **6**(1987), 409.

10 Slanina, Z. and Adamowicz, L., *Thermochim. Acta,* **177**(1991), 101.

11 Curl, R. F. and Smalley, R. E., *Science,* **242**(1988), 1017.

12 Dayton, L. and Johnson, J., *New Sci.,* 1991, No. 1776: 26.

13 Bakowies, D. and Thiel, W., *J. Am. Chem. Soc.,* **113**(1991), 3704.

14 Slanina, Z., Adamowicz, L., Bakowies, D. *et al., Thermochim. Acta,* **202**(1992), 249.

15 Berry, R. S., *Large Finite Systems* (eds. Jortner, J. *et al.*) Reidel, Dordrecht, 1987.

Anti-mutagenic Effects of Kiwi Fruit Drink on Benzo(a)-pyrene and Benzene*

XU Hou'en, CHEN Jidi, ZHOU Zongcan, SONG Yanjun and GAO Guanghua

(*Department of Toxicology, Beijing Medical University, Beijing* 100083, *China*)

Abstract To observe the antimutagenicity and detoxification of kiwi fruit drink on benzo(a)pyrene (BaP) and benzene, Ames test, micronucleus test, sister chromatid exchange (SCE) and improved micronuclear assay in population were studied.

I. Materials and Methods

1. *Ames Test*

Salmonella typhimurium tester strain TA 98 and TA 100 were kindly provided by Professor Bruce Ames, University of California, Berkeley.

In this assay, Genotypes of tester strains were confirmed. The concentrated drink, the *S. typhimurium* tester strain, the mutagen and liver homogenates (S9) from rats pretreated with Aroclor 1254, were mixed and incorporated into an agar overlay. After incubation at 37°C for 2 days, revertant colonies were counted. All testing was done in duplicate.

2. *Micronucleus Test*

The effect of kiwi fruit drink on the micronuclei formation of benzene was studied by a micronucleus test in mice. A test consisted of the use of 10 animals (Kunming mice) per sex. The 5 test groups included a positive control group exposed to benzene, a group drinking Vitamin C, a group drinking kiwi drink, a group drinking kiwi plus Chinese herb juices and a negative control group drinking water. The positive control group and all of the experimental groups were exposed to 100 ppm benzene for 2 h in two days after drinking different drinks for 14 days.

A bone-marrow preparation was done about 24 h after the last application and 1000 polychromatic erythrocytes (PCE) were counted per animal for the presence of micronuclei (Mn).

* The project was supported by the Natural Science Foundation of China and Guangdong Jianlibao Sports Drink Co. LTD.

3. *Population Study*

SCE Assay We chose 7 bank staff who had lived in a polluted area for more than 5 years and did not smoke or were exposed in a chemical occupation, as subjects. Their mean SCE per cell and urinary BaP were 10.51 ± 0.99 and 0.0027— 0.0066 μg/L respectively. Their diet was supplemented by kiwi fruit drink at the rate of 710 ml daily per subject for 5 days.

Blood samples were drawn from the bank staff members and from six control residents. Replicate cultures containing 0.3 ml heparinized whole blood in 5 ml RPMI 1640 medium (Gibco) containing 15% (v/v) fetal calf serum, 1% glutamine, 100 units/ml penicillum, 100 μg/ml streptomycin 1% PHA-m (Gibco), 20 μm Brdurd, and supplements were incubated at $37°C \pm 0.1°C$ in the dark with no agitation for 72 h. Four hours before the end of the incubation, 0.1 ml of 10^{-5} mol/L colcemid was added (final concentration 2×10^{-7} mol/L). The cells were harvested in the usual manner and the slides were stained with the fluorescence plus Giemsa technique of Perry and Walff.

The slides were coded and cells in the metaphase containing 44, 45 or 46 chromosomes were counted for the number of SCE in 20 cells per sample.

Urinary BaP Analysis Polyurethane foam was cut into cylinders of diameter 2.8 cm which were treated with cyclohexane and acetone respectively, and then packed into a glass column of diameter 2.8 cm.

Each urine sample was heated to $75 \pm 5°C$ and passed through the column using a flow rate of 60 ± 10 ml/min. The foam cylinder was taken out of the column and dried overnight at 4°C.

The dried foam cylinder, loaded with BaP, was extracted four times with cyclohexane and the solution concentrated to 0.1 ml. The BaP was determined by a paper chromatography method.

Improved Micronuclear Assay Seven workers exposed to benzene were surveyed to determine the effect of kiwi drink supplementation on cytogenetic damage. The range of cells with Mn in the workers was 7— 14%. The workers drank 500 ml of kiwi fruit drink B daily for six days.

We adopted the cytokinesis-block method to measure the rate of cells with Mn (Fenech, Metal 1985). Blood samples were drawn from the seven workers exposed to benzene. Replicate cultures containing 0.3 ml heprinized whole blood in 4 ml RPMI 1640 medium (Gibco) were incubated at 37°C in the dark with no agitation. Cytochalasin B was added after 44 h (final conc. 4.6 μg/ml). The cultures were stopped at 72 h. Cytocentrifuge preparations of the cells on slides were made for each subject.

The micronuclei in 1000 binucleate cells were counted per sample.

II. Results

The results from the Ames test showed that kiwi fruit drink could inhibit the mutagenicity of BaP (Table 1)

Table 1 Effects of Kiwi Fruit Drink on Matagenicity of BaP

Dose of Concentrated Drink (1 plate)	Revertants Per Plate (TA98)
0	2983±678.0 (100 %)
0.03ml	2465±384.5 (82.6 %)
0.15ml	675±92.3 (22.0 %)
0.03ml	25±4.9 (0.8 %)

Bap, 10 μg/plate; Negative control TA98, 25±8.0/plate.

In the micronucleus test, the results showed that the formation of micronuclei in PCE induced by benzene exposure can be decreased by drinking vitamin C drink and kiwi fruit drink. A mixed kiwi-Chinese herb drink had a more significant effect (Table 2).

Table 2 Effect of Kiwi Drink on Micronuclei Formation of Benzene

Group	Animal Number	Number of PCE	No. of Cell With Mn	Cell With Mn (‰)	P
Drinking water 14 days +Benzene exposure (100 ppm)	20	20000	100	5.0	
Drinking Vc (45 mg/100 ml)14 days +Benzene exposure (100 ppm)	20	20000	46	2.3	<0.01
Drinking kiwi Drink 14 days	20	20000	36	1.8	
Drinking kiwi-Chinese Herb Juice 14 day +Benzene Exposure (100 ppm)	20	20000	25	1.25	
Drinking water contral	20	20000	24	1.2	

Average amount of daily intake was 10 ml; PEC/NCE>0.1.

After supplementation of their diet with 710 ml of kiwi fruit drink daily for five days, the mean SCE per cell in seven individuals exposed to air pollution decreased from 10.51±99 to 8.06±1.48, and urinary BaP decreased from 0.0027— 0.0066 μg/l to <0.002 μg/l (Table 3).

After supplementation of their diet with 500 ml of kiwi fruit drink B daily for six days, the rate of cells with Mn in seven workers exposed to benzene was decreased from 10.4±2.8‰ to 5.7±2.8‰ (Table 4).

III. Summary

Kiwi fruit drink is made mainly from a wild fruit (*Actinidia chinensis* Planch) with

Table 3 Effect of Kiwi Fruit Drink Supplementation on SCE and Urinary BaP

Subject Code Number	Sex	Age	SCEs/Cell Before supplementation	SCEs/Cell After supplementation	Urinary BaP (μg/l) Before supplementation	Urinary BaP (μg/l) After supplementation
1	M	29	10.05	6.45	0.0036	<0.002
2	F	27	10.65	6.25	0.0061	<0.002
3	F	29	10.05	9.10	0.0066	<0.002
4	F	36	12.05	9.30	0.0034	<0.002
5	F	27	11.20	9.70	0.0063	<0.002
6	F	30	8.90	7.50	0.0027	<0.002
7	M	28	10.65	7.65	0.0058	<0.002
$\overline{X}\pm SD$			10.51±0.99	8.06±1.48		
t				5.01		
P				<0.005		

710 ml daily intake per subject for 5 days.

Table 4 Effect of Kiwi Fruit Drink on Micronuclei Formation of Benzene

Subject Code No.	Sex	Age	Rate of Cells With Mn (‰) Before supplementation	Rate of Cells With Mn (‰) After supplementation
1	F	35	11	7
2	F	32	14	5
3	F	31	10	8
4	M	30	8	8
5	F	31	14	8
6	M	30	7	2
7	M	20	9	2
$\overline{X}\pm SD$			10.4±2.8	5.7±2.8
P			<0.01	

500 ml daily intake per subject for 6 days.

extracts of a natural food with abundant trace elements. This drink possesses anti-mutagenic effects on BaP and benzene. However, the mechanism of the antimutagenic effects of kiwi fruit drink on BaP and benzene awaits further study.

References

Xu, H. E, Chen, J. D. *et al., Chinese Journal of Sports Medicine,* **9**(1990), 3:129.

Fenech, M and Morley, A. A., *Mutation Research,* **147**(1985), 29.

Chen, J. D. *et al., The Journal of Sports Medicine and Physical Fitness,* **30**(1990), 2:181.

Urinary 1-Hydroxypyrene as an Index for Human Exposure to Ambient PAH

ZHAO Zhenhua, QUAN Wenyi and TIAN Dehai

(Beijing Municipal Research Institute of Environmental Protection, Beijing 100037, China)

Abstract The levels of urinary 1-hydroxypyrene in residents living in five Chinese cities and in different functional areas of Beijing were determined. Statistical analysis shows that the concentration of 1-hydroxypyrene in human urine is significantly correlated with the level of organic matter and mutagenicity in airborne particulates.

The urinary 1-hydroxypyrene of traffic policemen, road cleaning workers and bank employees was determined and analyzed. An increase of urinary 1-hydroxypyrene is observed when coal ranges are used for heating in winter. All the results suggest that urinary 1-hydroxypyrene is a specific, sensitive index for human exposure to ambient PAHs and may be useful in the risk assessment of environmental and human health hazards.

Polynuclear aromatic hydrocarbons (PAHs) are important carcinogens in the environment[1]. There exists an etiologic link between lung cancer and pollution by PAHs due to coal burning[2, 3]. A sensitive, specific and practical index for human exposure to ambient PAHs is of significant importance for the assessment of the health risk arising from human exposure to PAHs, and is valuable in the process for eventually establishing effective ways to monitor endogenous exposure to environmental hazardous pollutants. Pyrene is a major component in ambient PAHs. It has been found that the concentration of pyrene is in fairly constant proportion to that of PAHs. The percentage of pyrene in the total amount of PAHs varies over a fairly narrow range despite the diversity of sample sources in coal-burning environments[4]. Therefore, the concentration of pyrene in the ambient air was representative of PAHs pollution. Urinary 1-hydroxypyrene, which is a major metabolite of pyrene, has been suggested as a biological monitoring index for human exposure to ambient PAHs[4－6]. In this paper, the urinary 1-hydroxypyrene concentrations of several populations who lived in different areas were determined by HPLC[7]. The method was based on the enzymic hydrolysis of conjugated metabolites, followed by concentration and extraction of the metabolites. The results obtained are discussed in view of pollution by ambient PAHs.

---

* Project supported by the National Natural Science Foundation of China, and partially by the Beijing Municipal Environmental Protection Bureau.

1. *Measurements of Urinary 1-Hydroxypyrene for the Populations Who Live in Different Social Functional Areas in Beijing*

Volunteers in each population were chosen who lived in the same residential environment, had the similar dietary habits and the same professional occupation, exc pt for the group of coke oven workers. Six locations in different social functional districts were selected and the urine samples of each volunteer from those areas were collected respectively in winter and in summer. Details of the determined concentrations of 1-hydroxypyrene and the *t*-tests are listed in Table 1.

For the samples from the coke oven, industrial area and tourist area (control) volunteers, 1-hydroxypyrene content is higher in summer than in winter. *t*-Tests also indicate that urinary 1-hydroxypyrene in summer is significantly higher than that in winter for both the industrial area and tourist area, but the difference is not significant for coke oven workers. For the samples from the steel plant, commercial and residential areas, the concentration of urinary 1-hydroxypyrene is higher in winter than in summer, and *t*-tests show significant difference for the commercial area, but no significant difference was found for either the steel plant or the residential area. According to the sum of the average concentrations for summer and winter (Fig. 1), the level of 1-hydroxypyrene in urine for coke oven workers is the highest (about 7—18 times higher than other groups). It declines in the following order: industrial area, commercial district, residential area, followed by the tourist area (control). The level of PAHs in the atmosphere decreases in the same order.

Table 1 Statistics of Urinary 1-OH-pyrene Content of Beijing Residents and Results of *t*-Tests (Sampled in June and December, 1988)

Social Function	Sampling Location	Season	Number of Volunteers	1-OH-pyrene (μmol/mol creat.) Geometric mean	95% confidence interval	*t*-Tests Results *t*	D_f	P	Significance
Coke oven		Summer	20	6.51	1.21—34.99	1.747	28	0.092	−
		Winter	10	3.64	0.680—19.61				
Steel plant		Summer	38	0.711	0.154—3.281	1.198	56	0.236	−
		Winter	20	0.906	0.265—3.102				
Industrial area	Shijingshan District	Summer	20	0.795	0.330—1.912	2.440	59	0.018	+
		Winter	41	0.533	0.146—1.943				
Commercial district	The East District	Summer	20	0.370	0.110—1.246	4.450	38	<0.001	++
		Winter	20	0.766	0.358—1.636				
Residential area	The West District	Summer	19	0.329	0.110—1.021	1.250	39	0.227	−
		Winter	22	0.399	0.170—0.933				
Tourist area	The Ming Tombs	Summer	19	0.448	0.231—0.869	4.515	34	<0.001	++
		Winter	17	0.145	0.021—1.026				

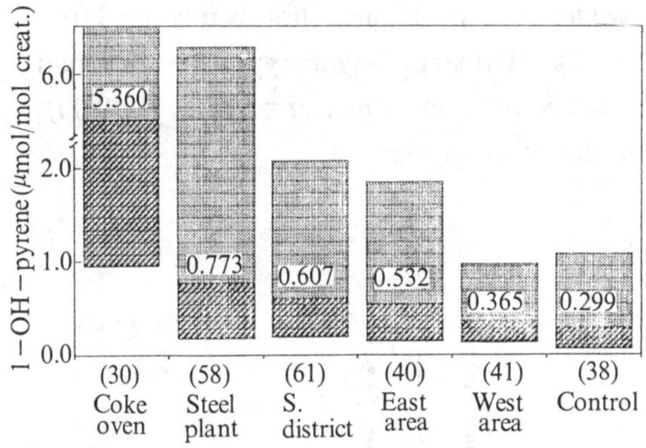

Fig. 1 1-Hydroxypyrene in urine from different sampling locations in Beijing. Numbers in columns are the geometric mean of 1-OH-pyrene, numbers in paren-theses are the sample size.

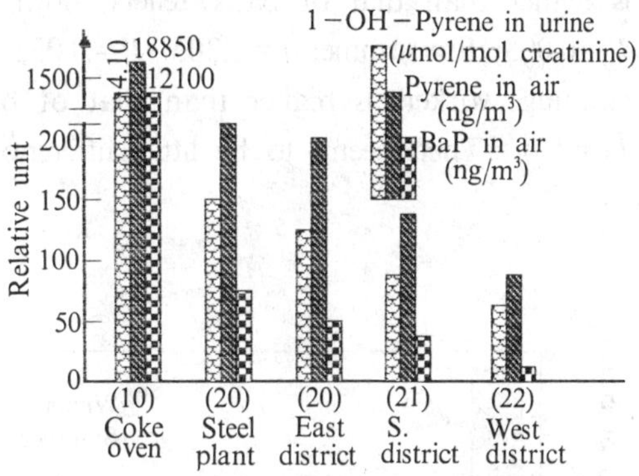

Fig. 2 Correlation of urinary 1-OH-pyrene with ambient pyrene and benzo(a)pyrene in Beijing. Numbers in parentheses are sample size.

Post-hoc tests indicate that there is no significant difference among the steel plant, industrial area, and the business district. The urinary 1-hydroxypyrene level in those three areas is significantly higher than the tourist area, while there exists no significant difference between the residential and tourist areas. However, the correspondence between the urinary 1-hydroxypyrene and the concentration of PAHs collected in personal samplers carried by volunteers is obvious for all the sampling locations. Fig. 2 shows the histogram of urinary 1-hydroxypyrene and the contents of pyrene and benzo(a)pyrene in the atmosphere from personal samplers in Beijing.

2. *1-Hydroxypyrene in Urine of Different Populations in Beijing*

Volunteers were road cleaning workers, traffic policemen and bank tellers from the same area in the West Beijing. The control group was from herdsmen living on the Inner-Mongolian grassland where the refreshing atmosphere is not yet polluted by either industry or coalburning. Concentrations of 1-hydroxypyrene in urine samples which were collected respectively in summer and in winter were determined. Fig. 3 shows the number of volunteers, the geometric means and standard deviation of urinary 1-hydroxypyrene for the four groups. It reveals that the highest concentration of 1-hydroxypyrene is from road cleaning workers in winter, but in summer the highest concentration appears in the samples from traffic policemen. The paired *t*-tests indicate that for road cleaning workers, urinary 1-hydroxypyrene in winter is very significantly higher than in summer ($n=29$, $t=5.42$, $P<0.001$); for traffic policemen the situation is similar ($n=31$, $t=2.291$, $P=0.029$); but for bank tellers the difference between winter and summer is not significant ($n=23$, $t=0.056$, $P=0.956$). The level of 1-hydroxypyrene for bank tellers is very close to that of the control group. The road cleaning workers and traffic policemen stay in the streets for about ten hours a day, so the high levels of urinary 1-hydroxypyrene in winter may be attributed to seirous pollution of the ambient air by PAHs. Moreover, *t*-tests show that urinary 1-hydroxypyrene for traffic policemen is higher than that of bank tellers, both in winter and in summer (for winter $t=3.084$, $P=0.003$; for summer $t=2.305$, $P=0.025$, $D_f=52$). Urinary 1-hydroxypyrene for road cleaning workers is higher than that of bank tellers only in winter ($t=5.862$, $P<0.001$, $D_f=50$). There seems to be little difference for the other groups.

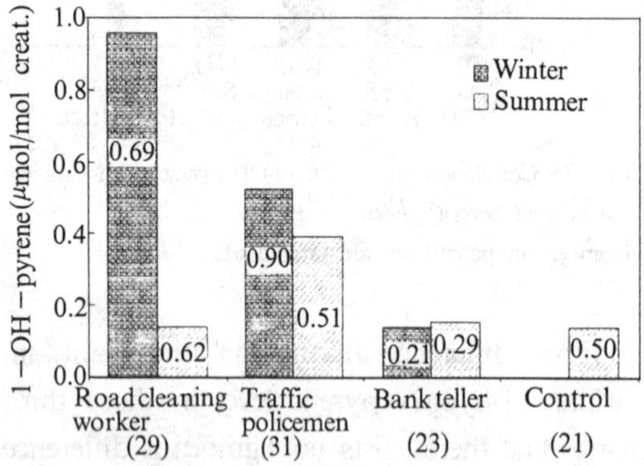

Fig. 3 Geometric mean of urinary 1-OH-pyrene of volunteers from Beijing.
Numbers in columns are the standard deviation, numbers in parentheses are the numbers of volunteers.

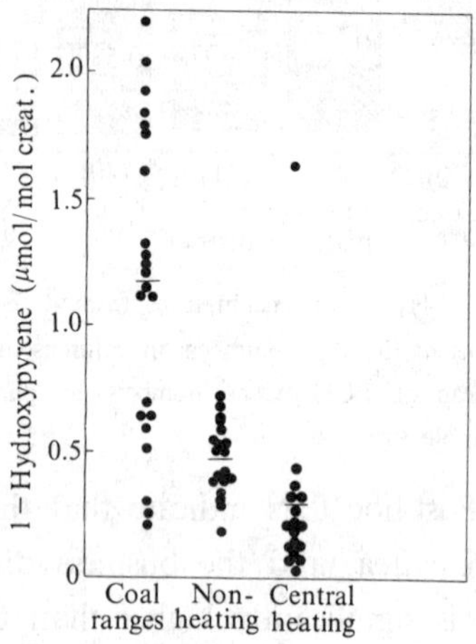

Fig. 4 1-Hydroxypyrene in urine of several population groups.

The results reported here show that the high urinary 1-hydroxypyrene of traffic policemen in summer is a result of PAH pollution by traffic exhaust. In winter, serious pollution of the city air by coal-burning results in an increase in the urinary 1-hydroxypyrene of road cleaning workers. To investigate the effect of indoor heating with a coal range, the urinary 1-hydroxypyrene of the volunteers who used coal ranges or central heating in the heating period was determined in comparison with the measurements in non-heating seasons. Fig. 4 shows that the level of urinary 1-hydroxypyrene of the persons using coal ranges for indoor heating is higher than that for those with central heating or that in the non-heating season.

Six volunteers living in the same kind of apartment rooms were also tested for their urinary 1-hydroxypyrene levels. In winter they used coal ranges for indoor heating and the breathing zone was seriously polluted by PAHs. The results of the determination show that urinary 1-hydroxypyrene during winter is significantly higher than that in summer (the mean being 1.20 μmol/mol creat. In winter and 0.48 μmol/mol creat. in summer; $t=3.178$, $P<0.025$).

3. *Determination of Urinary 1-Hydroxypyrene and Mutagenicity of Airborne Particulates in Different Cities*

Samples of urine were collected from the housewives living respectively in Beijing,

Taiyuan, Shenyang, Wuhan and Shanghai. Airborne particulates were collected with Andersen high-volume samplers in the five cities and biochemical analysis was done separately. The extraction of air particulates with CH_2Cl_2 was taken as the tota organic matter in particulates, and used in the mutagenicity assay. The sister chromatic exchange (SCE/CHO cell) assay was performed as described in reference[8]. The Ames test[9] was also conducted with salmonella typhimurium TA98. The histograms of urinary 1-hydroxypyrene, organic matter, SCE/CHO cell, Ames test (TA98+S9) and benzo(a)-pyrene for those cities are shown in Fig. 5. Statistical analysis (Table 2) indicates that the concentration of 1-hydroxypyrene in the urine of residents is positively correlated with the organic matter, SCE/CHO cell and benzo(a)pyrene in air particulates at a high level of confidence for four of the cities (the air samples of Shanghai were too contaminated for mutagenicity assay). Despite high values of the correlation coefficient between 1-hydroxypyrene and Ames test, correlation is not yet significant because of the small size of the samples.

Table 2 Regression of Urinary 1-OH-pyrene With Airborne Organic Matter and Mutagenicity

Y	X	Regression	r	P	Significance
Organic matter ($\mu g/m^3$)	Urinary1-OH-pyrene (μmol/molcreat.)	$Y=0.20+0.01\sqrt{X}$	0.9978	<0.01	+
SCE/CHO cell/m^3	ditto	$Y=0.50+0.50\sqrt{X}$	0.9762	<0.05	+
Ames test (TA98+S9,R/m^3)	ditto	$Y=0.50+0.50\sqrt{X}$	0.8936	>0.05	−
Ambient BaP ($\mu g/100m^3$)	ditto	$Y=0.54+0.52\sqrt{X}$	0.9963	<0.01	+

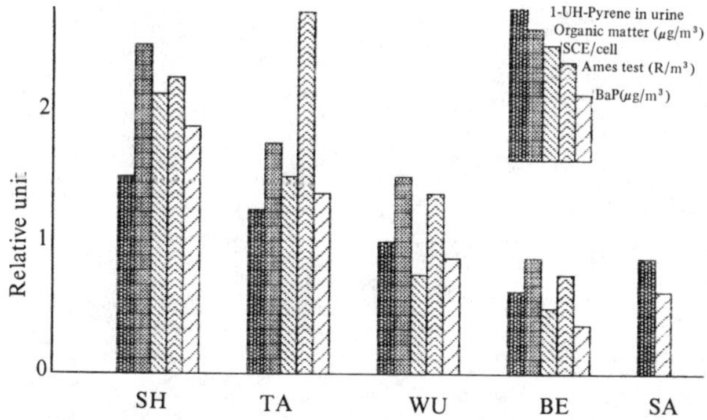

Fig. 5 Correlation of 1-OH-pyrene with organic matter & mutagenicity in air particulates from different cities.

4. *Closing Remarks*

It has been demonstrated that 1-hydroxypyrene in human urine is correlated at a high level of significance with the levels of pyrene and benzo(a)pyrene in ambient air[10] and the influence of sex, age, and smoking on urinary 1-hydroxypyrene is statistically insignificant[11]. In this work samples under various conditions were determined. All of those facts suggest strongly that urinary 1-hydroxypyrene could be used as an index of human exposure to ambient PAHs.

The authors are grateful to Professors Shouren Cao, Shuyi Yu and Mr. Bingcheng Zhao (engineer) for conducting the mutagenicity assays.

References

1 International Agency for Research on Cancer, *Polynuclear Aromatic Compounds*: Part 1, Environmental and Experimental Data (IARC monograph volume 32), Lyon, 1983.

2 Mumford, J. L. *et al.*, *Science*, **235**(1987), 217.

3 Dept. of Epidepiology, *Tianjin Cancer Inst. J. Environ. Health* (China), **6**(1989), 6:1.

4 Zhao Zhenhua *et al.*, *Sci. Total Environ.*, **92**(1990), 145.

5 Jongeneelen, F. J. *et al.*, *Scand. J. Work. Environ. Health*, **12**(1986), 137.

6 Clonfero, E. *et al.*, *Int. Arch. Occup. Environ. Health*, **61**(1989), 363.

7 Zhao Zhenhua *et al.*, *Environ. Monitoring in China*, **6**(1990), 4:37.

8 Qin Yuhui, *Research in Health*, **136**(1984), 14.

9 Ames, B. N. *et al.*, *Mut. Res.*, **31**(1975), 347.

10 Zhao Zhenhua *et al.*, *Sci. Total Environ.* (in press).

11 Zhao Zhenhua *et al.*, *J. Environ. Sci. Health* (in press).

The Examination of Intermolecular Weak Interaction Between Bases of DNA by Using Fast Atom Bombardment Mass Spectrometry (FAB-MS) and Surface-enhanced Raman Scattering (SERS)*

LONG Yaoting,

(*Research Center for Eco-Environmental Sciences, Chinese Academy of Sciences, Beijing* 100085, *China*)

MO Yujun

(*Institute of Physics, Chinese Academy of Sciences, Beijing* 100080, *China*)

and CAO Enhua

(*Institute of Biophysics, Chinese Academy of Sciences, Beijing* 100080, *China*)

Abstract The intermolecular hydrogen bonding between nucleoside and/or bases was examined by FAB-MS and the dynamic process of hydrogen bonding between the bases was observed by SERS. The experimental results from FAB-MS show the formation of guanine-thymine, adenosine-cytosine and cytosine-cytosine pairs in solution with hydrogen bonding being the likely force holding the molecules together. The experimental results by SERS show that explicit spectra of the bases could be obtained on an Ag mirror substrate at 514.5 nm. The present work indicates that the dynamic process of intermolecular interactions could be investigated by SERS. The kinetic constant between guanine and cytosine is 2.7×10^{-2}.

I. Introduction

Knowledge of the intermolecular interaction between DNA bases is being accumulated. In the past decade extensive studies have shown that carcinogens are complexed to DNA via intercalation, groove binding or covalent bonding and/or hydrogen bonding. The main aspect of the problem is how to obtain further information from trace biological samples.

Fast atom bombardment mass spectrometry (FAB-MS) is a powerful technique that permits the analysis of polar and nonvolatile substances at micro-quantitative level by transferring them from a liquid matrix directly into the vapor phase[1]. A prominent feature of FAB mass spectra is the formation of cluster ions with hydrogen bonding being the likely force holding the clusters together. Analyte-analyte clusters have also been detected by FAB-MS. Ions reflecting intermolecular associations have also been reported by Williams *et al.*[2] in two examples of the FAB spectra of binary peptide mixtures.

* Project supported by the National Natural Science Foundation of China.

Meijers *et al.*[3] showed that cluster formation is a common phenomenon of the FAB mass spectra of porphyrins and suggested that such cluster formation may be important in the tumor localization process. Hydrogen bonding was invoked to explain the occurrence of dimers between imidazole and trimethyl phosphate system[4] and between pyridinium ions and other electron donors[5].

Michaud *et al.* [5] assessed the use of FAB-MS for the study of intermolecular associations in solutions. Conventional electron impact MS, which is typically preceded by a thermal vaporization step, is not suitable for a study of phenomena governed by relatively weak (<10 kcal/mol) noncovalent bonds. In contrast, FAB-MS is a low-energy process. There is significant evidence that an FAB mass spectrum adequately represents the established equilibrium in the liquid state[7].

One part of this report focuses on the investigation by FAB-MS of ligand-ligand interactions involving several biologically significant compounds: a nucleoside (adenosine (A')) and bases (guanine (G), adenine (A), cytosine (C), and thymine (T)). Intermolecular interactions are indicated by the presence of peaks above the molecular ion peak of the monomeric species in the mass spectrum. In the case of two compounds, there is the possibility of mixed-association as well as self-association. The extent of mixed-association can be used to study the interaction of biologically important molecules. Another part of this report concentrates on exploring the use of surface enhanced Raman Scattering (SERS) for the study of dynamic processes or intermolecular association in aqueous solution.

Surface enhanced Raman scattering has received considerable attention since it was first reported in 1974 by Fleishmann and coworkers[8]. As the technique has matured, attention has shifted to the application to SERS in analytical chemistry and other fields.

Although the SERS spectra of nucleic acids, nucleosides and bases have been extensively studied because of their biological importance[9], these studies have been done only under limited experimental conditions and have not always been attributed to an explicit adsorption structure. Also, until now, SERS has almost only been employed to obtain non-dynamic process information. In this study we measured the SERS spectra of G, C, A and T adsorbed on an Ag mirror, which was developed by one of the authors and his coworkers[9], and explored the possibility of using SERS as a technique to permit the observation of the dynamic process of intermolecular interactions between bases. The experimental results will be described and discussed in detail in the following paragraphs.

II. Experimental Section

FAB-MS spectra were obtained by using a KYKY-1 mass spectrometer. The target surface was bombarded by a beam of energetic Argon atoms produced by an FAB gun operated at B keV and 1 mA. During all the experiments, the ion source was maintained at room temperature.

Nucleoside and bases solutions were prepared in a concentration of 10 mmol/L and used with the matrix glycerol or p-nitro-benzyl-alcohol.

Spectra were acquired at a rate of 5 s/decade, 1 second interscan time, and at nominal mass resolution. No significant variations in the spectral patterns were observed over a period of several minutes.

Raman spectra were measured on a Laser Raman Spectrophotometer model SPEX 1403 with a detector of RCA-31034, a programmable data acquisition and processing, and a datamate computer data system was used for data acquisition. The incident power on the sample was 40 mW. A solution of 10 mmol/L of each base was put into a cylindrical optical cell of 18 diameter.

III. Experimental Results and Discussion

FAB-MS The occurrence of an association between guanine (MW 151.15) and cytosine (MW 111.10) is shown in Fig. 1a. In this case an approximately 1:1 molar mixture of G to C was examined. The association between the two bases is evidenced by the peak at m/z 263.25 (151.15+111.10+1) corresponding to the protonated complex. The molecular interaction between G and C consists of a three-site complexation.

In the adenine-thymine complex a two-site interaction is expected. The protonated complex (m/z 262) is clearly present in the spectrum obtained when the two components are dissolved together (Fig. 1b).

The data presented above demonstrate that the FAB-MS spectra of bases obtained with Argon gas are similar to those with Xenon gas[5]. Besides these, we also observed the peak at m/z 278 (151.15+126.11+1) corresponding to a protonated complex of guanine-thymine (Fig. 1c).

In the examination of the interaction between adenosine and bases, the peaks at m/z 378, m/z 394, respectively corresponded to the protonated complexes of A′-C and A′-T, which were observed in their FAB mass spectra (Fig. 2a, b). It should be noted that the protonated self-association ion of cytosine (m/z 223) also appeared in the corresponding FAB mass spectrum (Fig. 1b, Fig. 2a, b). Significantly, according to the ratio of the intensity of the dimer to the mixed-association complex, the latter is preferred to self-association. This evidence indicates that they are more likely to occur in aqueous solution, although this kind of mismatch has not been mentioned in biological literature to date. The results presented here show that FAB-MS may be used not only to determine the presence of intermolecular complexes in solution but also to probe the selectivity of

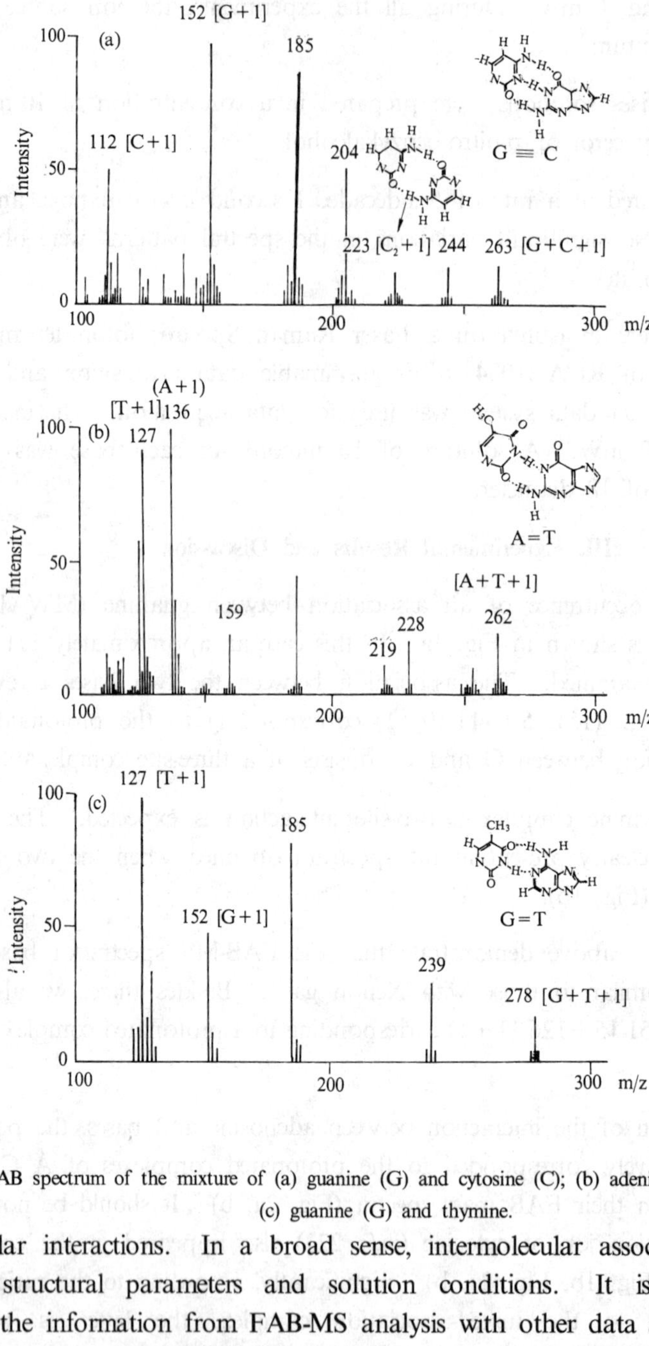

Fig. 1 FAB spectrum of the mixture of (a) guanine (G) and cytosine (C); (b) adenine (A) and thymine (T); (c) guanine (G) and thymine.

intermolecular interactions. In a broad sense, intermolecular associations may be influenced by structural parameters and solution conditions. It is envisioned that by combining the information from FAB-MS analysis with other data and techniques, it may be possible to evaluate the relative contributions of these parameters. FAB-MS can provide sensitive and rapid screening for such features.

SERS Figure 3a gives the SERS spectrum of cytosine excited at a wavelength of 488 nm. Fig. 3b shows the SERS spectrum of cytosine where the wavelength of

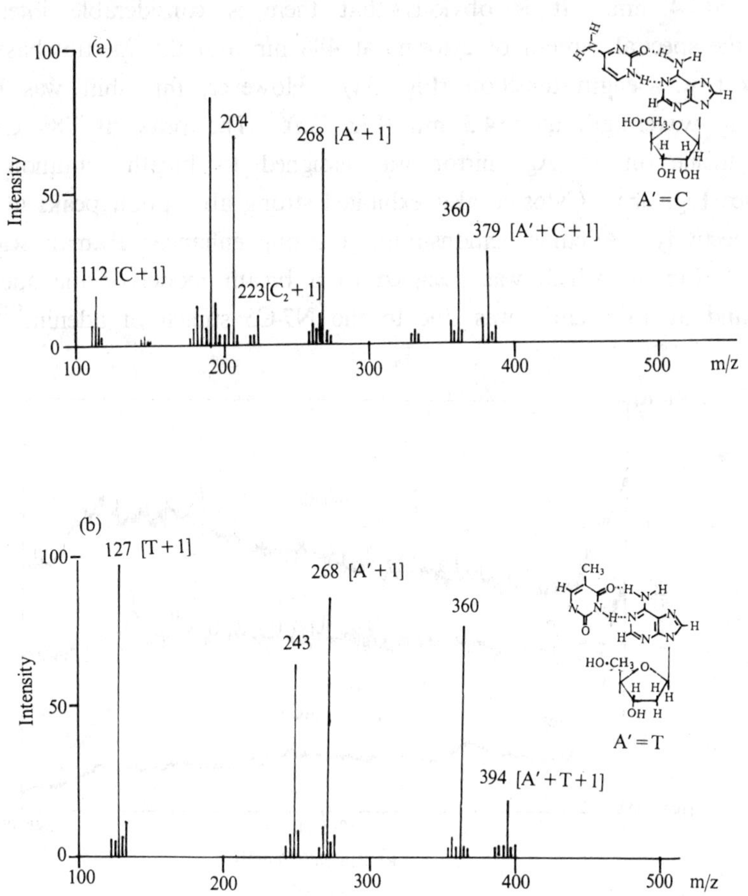

Fig. 2 FAB spectrum of the mixture of (a) adenosine (A') and cytosine (C); (b) adenosine (A') and thymine (T).

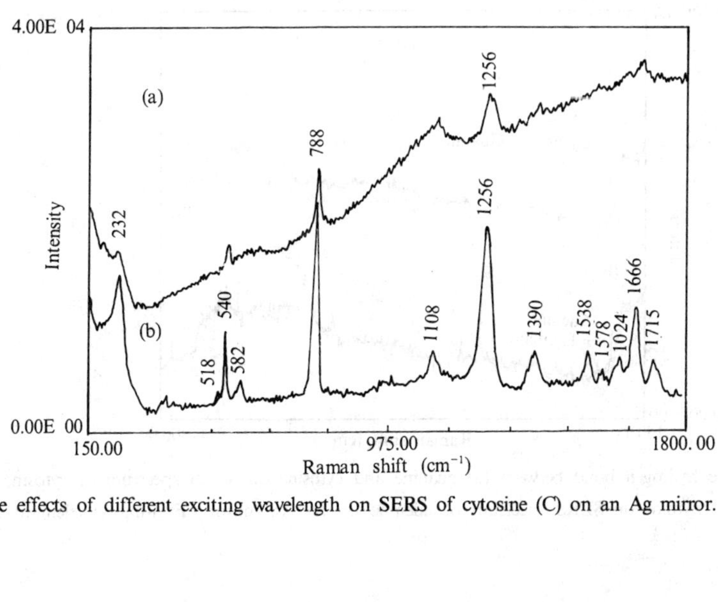

Fig. 3 The effects of different exciting wavelength on SERS of cytosine (C) on an Ag mirror. (a) 488 nm; (b) 514.5 nm.

excitation was 514.4 nm. It is obvious that there is considerable interference by fluorescence in the spectral pattern of cytosine at 488 nm and the spectral base line shifts upwards in short wavelength direction (Fig. 3a). However, this shift was reduced by using an exciting wavelength at 514.5 nm (Fig. 3b). The peak at 788 cm^{-1} in the spectrum of cytosine on an Ag mirror wa assigned to breath vibration model of Cytosine-ring (see Fig. 3b). Cytosine also exhibited strong absorption peaks at 540, 1256, 1666 cm^{-1}, respectively. Adenine demonstrated a strong enhanced Raman scattering signal at 730 cm^{-1} (Fig. 4), which was assigned to a breath model of the adenine-ring[10]. The spectral band at 1326 cm^{-1} was due to the N7-C5 stretch of adenine[11]. Fig. 4b

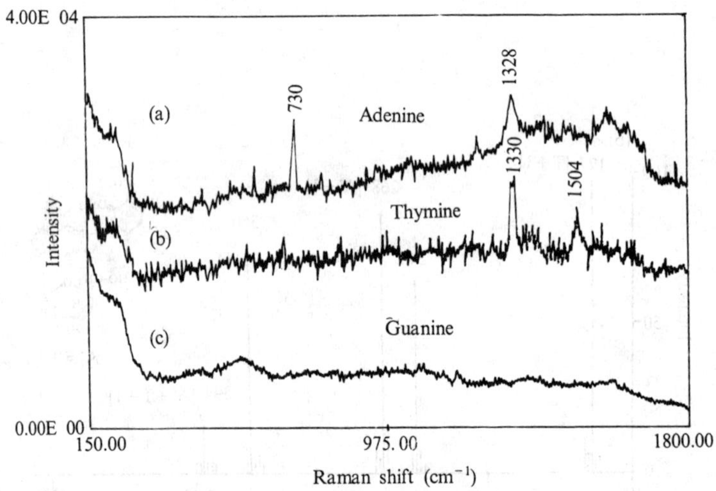

Fig. 4 The SERS spectra of (a) adenine (on an Ag mirror, 514.5 nm); (b) thymine (on an Ag mirror, 514.5 nm); (c) guanine (on an Ag mirror, 514.5 nm).

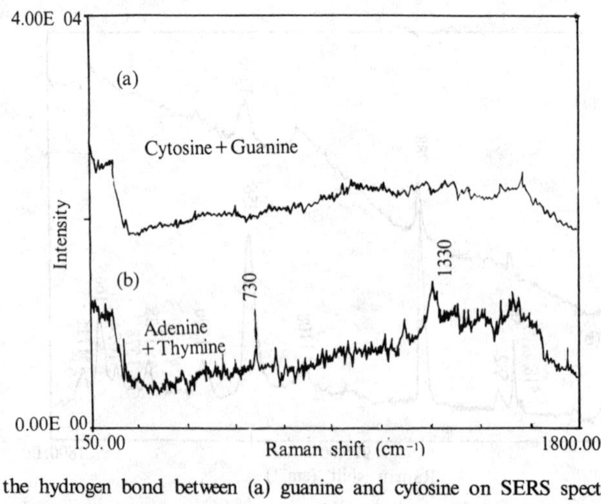

Fig. 5 The effects of the hydrogen bond between (a) guanine and cytosine on SERS spectrum of cytosine on an Ag mirror; (b) adenine and thymine on SERS spectrum of adenine on an Ag mirror. Exciting wavelength: 514.5nm.

gives the SERS spectrum of T on an Ag mirror and the SERS spectrum of G is shown in Fig. 4c. It is obvious from Fig. 4c that the enhanced effect of G on an Ag mirror, in contrast with other bases, is so low that it can be neglected. Significantly the SERS spectrum of C almost completely disappeared when G is present with C in aqueous solution (Fig. 5a), a "quench" phenomenon appeared. This suggested that a stronger interaction occurred between C and G then between C or G and Ag, so that adsorption of C on the Ag surface was destroyed by G. Adenine and T behave similarly (Fig. 5b), but their interaction was not so strong as that between C and G. This fact can be explained by hydrogen bonding between the bases in solution. That can be explained by three-fold hydrogen bond association for G-C and two-fold for A=T. It is also reasonable to propose as a working hypothesis, a model of an Ag-Cl-(hydrogen bond)-cytosine complex. According to this model, the Cl′ ion would react with the Ag on an Ag mirror to form an AgCl film on which hydrogen bond is formed between the Cl of AgCl and the strong electrophilic group of cytosine. This model accounts for why Cl′ is necessary in the Ag-substrate system.

When G was added into the aqueous solution, the N- or O-containing group of cytosine, which was adsorbed on Ag surface, was detached from the Ag surface by strong multi-site hydrogen bonding so that its enhanced effect disappeared. Fig. 4c shows that the enhanced effect of G on the Ag substrate is so weak that it can be neglected. It demonstrates that the adsorption of guanine on the Ag film is also very weak. Fig. 6 is

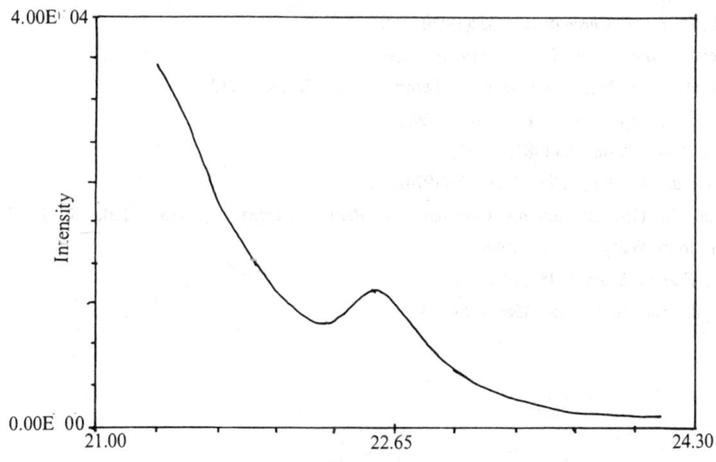

Fig. 6 Dynamic trace of the hydrogen bonding interaction between cytosine and guanine on an Ag mirror film. Exciting wavelength: 514.5 nm.

a dynamic trace of the spectral "quenching" of C by G. It was obtained by monitoring the spectral band of C at 788 cm^{-1}. The sampling interval was 0.1s. This interaction of C and G, leading to quenching of the cytosine spectrum, follows secondary order kinetics according to the following equation:

$$-dc/dt = k(c)\ (G),$$

where c is the concentration of cytosine in aqueous solution, G is the concentration of guanine in aqueous solution, and k is the kinetic constant. The experimental results show that the association process of formation of the hydrogen bond took about 2.5 s, and the kinetic constant k was 2.7×10. In the case of adenine and thymine, the dynamic process took slightly longer, about 3. It should be noted that there was a peak in the dynamic trace about 2 s after the beginning of the interaction which disappeared half a second later. This suggests that probably an unknown intermediate was formed during the dynamic association process. The experiment was reproducible. Adenine and thymine showed similar curves; however, no peak was observed in their dynamic traces, and the extent of quenching of their SERS signal was less than that for C and G. A more in depth experimental study is underway.

The authors thank the National Natural Science Foundation of China for financial help.

References

1 Barber, M. *et al.*, *J. Chem. Soc.*, Chem. Commun., 1981, p. 325.

2 Williams, D. H. *et al.*, *J. Am. Chem. Soc.*, **103**(1981), 5700.

3 Meijers, J. C. M. *et al.*, *J. Chromatogr.*, **352**(1986), 231.

4 Clark, J. H. *et al.*, *J. Ame. Che. Soc.*, **106**(1984), 4056.

5 Broen, S. J. and Miller, J. M., *J. Chem. Soc.*, Perkin Trans., **2**(1987), 1129.

6 Michaud, D. P. *et al.*, *Anal. Chem.*, **62**(1990), 1069.

7 Cupriolai, R. M., *Anal. Chem.*, **55**(1984), 2387.

8 Fleishmann, M. *et al.*, *J. Chem. Phy. Lett.*, **26**(1974), 163.

9 Minami, K. *et al.*, In 11*th International Conference on Raman Spectroscopy* (eds. Clark, R. J. H. and Long, D. A.), Section 4.16, John Wilty & Son, 1988.

10 Kohlin, E. *et al.*, *Surface Science*, **158**(1985), 370.

11 Watanabe, T. *et al.*, *Surface Science*, **158**(1985), 341.

The Cytogenetic, Morphological and Clinical Study of M2/*t*(8:21) Acute Nonlymphocytic Leukemia (ANLL)

CHENG Fanjun,* YANG Aide and FEI Hongbao

(Research Unit of Hematological Genetics, Institute of Hematology, Union Hospital, Tongji Medical University, Wuhan 430022, China)

Abstract In 87 cases of ANLL-M2, clinical and bone marrow studies including morphology, morphometry and ultrastructure were performed. Among the cases, 35 (41%) were of M2/t (8; 21) and 23 (26%) were of M2/NN.

The morphologic study of M2/*t* (8; 21) showed a higher degree of differentiation and maturation and predominence of cell type II myeloblast cell. The ultrastructural study showed that the organs of the leukemic cells were well developed but often swollen and denatured. The morphometric data reflect the disturbance in the development of cell and the nuclear membrane as well as the cytoplasma and the nucleus. Most of the cases of M2 (8; 21) were young males with acute disease and severe anemia and thrombocytopenia. The incidence of leukemic cell infiltration was shorter and the prognosis was poor in patients with M2 (8; 21) and especially in those with loss of a sex chromosome.

According to the criteria of FAB (1985)[1] and Tianjin (1986)[2] for acute leukemia, M2 is found to be the most common subtype (30—80%) in acute nonlymphocytic leukemia. Rowley J.D. observed that *t* (8;21) (q22;q22) was specific for ANLL type M2 (ANLL-M2) by using the quinaorine fluoresoence technique[3]. About 90% of patients with *t* (8; 21) were M2, 5% were M4 and 5% were M1[4]. For the further understanding of the biological behaviour of leukemic cells in cases of ANLL-M2 with 8/21 translocation (M2/*t* (8;21))[5], cytologic, morphologic, morphometric, ultrapathologic and clinical studies were performed in an M2/*t* (8; 21) group and an M2/NN group (M2 with normal karyotype).

I. Patients and Methods

From Jan. 1981 to Dec. 1989 cytogenetic analysis was performed on 97 patients diagnosed as having *de novo* ANLL-M2 by using a high resolution technique. Blood and bone marrow smears were prepared by using Wright's stain and by cytochemical staining including peroxidase and nonspecific esterase stains, etc.

Morphometric studies were performed on 40 patients with 20 patients in each of the M2/*t* (8;21) and M2/NN groups. Bone marrow cells were used for the study and 50

* Postgraduate: Now he is working in Center Hospital of Second Automobile Works.

cells were measured using ASM 68k auto-morphometry for each kind of leukemic cell in each case.

A modified method described by Ticot was used in the ultrastructural study[6]. 4 cases of M2/*t* (8; 21), 2 cases of M2/NN and 2 normal persons were studied.

II. Results

1. *Cytogenetic Study*

In total, 87 cases were successfully studied; *t* (8; 21) was found in 35 cases (41%, male 26, female 9), other chromosomal abnormalities in 29 cases (33%) and normal karyotype in 23 cases (26%).

2. *Cytologic Study*

(1) The bone marrow showed high cellularity (Table 1) with a low percentage of nonerythroid cells (NEC) (Table 2).

Table 1 Cellularity of Two Subtypes of M2

	M2/*t* (8; 21) $n=35$		M2/NN $n=23$		*P*
	case	%	case	%	
Hypocellularity	0		2		
Normal cellularity	1		3		
Significant ↦ Hypercellularity	18	51.4	14	60.8	< 0.05
Extreme ↦ Hypercellularity	18	45.7	4	7.4	<0.001

(2) The percentage of early myeloid precursors in NEC (nonerythroid cells) of M2/*t* (8; 21) was higher than that of M2/NN.

Table 2 The Percentage of Early Myeloid Precursors in NEC

	M2/*t* (8; 21)	M2/NN	*P*
Myeloblast	42.68%	63.67%	<0.005
Premyelocyte	18.86%	11.87%	<0.05
Neutrophilic myelocyte	9.0%	4.13%	<0.05

(3) The percentage of type I myeloblasts was about 20% and that of type II myeloblasts was about 80% in all myeloid cells in M2/*t* (8; 21). On the other hand, the percentages of type I and type II were about 90% and 10% respectively in M2/NN.

(4) The deformity of the leukemic cells and especially of their nuclei was more evident in the M2/*t* (8;21) group than that in the M2/NN group. The deformed nuclei in the myeloblasts of M2/*t* (8;21) was about 50% and that in M2/NN was about 10%. Nucleocytoplasmic asynchrony was more easily found in M2/*t* (8;21).

(5) Dysmegakaryocytopoiesis and dyserythropoiesis were more obvious in bone marrow cells in the M2/*t* (8; 21) group (about 70%) than that in the M2/NN group (20%), $P<0.05$.

3. *Morphometric Study*

Table 3 The Morphometric Values in Two Space Type M2 Patients and Normal Persons

	Normal	M2/*t* (8; 21)	M2/NN	*P*
Myeloblast:				
Ac	155.4±40 μm^2	165.1±42 μm^2	144.77±35 μm^2	<0.01
Fc	97±0.04	0.948±0.09	0.949±0.07	>0.05
An	117.67±25 μm^2	115.2±28 μm^2	110±23 μm^2	<0.01
Fn	0.95±0.05	0.92±0.08	0.96±0.04	<0.01
N/P	0.7688±0.08	0.7057±0.06	0.768±0.07	<0.01
Promyelocyte:				
Ac	239±53 μm^2	226.5±48.7 μm^2	200.5±56.8 μm^2	<0.01
Fc	0.98±0.04	0.956±0.06	0.937±0.08	<0.01
An	129.3±29 μm^2	129.8±275 μm^2	121.19±30 μm^2	<0.01
Fn	0.94±0.05	0.88±0.11	0.911±0.08	<0.01
N/P	0.546±0.08	0.575±0.08	0.61±0.09	<0.01

Ac is the plane surface area of the cell, Fc is the form factor of the cell, An is the plane surface area of the nuclei, Fn is the form factor of the nuclei and N/P is the ratio of the nucleus to the cytoplasma.

4. *Transmission Electron Microscopy*

In this investigation, the ultrastructural features of all four cases of *t*(8;21) ANLL-M2 were shown to be: nuclear blobs, nucleocytoplasmic asynchrony in the early myeloid precursors, Auer rods, giant granules, hypogranular PMN (polymorphologic nuclear leukocyte), PMN lacking secondary granules, absence of a hiatus leukemicus, and the cell's organs being well developed but often swollen and denatured.

5. *Clinical Data*

In 35 cases of M2/*t* (8;21) patients, there were 26 male (75%) and 9 female (25%). The mean age of the M2/*t* (8;21) patients was 19.8—16.8 years: The male/female ratio of the M2/NN patients was 1 and the mean age was 28.6±17 years. The symptoms, signs and laboratory data are presented in Tables 4, 5 and 6.

III. Discussion

In our study, *t* (8; 21) was observed in about 40% of patients with M2[5]. Four

Table 4 The Clinical Data of Two Types of M2 Patients

	M2/*t* (8; 21) $n=35$		M2/NN $n=23$		*P*
	case	%	case	%	
Anemia	29	82.8	11	47	<0.01
Bleeding	27	77.1	17	74	>0.05
Infection & fever	16	45.7	10	43.4	>0.05
Infiltration	30	85.7	11	47	<0.01
Liver spleen & lymphonodi	22	60	10	43.4	<0.05

Table 5 First Peripheral Blood Test of Two Subtypes of M2 Patients

	M2/*t* (8; 21)		M2/NN		*P* value
	case	X±SD	case	X±SD	
Hb (g/l)	30	45.2±15.4	21	69±21.8	<0.01
WBC (10^9/l)	28	12.5±94	22	21.5±246	<0.01
BPC (10^9/l)	22	69.8±28.7	20	98.7±25.3	<0.01
Myeloblast%	35	28.5±22	23	40.1±28.5	<0.01

Table 6 The Prognosis of Two Subtypes of M2 Patients

	M2/*t* (8; 21)		M2/NN	
	observed case	mean	observed case	mean
CR rate %	9	56	13	30
MST (week)	9	22.8	13	22.8
CR period (w)	5	26.7	2	69
MST of CRs (w)	5	36.1	2	92.5

CR: complete remission rate, MST: mean survival time.

kinds of chromosomal abnormalities were seen.

(1) *t* (8;21) only;

(2) *t* (8;21) and loss of a sex chromosome (−x or −y);

(3) mosaic of *t* (8;21) and normal karyotype;

(4) *t* (8;21) and other chromosomal abnormalities.

The abnormal expression of oncogenes located at or near the breakpoint (8q22, 21q22) may play an important role in the pathogenesis of ANLL-M2[4,7,9] (Table 7).

The bone marrow showed high cellularity and some degree of granulocytic maturation and differentiation in patients with M2/*t* (8; 21). In our study, a lower percentage of myeloblasts in NEC and all nuclear cells (ANC), a lack of leukemic hiatus, and the predominance of type II myeloblastic cells were observed in the M2 (8;21) group.

Table 7 *t* (8; 21) and its Relatively Oncogenes

Name	Location	Effects
C-mos	8q22	cell differentiation disturbance
c-myc	8q22	cell multiplication free from the control of CGF
Cets-2	21q22	maligeneous cell
SOD-1	21q22	Increase in the production of Azurophilic granules

Besides the evident deformity of the shape of the cells and the nuclei. Auer rod and nucleocytoplasmic asynchrony were easily found in leukemic cells.

The bone marrow revealed obvious dysmegakaryocytopoiesis and dyserythropoiesis, which would be related to the poor prognosis of the M2/*t* (8; 21) patients.

Our study shows that a morphometric technique with a mathematical analysis of the results and a morphologic study of leukemic cells are useful for diagnosis, classification and prognosis of patients with ANLL-M2[8]. In this research we found that the plane surface area could indicate the growth of both the cell (Ac) and the nucleus (An). The ratio of the cytoplasma to the nucleus (N/P) was found to represent the relative growth of nucleus and cytoplasma, and the form factor (F) was found to reflect the degree of deformity of the cell and the cell nucleus. The lower the value of the F factor, the more striking the irregularity of the body cells and the nucleus. From the cytological point of view, the F-factors were influenced by the surface area of the cell membranes and nuclear membranes. In contrast, in patients with M2/NN, the higher the plane surface area of the cell and the nucleus, the lower the F-factor and the N/P value. Thus, these values could reveal the development of leukemic cells.

The ultrastructural features of leukemic cells in the M2/*t* (8; 21) also indicate the changes resulting from the development of leukemic cells.

The most striking clinical findings of patients suffering from M2/*t* (8; 21) were high infiltration rates, severs anemia and thrombocytopenia, and a relatively low count of peripheral and bone marrow blast cells. Some authors have reported that the M2/*t* (8; 21) leukemia had a higher complete remission rate (CR) and a longer survival time (MST)[10, 11], but those findings were not verified by this research. The prognosis was poor especially for the patients with the loss of one sex chromosome.

References

1 Bennett, J.M. *et al., Annals of Inter. Med.,* **103**(1985), 620.

2 Wang, Z. C., *Chinese J. of Hematopathology,* **8**(1987), 3: 181.

3 Rowley, J.D., *Annals de Genetique* (Paris), **16**(1973), 109.

4 Fenaux, P. *et al., Bri. J. Heamatol.,* **73**(1989), 61.

5 Second MIC cooperative study group, *Cancer Genet. Cytogenet.,* **30**(1988), 1.

6 Tricot, G. *et al., Cancer,* **53**(1984), 453.

7 Berger, R. *et al., Blood,* **59**(1982), 1: 171.
8 Tosi, P. *et al., Pathol-Res-Pract.,* **182**(1987), 3: 416.
9 Koeffler, H.P., *Annals of Inter, Medicine,* **107**(1987), 748.
10 Nakamura, H. *et al., Jpn. J. Hematol.,* **30**(1989), 6: 806.
11 Bian, S. G. *et al., Chinese J. of Hematopathology,* **9**(1988), 1: 10.

Transcription and Methylation of Epidermal Growth Factor Receptor Genes and Ribosomal RNA Genes in Melanoma Cells During Differentiation Induced by Differentiating Agents

YAN Yongshan

(*Institute of Genetics, Academia Sinica, Beijing* 100101, *China*)

Abstract A human melanoma cell line has chromosome aberrations including one or two marker chromosomes with an active nucleolar organizer region (NOR). Treatment of this cell line with retinoic acid (RA) both induces the morphological differentiation and reduces the cellular saturation density together with a significant decrease in Ag-NOR activity, and eliminates its cloning capacity in soft agar. RA-treated cells grown in the absence of this differentiating agent display a return to normal Ag-NOR activity, indicating that the effect of RA on the transcription on ribosomal genes in reversible.

With the v-erb B oncogene as a probe, the slot-blot hybridization of genomic DNA from the untreated cells do not show amplification of the epidermal growth factor (EGF) receptor gene as compared with the normal diploid fibroblasts. Analyses of RNAs from the R A-treated and RA-untreated cells show essentially no difference, indicating that the RA treatment does not modulate the EGF receptor gene transcription. Our results suggest that the RA-induced changes in the transformation phenotype may be independent of the EGF receptor-mediated pathway in the cell line.

I. Introduction

Cancer cells are characterized by the loss of the normal growth mechanisms. Numerical and/or structural alterations of the cell surface receptors are probably associated with maligment transformation. Increased levels of the cell surface receptors for the epidermal growth factor (EGF) have been found in several kinds of tumors. The EGF receptor gene is the v-erb B protooncogene (Downward *et al.* 1984). Overexpression of the EGF receptor gene has been shown to result from gene amplification in a human carcinoma cell line. DNA methylation at specific sites is causally related to gene inactivation. It is unknown whether DNA methylation directly constitutes a signal modulating specific DNA-protein interaction by eliciting or stabilizing structural changes in DNA or not. Changes in the DNA methylation patterns of specific genes may be responsible for the specific gene expression. Since the actively dividing cells require the synthesis of ribosomal RNA (rRNA), the amplification or enhanced expression of rDNA might provide a selective growth advantage in tumor cells. Structural rearrangements involving nucleolar organizer regions (NORs) containing rRNA genes could result in the activation of genes placed in juxtaposition to NORs and be biologically important in determining tumorigenic properties. Gene mutation or transposition resulting from chromosoms rearrangements may serve to disrupt normal regulatory mechanisms and lead to neoplastic growth. It has been reported that c-abl oncogenes in a leukemia cell line appeared to be activated as a result of the translocation of an NOR (Takahashi *et al.* 1986). Many agents have been demonstrated to induce cellular differentiation and to modulate gene expression including rRNA synthesis in tumor cells (Marks *et al.* 1987). *In situ* DNA/RNA hybridization studies (Hsu *et al.* 1975; Call *et al.* 1969) have shown that the silverstained NORs (Ag-NORs) are believed to be the sites of genes coding for 18s and 28s rRNA on chromosomes, and the Ag-NOR number could be used to test the transcription level of the rRNA genes (Goodpasture *et al.* 1975; Jhanwar *et al.* 1981).

In the present study, we report the effect of treatment of a human melanoma cell line with differentiating agents on the following factors: morphological differentiation; gene copy number; gene methylation; the amounts of mRNA of EGF receptor gene; insertion of an active NOR to a marker chromosome and NOR activity.

II. Materials and Methods

1. *Cell Culture and NOR Analysis*

The cell line was established from a human melanoma with metastases to the leg. The cells were grown in a DMEM medium with 15% fetal calf serum. Morphological differentiation was induced in the cells by treatment with retinoic acid (RA), retinol (Rt) and dimethylsufoxide (DMSO).

To obtain growth curves, 5.8×10^6 cells were seeded into 35-mm dishes containing 1.0 ml medium with or without RA (1.0×10^{-5} mol/L). The cell number was determined by hemocytometer counts of trypsinized cells at different time intervals. In the RA-treated group, the cells were grown in an RA-containing medium for 27 days prior to seeding.

For the NOR analysis, cell cultures were treated with 0.01 μg/ml colcemid for 45 min before the cells were harvested. Slides were prepared and air-dried. The 2 — 6-day old slides were treated with 6 drops of 50% $AgNO_3$ and one drop of 3% formalin. The slides were covered and incubated in a moisture chamber at 37°C for 20 h before being washed with distilled water and with Giemsa (Yan *et al.* 1983). The number of Ag-NORs per cell and the chromosomes bearing Ag-NORs were recorded and statistically analyzed by student's *t*-test.

Cloning in soft agar was done by the Stoker method. The cells (2.0×10^2— 1×10^3) were suspended in 0.33% agar (Difco) in DMEM medium with or without 2.0×10^{-5} mol/L RA and added to 60-mm dishes containing a base layer of 0.5% agar. The culture was incubated for 26 days at 37°C.

2. *Preparation of DNA and Total RNA*

High molecular weight genomic DNA was isolated by using a modification of the procedure described by Hunts. The cells were lysed overnight at 37°C in a buffer (150 mmol/L NaCl, 20 mmol/L Tris HCl pH 8, and 10 mmol/L EDTA) containing 1% sodium dodecylsulfate (SDS) and proteinase K (200 μg/ml). The lysate was extracted once with the buffer-saturated phenol containing 0.1% 8-hydroxyquinoline and once with chloroform: isoamyl alcohol (24:1). One-tenth volume of 3 mol/L sodium acetate was added, and the DNA was precipitated with 2 V of cold ethanol. After centrifugation, the DNA pellet was dissolved in 10 mmol/L Tris-HCl at pH 7.5, retreated with the buffer-saturated phenol, phenol: chloroform, and chloroform-isoamyl alcohol, reprecipitated and redissolved.

The RNA was extracted by the guanidinium hot phenol procedure (Maniatis *et al.* 1982). Cells were lysed in 4 mol/L guanidinium isothiocyanate containing 0.3% sodium lauryl sarkosinate and 12 mmol/L EDTA at 60°C. The lysate was extracted with phenol at 60°C. To this extract was added 0.5 V of 0.1 mol/L sodium acetate, 10 mmol/L Tris-HCl of pH 7.4, and 1 mmol/L EDTA. This solution was extracted once with chloroform: isoamyl alcohol (24:1) at 60°C and then cooled in ice and reextracted once with phenol: chloroform and twice with chloroform. The RNA was precipitated with cold ethanol overnight at −20°C. The RNA pellet was dissolved and incubated with 0.1 mol/L Tris-HCl of pH 7.4, 50 mmol/L NaCl, 10 mmol/L EDTA containing 0.2% SDS and proteinase K (200 μg/ml) for 2 h at 37°C. The RNA was extracted with phenol at 60°C and then twice with chloroform: isoamyl alcohol (24:1), and precipitated with ethanol.

3. *DNA and RNA Slot Blotting*

The slot blotting was performed as described by Meinkoth and Wahl for DNA and Williams and Mason for RNA. The DNA was denatured with 3 mol/L NaOH at 56°C for 1 h and then cooled to room temperature, neutralized with 2 mol/L ammonium acete (pH 7) and diluted with 10×SSC. Dilutions of DNA were blotted onto nitrocellulose or nylon filters using a Hybrislot manifold. RNA was dissolved in denaturation solution (0.06 mol/L glyoxal, 5 mmol/L Na_2HPO_4, pH 7) and diluted with 1% SDS for blotting onto the filters. All filters were dried for 2 h at 80°C under vacuum.

4. *Digestion of DNA With Restriction Endonuclease*

The DNA preparations were cleaved with EcoRI/Mspl. The fragments were separated by electrophoresis on 1.5% agarose slab gel, transferred to nitrocellulose or nylon filtres by Southern blotting and visualized by hybridization with a ^{32}P-labeled v-erb B probe followed by autoradiography as described below.

5. *Prehybridization and Hybridization*

All filters were prehybridized by rehydration with $2\times$SSC followed by incubation with hybrisol containing 40% formamide for 1 h at 45°C. To the hybridization bag was added 1.0×10^7 com ^{32}P-labeled denatured v-erb B probe (Oncor). The filters were incubated at 45°C for 20 h and then washed three times for 15 min each in wash solution ($0.5\times$SSC; 0.1% SDS) and then for 1 h at 52°C. Dried filters were exposed to X-ray film for 9 days at -70°C in a cassette containing an intensifying screen. For RNA slot blots, the filters were treated in boiling 20.0 mmol/L Tris-HCl, pH 8, for 5 min, cooled to room temperature to remove glyoxal groups before prehybridization, and then treated as described previously.

III. Results

1. *Cell Growth Characteristics During the Differentiation*

Morphological changes were induced in the cell line following the treatment for 3—6 days with either RA, Rt or DMSO. These cells have a more flattened appearance and display extensive bipolar and branched dendritic processes characteristic of normal melanoma cells. Although the population-doubling kinetics during the log phase of the growth curve were parallel, the saturation densities during the plateau were markedly different. The cell density for untreated cells was 1.87×10^8 cells/cm^2, while the RA-treated cells had a density of 1.33×10^8 cells/cm^2, representing a 29% decrease.

When plated in the soft agar, the cells showed a high cloning efficiency of 55.6%, characteristic of tumorigenic cells, while the RA-treated cells showed a very low cloning efficiency of 0.36%.

2. *Transcription of rRNA Genes*

The untreated cells have an average of 6.22 Ag-NORs per cell, with 1.78 Ag-NORs identified on copies of the marker chromosome with an NOR insertion. Following the treatment with 1.0×10^{-6} mol/L RA for 72 h, there was a significant decrease in total Ag-NOR activity, but essentially no difference in the marker chromosome Ag-NOR activity. After 17 days treatment, the total Ag-NOR activity was decreased by 73% and that of the marker chromosome by 65%. After the treatment with 1.0×10^{-5} mol/L RA for 14 days, the total Ag-NOR activity was decreased by 86% and that of the marker chromosome by 85%. Treatment of the cells with 0.1% DMSO alone or with 1.0×1.0^{-5} mol/L Rt with DMSO significantly decreased the total Ag-NOR activity, but RA had no effect on the level. These results indicate that the decrease in transcription of the rRNA genes was dependent on the type of differentiating agents, dose, and length of the treatment. However, RA-treatment did not induce an irreversible suppression of NOR activity which remained low for a short period of time but then increased with the continued cultivation in the absence of the differentiating agent.

3. *Slot-blot Analyses of DNA and RNA*

It was found in the slot-blot hybridization of the v-erb B probe to genomic DNA extracted from the melanoma cells and normal human diploid fibroblasts that the hybridization signal from the melanoma cells was 0.63 times higher than that obtained from the normal cells, which is considered within the range of experimental error. This indicates that the EGF receptor gene is not significantly amplified in this melanoma cell line. The results from a slot blot of RNA extracted from the RA-untreated and RA-treated cells and hybridized with a v-erb B probe showed that the intensity of the hybridization signals (determined from densitometric measurements) from the RA-treated melanoma cells was 1.14 times that obtained from the untreated cells, indicating that RA does not significantly affect the amount of EGF receptor mRNA in the treated cells.

4. *Methylation of EGF Receptor Gene*

There were 5 bands with fragment sizes of 1.6 kp, 1.7, kp, 2.5 kp, 4.7 kp, and 22.4 kp, respectively, on the Southern blotting filters hybridized with a ^{32}P-labeled v-erb B probe for the EGF receptor gene of the normal fibroblasts and the untreated melanoma cells, but a band with a size of 22.4 kp was missing for the RA-treated melanoma cells with morphological differentiation. The failure of MspI to cause cleavage indicated that the methylation was induced at the 22.4 kp site by the differentiation.

IV. Discussion

The RA treatment essentially eliminates the anchorage-independent growth in soft agar, induces the distinct morphological changes and reduces the cellular saturation density, indicating RA could induce the morphological differentiation of the melanoma cells.

We did not detect gene amplification for the EGF receptor gene as compared with the normal diploid fibroblasts using the v-erb B oncogene as a probe in the slot-blot hybridization with genomic DNA. Analysis of EGF receptor specific mRNA as determined by RNA blot assays did not show a significant difference between RA-treated cells and untreated cells, indicating that the RA treatment did not alter the transcription of the EGF receptor gene. The RA-treatment could induce the methylation of the EGF receptor gene at 22.4 kp site.

Since the activation of some oncogenes following the translocation of an NOR (Takahadi *et al.* 1986) or the rearrangement and amplification of NOR (Shtromas *et al.*

1985) occurs, it is suggested that the chromosome aberrations involving NORs could be biologically important in tumor initiation and/or progression. In our case, the NOR on the marker chromosome may activate a gene(s) and thereby affect tumorigenic or metastatic properties. We first ascertained the effect of differentiating agents on these rDNA oci. RA, Rt and DMSO were all able to significantly reduce Ag-NOR activity on all chromosomes in a time- and dose-dependent manner. Our results suggest that Ag-NOR activity may provide a cytologic marker for the induced differentiation and facilitate further studies on the effect of gene modulation on the tumorigenic and/or metastatic phenotype in melanoma cells.

References

Downward, J. *et al.*, *Nature*, **307**(1984), 521.

Marks, P. A. *et al.*, *Cancer Res.*, **47**(1987), 659.

Shtromas, I. *et al.*, *Cancer Res.*, **45**(1985), 642.

Yan Yongshan *et al.*, *Theor. Appl. Genet.*, **68**(1983), 81.

Sections C and D

Reaction Metabolic Fate and Control of Chemical Carcinogens; Promoter, Inhibitor of Carcinogenesis

Structure-Carcinogenic Activity Relationship, Other Structure-Activity Relationship Related to Cancer Research

Bionic Catalysis of Polycyclic Aromatic Hydrocarbons With Metalloporphyrins

ZHAI Fudong, WANG Xiaoyi, MA Binglun, LI Tingshu and DAI Qianhuan
(Department of Chemistry and Environmental Engineering, Beijing Polytechnic University, Beijing 100022, China)

Abstract Two kinds of biomimetic oxidative catalysts, MnTPPCl and FeTPPCl, have been synthesized for use in the effective NaOCl/MnTPPCl system for the oxidation of anthracene and phenanthrene. The structures of their four oxidized products are analyzed by GC-MS and LC-MS. This work is the first success in biomimetic oxidation of PAH at room temperature.

In the recent development of the use of metalloporphyrins as biomimetic catalysts to mimic cytochrome P-450 in oxidation reactions, work has been focused on alkenes[I-II] which can easily be oxidized, while the study of the oxidation of PAH has not been reported.

The practical goal of this research is an attempt to find catalysts, which might eliminate harmful PAH at room temperature.

I. Experimental

1. *Reagents*

anthracene (c. p.); phenanthrene (c. p.);
5% aqueous sodium hypochlorite; chloroform (c. p.);
tetrabutylammonium bromide (TBAB) (A. R.);
5, 10, 15, 20-tetraphenylporphyrin (TPP);
MnTPPCl; synthesized FeTPPCl (synthesized).

2. *Instruments*

Shimadzu GC-16A (FID),
Finnigan Mat 800 GCMS,
HP5988A LCMS,
78-1 magnetic stirrer.

3. *Syntheses of* TPP, FeTPPCl *and* MnTPPCl

We used Ader's methods to synthesize TPP and the improved method of Fleischer's[12] to synthesize FeTPPCl and MnTPPCl.

According to the method of Fleischer, 0. 4 g $FeCl_2 \cdot 4H_2O$ and 1 g TPP were dissolved in 100 ml DMF. After refluxing for about 6 h with stirring and while controlling the temperature between 140 and 150°C, the reaction solution was examined on TLC until the TPP completely disappeared. Reflux was discontinued and the solution was allowed to cool. The solution was concentrated to a small volume, allowed to crystallize, then filtered. Dull purple crystals having a metallic shean were obtained. They were first washed with a small quantity of chloroform, then with 6*N* hydrochloric acid, distilled water and methanol for several times. The resulting crystal was air-dried and analysed by TLC. The *Rf* value of the crystals was exactly the same as that of the standard FeTPPCl. Further, the elemental analysis of the crystals was satisfactory.

The synthesis of MnTPPCl was similar to that of FeTPPCl except for the solvent and the temperature. Also $MnCl_2 \cdot 4H_2O$ was used instead of $FeCl_2 \cdot 4H_2O$.

The resulting dull green crystals with a metallic sheen were examined on TLC. Their *Rf* value was exactly the same as that of standard MnTPPCl and the elemental analysis of the crystals was satisfactory.

4. *Procedure for the Oxidation of PAH by the Biphasic System*

The oxidation of anthracene and phenanthrene by the metallo-porphyrin catalysts was carried out under the following conditions: to 0.044 mmol of biomimetic catalyst and 10 mg of tetrabutylammonium bromide were added 20 ml of dichloromethane and 0.280 mmol of PAH; finally 20 ml of 5% aqueous sodium hypochlorite solution was added and the mixture was stirred at room temperature. After the required time, GC was used to analyze the solution.

II. Results

1. *Oxidation of* PAH *by the* NaOCl/MnTPPCl *or* NaOCl/FeTPPCl *Systems*

Anthracene and phenanthrene are aromatic compounds, and therefore they are not so easily oxidized as alkenes. Although the 9, 10 positions are active, they are oxidized to quinones only with concentrated sulphuric acid and potassium dichromate. In this research, we have used a biphasic system, with sodium hypochlorite as a "single-oxygen-donor", in the presence of a phase transfer reagent, and with FeTPPCl or MnTPPCl as bionic catalysts. With these systems anthracene and phenanthrene can be oxidized under mild conditions. The conversion rates are satisfactory (see Table 1).

From Table 1, it can be seen that both substrate peaks have disappeared after 150 min. Thus, there was complete conversion after this time with MnPPCl. For phenanthrene, 64.46% was oxidized after 150 min with MnPPCl.

To follow the reaction more closely, the reaction solution was analyzed every 30 min or 60 min. The results are listed in Table 2.

Table 1 PAH Conversion Rate in NaOCl/Porphyrins System

No.	Catalyst (mmol)	Substrate (mmol)	Reaction time (min)	t_r (min)	Substrate area	Conversion rate	Product area
950	MnTPPCL 0.043	anthracene	0	7.803	1365,112		
951	TBAB (10 mg)	0.280	150	10.675 16.322	0	100%	6,104 22,978
952	MnTPPCL 0.044	phenanthrene	0	7.430	1537,767		
953	TBAB (10 mg)	0.280	150	5.191 9.288	0	100%	30681 128,773
960	FeTPPCL 0.044	anthracene	0	8.136	962,676		
961	TBAB (10 mg)	0.280	150	10.318 15.988	0	100%	44,550 72,725
962	FeTPPCL 0.044	phenanthrene	0	7.790	1169,517		
963	TBAB (10 mg)	0.280	15	7.711	753,904	64.46%	

GC condition: OV101, 25 m capillary coln.; t_r, retention time of substrate or oxidation products; Inj. temp. 270°C, Det, temp. 270°C; Coln. temp. $180°C \xrightarrow{5°C/min} 250°C$.

Table 2 PAH Conversion Rate at Different Times

No.	Catalyst (mmax)	Substrate (mmol)	Reaction time (min)	t_r (min)	Substrate area	Conversion rate	Note
406			0	22.460	224,433		GC
407	MnTPPCL		60	22.667	161,153	28.2%	Coln. temp.
408	0.019	anthracene	90	22.928	53,621	76.1%	$120°C \xrightarrow{5°/min} 200°C$
409	TBAB	0.057	120	23.006	46,354	79.3%	
410	(5 mg)		150	– –	32	100%	$200°C \xrightarrow{3°C/min} 250°C$
411			180	– –	49	100%	
924	MnTPPCL		0	5.562	157,351		GC
925			60	5.356	147,364		Coln. temp.
926	0.023	phenanthrene	120	5.403	14,645	90%	
927	TBAB (6 mg)	0.056	180	6.067	16,375 52,413		$200°C \xrightarrow{3°C/min} 250°C$
512	FeTPPCL	anthracene	0	5.300	84,672		GC
513	0.019	0.057	60	5.513	63,191		Coln. temp.
514	TBAB		90	5.466	53,980	54.1%	$200°C \xrightarrow{3°C/min} 250°C$
515	(5 mg)		120	5.570	38,891	65.9%	
808			0	5.668	180,078		GC
809	FeTPPCL		60	5.605	169,705	5.8%	Coln. temp.
813	0.019	phenanthrene	90	5.668	145,618	19.1%	
812	TBAB	0.056	120	6.008	77,502	57.0%	$200°C \xrightarrow{3°C/min} 250°C$
811	(5 mg)		150	5.93	53,382	70.3%	

From Table 2, it can be seen that after 3 h, the anthracene was completely oxidized and the phenanthrene was oxidized too by using MnTPPCl. However, the results with FeTPPCl were not satisfactory.

From these experiments we found that MnTPPCl is a better catalyst for PAH oxidation than FeTPPCl, and anthracene phenanthrene is more readily converted at room temperature than phenanthrene.

2. *Identification of the Oxidized Products of Anthracene and Phenanthrene*

With the superior NaOCl/MnTPPCl system, some of the oxidized products of anthracene and phenanthrene were separated by GC as peaks A1, A2 and P1, P2. The structures of these products were analyzed by GC-MS (A1, A2) and LC-MS (P1, P2).

Spectrum I (Fig. 1) is the MS of A1. In the spectrum, in addition to $M^{\rceil +}$ m/e 208, we can see m/e $180^{\rceil +}$, m/e $152^{\rceil +}$ and m/e $76^{\rceil +}$ fragments. They are possibly due to the following ions:

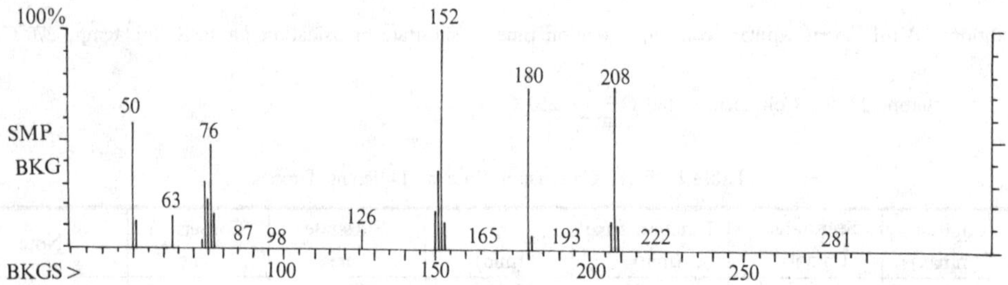

Fig. 1 Spectrum I.

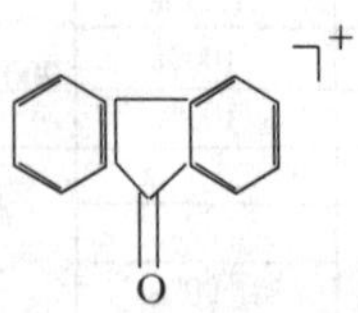

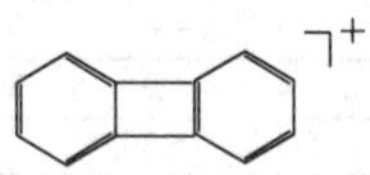

and

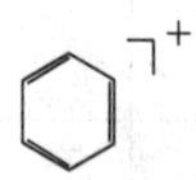

From these results and the behavior on TLC, we were able to identify A1 as anthraquinone. The computer showed 95% similarity to the storage spectrum in data system, which implies 100% identity by considering the condition difference.

Spectrum II (Fig. 2) is the MS from A2. The $M^{\rceil +}$ is 254 and we can see m/e 225^{+}, m/e 197^{+}, m/e 181^{+}, m/e $152^{\rceil +}$ fragments. With the substrate anthracene we believe that the original structure may be that shown in Fig. 3. This compound reacted with CHO (in solution) and produced the observed structure.

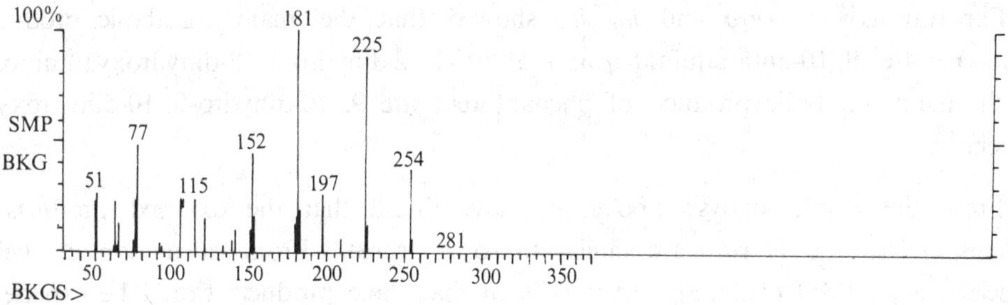

Fig. 2 Spectrum II.

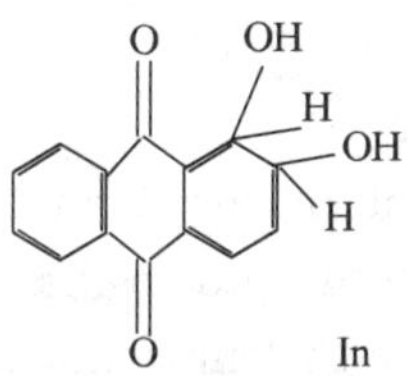

Fig. 3

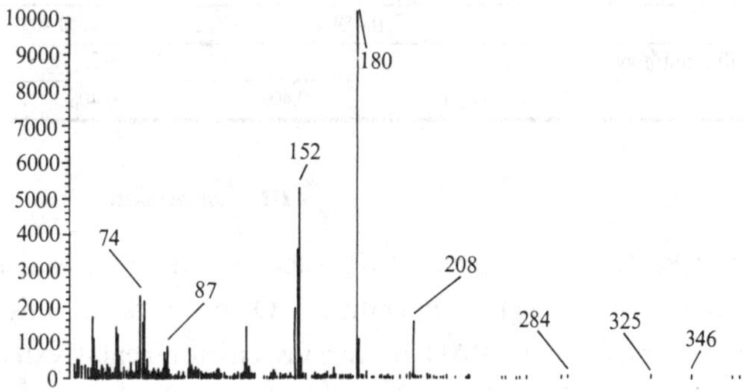

Fig. 4 Spectrum III.

Spectrum III (Fig. 4) is the MS from P1. In addition to $M^{>+}$ 208, we can see m/e $180^{>+}$, m/e $152^{>+}$ and m/e $74^{>+}$ fragments. From these results combined with the behavior on TLC, we could identify P1 as 9, 10-phenanthrenedione. The computer showed a similarity of 93% to the storage spectrum in data system, the anthentic sample got the same spectrum and the same similarity.

Spectrum IV (Fig. 5) is the MS from P2. The structure assigned is shown in Fig. 6. which gives a similarity of 81% to the spectrum stored in the data system.

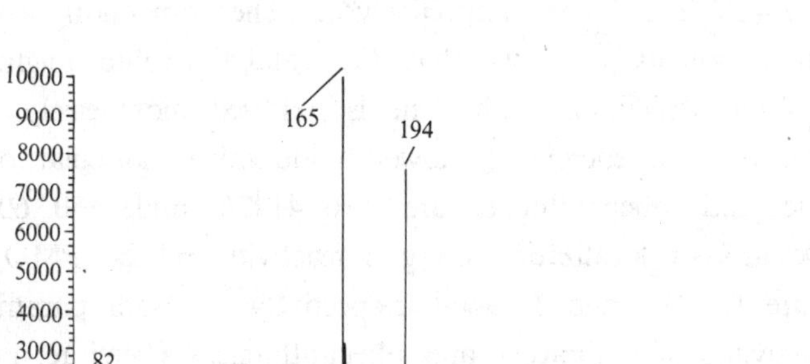

Fig. 5 Spectrum IV

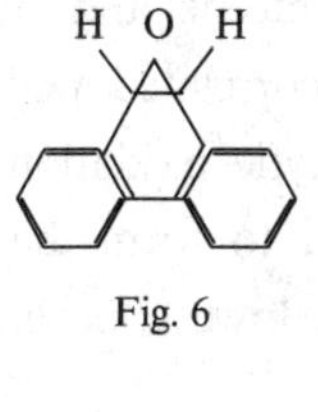

Fig. 6

Experiments[13] *in vitro* and *in vivo* showed that the main metabolic products of anthracene are 9, 10-anthraquinone and *trans* -1, 2-dihydro-1, 2-dihydroxyanthracene[14-18], and the main metabolic products of phenanthrene are 9, 10-dihydro-9, 10-dihydroxyphenanthrene[19].

From the simple analysis above, we have found that the oxidized products from reactions *in vivo* and *in vitro* are similar to some degree. From calculation of their free valencies using HMO (Table 3), it can be seen that these products would be expected.

Table 3 Free Valence

Anthracene	1	2	9
	0.459	0.409	0.520

Phenanthrene	1	2	3	4	9
	0.450	0.402	0.408	0.441	0.451

III. Discussion

1. Clearly, carcinogenic PAH such as those in water, food oil or air cannot be destroyed even at high temperature. Other work in this laboratory helped realize the catalytic elimination of PAH in various environmental exhausts[21] at high temperature. It is very interesting to find catalysts which are effective in eliminating harmful PAH at room temperature. Previous work related to biomimetic catalytic oxidation achieved only the oxidation on olefins of relative lower activation energies, while this paper attains for the first time, the biomimetic catalytic oxidation of PAH with high activation energies at room temperature. Therefore, this work not only would be a theoretical advance in biomimetic catalytic oxidation, but also would have obviously practical significance. NaOCl, the weak oxidation agent, has analogous oxidation potential with oxygen itself, and now, the biomimetic catalytic oxidation of PAH with oxygen or air, is undertaken in this laboratory.

2. MnTPPCl is a better biomimetic catalyst than FeTPPCl, and the first ionization potentials of Mn and Fe are 7.4 eV and 7.9 eV, respectively[22]. The correlation between catalytic activities and ionization potentials, shows that the catalytic route might be through free radical species. With MnTPPCl, anthracene is oxidized more easily than phenanthrene. It may be noted that the energies on lowest unoccupied molecular orbits (LUMO, HMO) of anthracene and phenanthrene, are -0.4142β and -0.6052β, respectively, and the lowest Dewar's or localization energies reactivity indices (PMO) on anthracene and phenanthrene are 1.2649β and 1.7960β, respectively[23]. Both parameters are correlated well with the reactivities of anthracene and phenanthrene. Therefore, in the catalytic oxidation process, the electron of free radical species at first enters the LUMO of PAH to form the activation complex; then the PAH free radical is formed at the position with lowest localization energy; thus the further oxidation would take place.

3. The active species in oxidation/MnTPPCl has been proposed to be Mn(v)=O[20]. From our results and the above discussion, it might be proposed that Mn (v) =Ȯ free radical combines reversibly with PAH to form a [O=Mn(v)PAH]˙ activation complex, which then reacts to produce the oxide of PAH according to the above-mentioned mechanism. The molecular mechanism summarized in discussion 2 and this paragraph, explains reasonably why the conversion of anthracene is quicker than that of phenanthrene. Energy of LUMO and lowest localization energy of PAH might be useful in prediction of the oxidation trend of PAH.

4. The localization energies in the positions of the projected angular ring in PAH are not the relatively low ones, while in general, the positions on L-region, L′-region as well as on K-region have relatively low localization energies. In chemical oxidation, the oxidation occurs superiorly in these positions with lowest localization energies, but not in the positions on the angular ring. However, in biological oxidation, an outstanding trend of oxidation occurs in the positions on the angular ring because the projected angular ring more easily enters the slit of the active center of the monooxygenase enzyme molecule[24]. The main metabolites of anthracene *in vivo* are *trans*-1, 2-dihydro-1,2-dihydroxyanthracene, 1, 2-dihydroxyanthracene and their conjugated products, which reflect the preferential trend of oxidation on the angular ring through the "lock-key" mechanism around the active center of enzyme. However, the products if this biomimetic catalytic process are brought from the positions with lowest energies on PAH. Obviously, the product A2, is just the further oxidation product of 9, 10-anthraquinone. The further experiments would prove that the difference between biomimetic catalysis with metalloporphyrins and enzymatic catalysis with cytochrome p-450, is that the former obeys the energy dependence and the latter depends on stereo requirement of "lock key" mechanism to some extent regardless of the analogues between the two.

5. Di-region theory, the new understanding of carcinogenesis, discovered that the carcinogenic PAH will produce two reactive centers during the metabolism[25]. In general, one center will be formed on the angular ring in bay-region through the intermediate of dihydrodiol-epoxide; the other will through the carbonium ion formed by epoxide on active K-region. The active K-region always has a position of lower localization energy, so the active K-region should be oxidized easily to form the detoxication products. Therefore, the chemical oxidation including the biomimetic oxidation with metalloporphyrin would destroy one of the reactive centers in the carcinogenic di-region and eliminate the carcinogenicity of the carcinogenic PAH. In practice, all the oxidation products of benz[a]pyrene, the 6, 12-, 1, 6-, and 3, 6-quinone of BaP, are non-carcinogens. The energies of LUMO of the common PAH in air, benz[a]pyrene (++++), pyrene (−), benz[a]anthracene (+/−), benz[e]pyrene (−), chrysene (+) and triphenylene (−), are −0.3711, −0.445, −0.452, −0.497, −0.520 and -0.684β,

respectively. It may be expected that the oxidation trend will be decreased approximatly along the above sequence, and the potent carcinoge, benz[a]pyrene, would be destroyed very easily by biomimetic oxidation with metalloporphyrins. The test and verification of the above prediction, now, are undertaken in this laboratory.

6. Whether the cheaper metalloporphyrin analogs, such as phthalocyanine pigment or other congeners, can be used as analogous catalysis, is very interesting from the practical consideration. Whether the metalloporphyrin catalysts can be used in the future time in the detoxication purification for cigarette smoking or in air conditioners, we will wait and see.

Acknowledgment: Prof. Zha Shen-ji, Department of Chemistry, Nankai University, who supplied standard samples of tetraphenylporphyrins.

References

1 Iwao Tabushi and Noboru Koga, *J. Am. Chem. Soc.*, **101**(1979), 2.
2 Iwao Tabushi and Akira Yazaki, *J. Am. Chem. Soc.*, **103**(1981), 7371.
3 Bernard Meunier *et al.*, *J. Mol. Catal.*, **41**(1987), 154.
4 Groves, J. T. *et al.*, *J. Am. Chem. Soc.*, **103**(1981), 2884.
5 Collman, J. P., *et al.*, *J. Am. Chem. Soc.*, **107**(1985), 2000.
6 Groves, J. T. *et al.*, *J. Am. Chem. Soc.*, **108**(1986), 507.
7 Tabushi, I. *et al.*, *Tetrahedron Letters*, **38**(1979). 3681.
8 Guilmet, E. and Meunier B., *Nouveau J. de Chimie*, **6**(1982), 11: 511.
9 Guimat, E. and Meunier, B., *Tetrahedron Letter*, **23**(1982), **24**, 2449.
10 Guilmat E. and Meunier, B. *J. Mol. Catal.*, **23**(1984), 115.
11 Groves, T. *et al.*, *J. Am. Chem, Soc.*, **101**(1979), 1032.
12 Fleischer, E. B., *J. Am. Chem. Soc.*, **93**(1871), 3162.
13 Jeffrey, A. M., Yeh, J. J. C., Jerina, D. M. *et al.*, *J. Am. Chem. Soc.*, **96**(1974), 6929.
14 Jeffery, A. M. and Jerina, D. M., *J. Am. Chem. Soc.*, **97**(1975), 4427.
15 Lavoie, E. J. *et al.*, *Carcinogenesis*, **6**(1986), 1483.
16 Boyland, E., *Biochem. J.*, **29**(1935), 2679.
17 Boyland, E., *Biochem. J.*, **30**(1936), 728.
18 Sims, P., *Biochem, J.*, **92**(1964), 621.
19 Boyland, E. and Eims, P., *Biochem. J.*, **84**(1962), 571.
20 Fontecave, M. and Dan Mansuy, *Tetrahedron*, **40**(1984), 21: 4279.
21 Zheng Qingying, Dai Qianhuan *et al.*, in this proceedings.
22 cf. Purcell, K. F. and Kotz, , J. C., *Inorganic Chemistry*, Saunders Company, 1977, Philadelphia, p. 62.
23 cf. Dai Qianhuan, *Theoretical Organic Chemistry*, BPU Press, 1989, Beijing.
24 Dai Qianhuan, *Scientia Sinica*, 1979, 10: 964; in *Polynuclear Aromatic Hydrocarbons, Mechanisms, Methods and Metabolism* (Eds. Cooke, M. and Dennis, A.) Battelle Press, Columbus, 1984, pp. 1045–1073.

Molecular Surface Areas of Polycylic Aromatic Hydrocarbons and Di-Region Theory

WANG Liansheng and WANG Xiaojiang

(*Department of Environmental Science, Nanjing University, Nanjing* 210008, *PRC*)

Abstract By using the approximate group contributions method, we have estimated the molecular surface areas of polycyclic aromatic hydrocarbons (PAHs). Based on the di-region theory, we have studied the relationship between the molecular surface areas (MSAs) and the carcinogenicity of PAHs and introduced MSA parameters into the di-region theory equation. The calculated carcinogencities of PAHs from the obtained equation show little difference from experimental results.

I. Introduction

It has been found by many researchers that the molecular surface areas (MSAs) of organic pollutants correlate with their physico-chemical properties such as octanol/water partition coefficients (K_{OW}), water solubilities (S_W) and boiling points[1]. Generally speaking, K_{OW} values increase with the increasing MSA, while S_W values decrease. MSAs have been used to predict physico-chemical properties because they can be obtained easily by calculation.

Although some workers believe that the MSAs of organic pollutants can exert an important effect on their toxicity[2], very little work has been done to study quantitatively the correlation between toxicity and MSA. This paper reports an investigation of the effect of MSAs on the carcinogenicity of PAHs based on the di-region theory.

II. Calculation of MSA

Hermann *et al.* have proposed an accurate method for calculating the MSAs of various kinds of organic compounds (cf. Ref. [1]). Their method can be used to calculate the MSAs of PAHs[3]. Since some of the relevant data needed for their method were not available, we used an approximate group contribution method based on the work of Yalkowsky[3]. It assumes that molecular surface areas are the sum of individual atomic or group surface area contributions. Relevant atomic and group surface areas for PAHs are listed in Table 1.

The values of MSAs calculated by Hermann's method, by Yalkowsky's method and by us are listed in Table 2. It can be seen from Table 2 that the MSAs calculated by us are more accurate than those by Yalkowsky's method if those calculated by Hermann's method are taken as standards. Since the improved group contribution method used by us is sufficiently accurate for most situations, it is suggested that it is useful for quick calculations of the MSAs of PAHs.

Table 1 Atomic and Group Surface Areas for PAHs

Group	Surface Area (Å^2)	
	Yalkowsky[a)]	This paper
$-CH_3$	33.2	31.2
$-CH_2$	18.1	23.1
$\langle$CH (aromatic)	18.2	18.2
$\langle$C− (aromatic)	4.1	4.5
$\langle$C=̈ (aromatic)	5.65	5.0

a) quoted from [3].

Table 2 MSA of PAHs

No.	Compound	MSA (Å^2)		
		Hermann	Yalkowsky	This paper
1	indan	151.5	135.3	151.1
2	naphthalene	155.8	156.9	155.6
3	1-methylnaphthalene	172.5	176.0	173.1
4	2-methylnaphthalene	176.3	176.0	173.1
5	1,3-dimethylnaphthalene	192.9	195.1	190.6
6	1,4-dimethylnaphthalene	189.2	195.1	190.6
7	2,6-dimethylnaphthalene	196.7	195.1	190.6
8	1,4.5-trimethylnaphthalene	200.9	214.2	208.1
9	biphenyl	182.0	190.2	191.0
10	acenaphthene	175.0	164.9	174.4
11	fluorene	193.6	183.2	187.7
12	phenanthrene	198.0	204.6	202.0
13	anthracene	202.2	204.6	202.0
14	2-methylanthracene	222.6	223.7	219.5
15	9-methylanthracene	215.1	223.7	219.5
16	pyrene	213.0	215.9	212.0
17	fluoranthene	218.0	215.9	212.0
18	1,2-benzofluorene	237.4	230.9	234.1
19	Chrysene	241.0	252.3	248.4
20	naphthacene	248.0	252.3	248.4
21	perylene	251.5	263.6	258.4
22	3,4-benzopyrene	256.0	263.6	258.4
23	3-methylcholanthrene	282.7	276.7	280.2
24	benzo [ghi] perylene	266.9	274.9	268.4

III. Relationship Between the Molecular Surface Areas and Carcinogenicity for PAHs

Although Dai and other researchers have agreed that the MSAs of PAHs exert an important effect on their carcinogenicity[2], no quantitative relationship between MSA and carcinogenicity has been presented so far. Prior to producing cancer, PAHs must be concentrated in the organism and pass through the cell membrane to react with its DNA. The ability of PAHs to bioaccumulate increases with increasing MSA, while its ability to enter the cell decreases due to steric hindrance. In addition, it is difficult for PAHs with large MSAs to have access to the microsome oxidases and DNA. Therefore, it is believed that there is an optimum value of the MSA for the greatest carcinogenic effect. According to theoretical estimates, this optimum MSA was considered to be 260. Based on the di-region theory, we have introduced a quantitative equation which links MSA with carcinogenicity.

$$\log K = 5.41 \Delta E_1 \cdot \Delta E_2^3 - 0.13\left(1.5n + \left|\frac{\mathrm{MSA}-260}{50}\right|\right), \tag{1}$$

where K is the carcinogenicity index of PAHs, ΔE_1 and ΔE_2 are the delocalization energies of the two electrophilic active centers, respectively, and n is the number of detoxification regions. The values of ΔE and n which we used are those adopted in Dai's paper[4—6]. The MSAs of the PAHs were calculated by the group contribution method described in this paper. According to Eq (1), there are five possible cases: (i) the PAHs with K values less than 6 were not carcinogenic; (ii) the PAHs with K values of 6— 15 were weakly carcinogenic; (iii) the PAHs with K values of 15— 45 were carcinogenic; (iv) the PAHs with K values of 45— 75 were markedly carcinogenic; (v) the PAHs with k values greater than 75 were strongly carcinogenic. The carcinogenicity of 77 PAHs was calculated. The results are listed in Table 3. The experimental carcinogenicities of the PAHs in Table 3 are quoted from Dai's paper.

Table 3 Experimental Values and Calculated Values of Carcinogenicity for PAHs

No.	Compound	MSA ($Å^2$)	ΔE_1 (β unit)	ΔE_2 (β unit)	n	Calculated Value		Experimental Carcinogenicity
						This paper	Dai's paper	
1	Dibenzo [a,l] pentacene	387.6	0.885	0.400	3	0.25 (−)	0.01 (−)	(−)
2	Benzo [rst] pentaphene	304.8	0.866	0.866	2	344 (++++)	327 (++++)	(++++/+++)
3	Dibenzo [h,rst] pentaphene	351.2	0.785	0.785	2	26.7 (++)	39.2 (++)	(++)
4	Dibenzo [b,def] chrysene	304.8	0.845	0.871	1	512 (++++)	376 (++++)	(++++/+++)
5	Dibenzo [a,j] naphthacene	341.2	0.818	0.400	3	0.31 (−)	0.01 (−)	(−)
6	Dibenzo [def,P] chrysene	304.8	0.800	0.713	1	18.1 (++)	17.20 (++)	(++/+++)
7	Dibenzo [a,c] naphthacene	341.2	0.787	0.787	3	19.0 (++)	32.17 (++)	(++)
8	Benzo [a] pyrene	258.4	0.794	0.833	1	192 (++++)	123.55 (++++)	(++++)
9	Benzo [a] anthracene	248.4	0.766	0.571	2	2.24 (−)	1.34 (−)	(−)
10	Dibenzo [a,h] anthracene	294.8	0.738	0.738	1	20.9 (++)	19.14 (++)	(++)

(to be continued on the next page)

(*continued*)

No.	Compound	MSA ($Å^2$)	ΔE_1 (β unit)	ΔE_2 (β unit)	n	Calculated Value This paper	Calculated Value Dai's paper	Experimental Carcinogenicily
11	Benzo [a] penthaphene	341.2	0.733	0.621	2	2.23 (−)	2.25 (−)	(−)
12	Dibenzo [a,j] anthracene	294.8	0.722	0.722	1	15.3 (++)	14.29 (≈++)	(++)
13	Benzo [b] triphenylene	294.8	0.722	0.545	2	1.42 (−)	0.837 (−)	(−/+)
14	Benzo [g] chrysene	294.8	0.719	0.667	1	7.39 (+)	6.94 (+)	(+)
15	Benzo [e] pyrene	258.4	0.714	0.400	0	1.75 (−)	1.65 (−)	(−)
16	Pentacene	294.8	0.709	0.400	0	1.43 (−)	0.007 (−)	(−)
17	Ditbenzo [fg, op] naphthacene	304.8	0.692	0.692	0	13.3 (−)	12.28 (+)	(+/−)
18	naphtho [8, 1, 2-Cde] naphthacene	304.8	0.971	0.691	1	26.4 (++)	23.28 (++)	(++)
19	triphenylene	248.4	0.664	0.664	1	6.71 (+)	5.61 (−)	(−)
20	Picene	294.8	0.662	0.662	1	5.67 (−)	5.45 (−)	(−)
21	Phenanthrene	202.0	0.658	0.658	1	4.66 (−)	5.14 (−)	(−)
22	Benzo [c] chrysene	294.8	0.648	0.623	0	5.72 (≈+)	5.55 (≈+)	(++)
23	Benzo [b] chrysene	294.8	0.647	0.581	1	2.50 (−)	2.11 (−)	(−)
24	Chrysene	248.4	0.639	0.639	0	7.44 (+)	6.20 (+)	(+)
25	Dibenzo [c, g] phenanthrene	294.8	0.638	0.638	1	4.08 (−)	3.89 (−)	(−)
26	Naphthacene	248.4	0.628	0.628	2	2.64 (−)	2.12 (−)	(−)
27	Hexaphene	341.2	0.600	0.600	3	0.80 (−)	0.80 (−)	(−)
28	Benzo [c] phenanthrene	248.4	0.600	0.600	0	4.69 (−)	6.20 (+)	(+)
29	Dibenzo [de, qr] naphthracene	304.8	0.559	0.400	1	0.76 (−)	0.23 (−)	(−)
30	anthracene	202.0	0.545	0.545	1	1.26 (−)	1.27 (−)	(−)
31	naphthalene	155.6	0.488	0.488	0	1.09 (−)	1.86 (−)	(−)
32	Dibenzo [Cd, lm] perylene	314.8	0.928	0.600	0	8.74 (+)	8.96 (+)	(+)
33	Benzo [ghi] perylene	268.4	0.826	0.713	0	39.6 (++)	26.45 (++)	(++)
34	1-Methylphenanthrene	219.5	0.682	0.639	0	7.21 (+)	7.01 (+)	(+/−)
35	2-Methylphenanthrene	219.5	0.658	0.526	0	2.59 (−)	2.85 (−)	(−)
36	3-Methylphenanthrene	219.5	0.685	0.572	0	3.88 (−)	4.04 (−)	(−)
37	2-Methylanthracene	219.5	0.628	0.577	1	2.25 (−)	2.03 (−)	(−)
38	9-Methylanthracene	219.5	0.978	0.503	0	3.70 (−)	3.90 (−)	(−)
39	1-Methylchrysene	265.9	0.648	0.662	0	10.0 (+)	7.82 (+)	(−)
40	2-Methylchrysene	265.9	0.762	0.639	2	4.68 (−)	3.57 (−)	(−)
41	4-Methylchrysene	265.9	0.786	0.639	0	12.4 (+)	9.43 (+)	(+)
42	5-Methylchrysene	265.9	0.839	0.724	0	51.0 (+++)	32.56 (++)	(++/+++)
43	6-Methylchrysene	265.9	0.672	0.719	0	21.7 (++)	15.37 (++)	(+)
44	5, 6-Dimethylchrysene	283.4	0.879	0.604	0	9.71 (+)	8.32 (+)	(+)
45	2, 3-Dimethylchrysene	283.4	0.898	0.649	4	3.07 (−)	2.61 (−)	(−)
46	2-Methylbenzo[c]phenanthrene	265.9	0.750	0.755	2	22.5 (++)	20.22 (++)	(+)
47	4-Methylbenzo[c]phenanthrene	265.9	0.825	0.648	0	15.8 (≈+)	11.65 (+)	(−/+)
48	5-Methylbenzo[c]phenanthrene	265.9	0.788	0.667	0	17.8 (++)	12.88 (+)	(++)
49	6-Methylbenzo[c]phenanthrene	265.9	0.788	0.625	1	6.77 (+)	5.05 (−)	(+)
50	1-Methylbenzo[a]anthracene	265.9	0.593	0.572	1	2.45 (−)	1.79 (−)	(−)
51	4-Methylbenzo[a]anthracene	265.9	0.647	0.583	0	4.77 (−)	4.06 (−)	(−)
52	6-Methylbenzo[a]anthracene	265.9	0.881	0.722	2	24.5 (++)	20.11 (++)	(++/+++)
53	7-Methylbenzo[a]anthracene	265.9	0.806	0.879	1	563 (++++)	335.32 (++++)	(+++/++++)

(*to be continued on the next page*)

(continued)

No.	Compound	MSA (Å^2)	ΔE_1 (β unit)	ΔE_2 (β unit)	n	Calculated Value: This paper	Calculated Value: Dai's paper	Experimental Carcinogenicily
54	10-Methylbenzo[a]anthracene	265.9	0.781	0.614	0	9.22 (+)	7.23 (+)	(+)
55	11-Methylbenzo[a]anthracene	265.9	0.766	0.602	0	7.74 (+)	6.44 (+)	(−/+)
56	12-Methylbenzo[a]anthracene	265.9	0.958	0.713	0	73.1 (+++)	44.64 (≈+++)	(+++)
57	4, 5-Dimethylbenzo[a]anthracene	283.6	1.006	0.722	1	61.9 (+++)	46.01 (+++)	(+++)
58	5, 12-Dimethylbenzo[a]anthracene	283.6	0.875	0.524	1	2.66 (−)	1.75 (−)	(−)
59	6, 7-Dimethylbenzo[a]anthracene	283.6	0.927	0.759	1	86.4 (++++)	64.37 (+++)	(+++)
60	6, 8-Dimethylbenzo[a]anthracene	283.6	0.926	0.738	1	57.2 (+++)	43.80 (≈+++)	(+++)
61	7, 8-Dimethylbenzo[a]anthracene	283.6	0.847	0.759	0	87.6 (++++)	57.48 (++)	(+++/++++)
62	7, 11-Dimethylbenzo[a]anthracene	283.6	0.806	0.759	0	97.9 (++++)	47.24 (+++)	(+++)
63	7, 12-Dimethylbenzo[a]anthracene	283.6	0.958	0.879	0	2875 (++++)	1233 (++++)	(+++/++++)
64	2-Methylbenzo[a]pyrene	275.9	0.794	0.833	2	113 (++++)	100.97 (++++)	(+++/++++)
65	3-Methylbenzo[a]pyrene	275.9	0.896	0.845	0	765 (++++)	370.17 (++++)	(+++/++++)
66	4-Methylbenzo[a]pyrene	275.9	0.875	0.775	0	99.0 (++++)	85.88 (++++)	(+++)
67	6-Methylbenzo[a]pyrene	275.9	0.794	0.880	0	769 (++++)	372.15 (++++)	(+++/++++)
68	8-Methylbenzo[a]pyrene	275.9	0.844	0.545	0	4.96 (−)	4.46 (−)	(−)
69	9-Methylbenzo[a]pyrene	275.9	0.833	0.691	0	27.9 (++)	20.22 (++)	(+)
70	11-Methylbenzo[a]pyrene	275.9	1.042	0.630	0	23.4 (++)	17.29 (++)	(+++/++++)
71	12-Methylbenzo[a]pyrene	275.9	0.858	0.800	0	217 (++++)	122.21 (++++)	high
72	fluoranthene	213.0	0.726	0.400	0	1.34 (−)	1.66 (−)	(−)
73	Benzo[ghi]fluoranthene	222.0	0.608	0.608	0	4.37 (−)	4.46 (−)	(−)
74	Benzo [j] fluoranthene	258.4	0.608	0.835	0	81.4 (++++)	48.1 (+++)	(+++)
75	Indeno [1,2,3-Cd] pyrene	268.4	0.770	0.617	0	9.04 (+)	7.0 (+)	(+)
76	Benzo [b] fluoranthene	258.4	0.569	0.400	1	1.00 (−)	0.24 (−)	(−/+)
77	cyclopento [c, d] pyrene	222.0	0.794	0.623	0	8.71 (+)	8.17 (+)	(+)

It can be seen from Table 3 that the calculated carcinogenicities of most PAHs are identical with the experimental values and approach the carcinogenicities calculated from Dai's equation. By means of a quantitative calculation, these results prove the correlation between the MSAs and the carcinogenicity of PAHs and provide useful information for further study of the structure-activity relationship of PAHs.

References

1 Wang Liansheng and Wang Xiajiang, *Environmental Chemistry* (in Chinese), **7**(1988), 13.

2 Chen Hong and Dai Qianhuan, *Environmental Chemistry* (in Chinese), **1**(1982), 253.

3 Yalkowsky, S. H. *et al., J. Chem. Eng. Data,* **24**(1979), 127.

4 Dai Qianhuan, *Scientia Sinica,* 1980, 4: 465.

5 Dai Qianhuan and Zhang Changyin, *Kexue Tongbao* (in Chinese), 1982, 11: 697.

6 Dai Qianhuan and Zhang Dunxin, *Scientia Sinica* (in Chinese), Series B, 1983, 8: 716.

Superoxide Radical in Human Esophageal, Gastric Cancer And Chronic Gastritis

WENG Qiliang, ZHANG Yulin, LIU Zhen, WANG Yinong, WANG Tianlang, NING Qilan, YANG Jianye, QIANG Yunyan and FENG Xinzheng

(*Analysis Center, Xi'an Medical University, Xi'an, Shaanxi 710061, China*)

Abstract In this paper, it is shown with a modified spectrophotometric method that superoxide radical $O_2^{\bar{\cdot}}$ levels (SOD) in the blood specimens of the patients with esophageal or gastric cancer, are significantly higher than that of normal people but the significant difference in SOD has not been found between the patients with chronic gastritis and normal people. So, the SOD level might be a reliable mark for the diagnosis of cancer.

It has been shown that free radicals are increased in animals implanted with cancer or treated with cancer-inducing chemicals[1, 2]. In this paper we report the use of a modified spectrophotometric method[3] with λ at 420 nm to assay the superoxide dismutase (SOD) levels in patients with gastric cancer (G.C.), esophageal cancer (E.C.) and chronic gastritis (C.G.) in order to study the relationship between $O_2^{\bar{\cdot}}$, SOD and those diseases.

I. Principle of the Method

The reaction scheme in Fig. 1 illustrates the principle of the SOD assay.

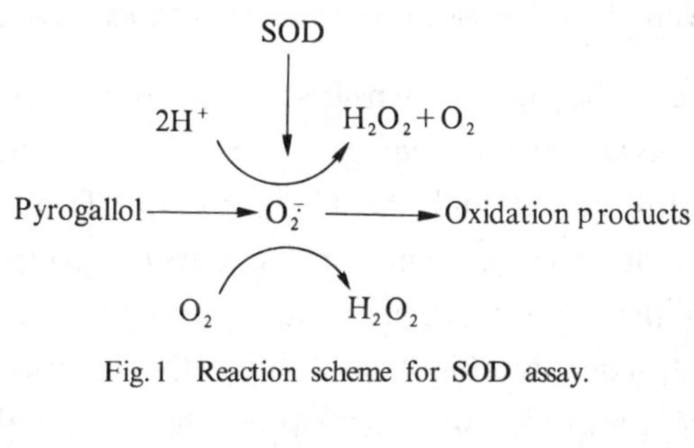

Fig. 1 Reaction scheme for SOD assay.

In this method pyrogallol was used as an agent to produce superoxide radicals $O_2^{\bar{\cdot}}$ and an SOD solution with known activity unit was used as a standard. The pH of the solution was adjusted to 8.25; the temperature was maintained at 25°C; then the change in optical density with time was measured at a wavelength of 420 nm.

II. Materials

(1) *Reagents* The superoxide dismutase was obtained from Sigma Chemical Co., the Triton X-100 from Karl Roth KG Chemische Farbrik Karlsruhe, the sodium cacodylik from Merck, the pyrogallol was A.R. and the diethylenetriaminepentaacetic acid and the tris were C.P.

(2) *Instruments* A Shimadzu UV-visible recording spectrophotometer was used together with an Rc5c Dupont centrifuge.

(3) *Blood specimens* The ages of the three groups of patients were similar to those of the reference group, all being between 45 and 55. Half of each group was male and half female. Venous blood samples were taken. Each sample was treated by separating and hemolyzing the red blood cells and adjusting the Hb concentration of 10%. To 0.5 ml of sample was added water (2 ml), alcohol (2 ml) and chloroform (0.6 ml). The mixture was centrifuged at 4°C and 15,000 g and the supernatant containing the extracted SOD was used for the assay.

(4) *Standard SOD solution* The SOD was dissolved in a water: alcohol: chloroform (2.5: 20: 0.6) solvent to give a concentration of 5 mg/100 ml.

III. Method[3]

The specimen extract (0.30 ml) was placed in a cell and solvent (0.70 ml) and triton X-100 (16% v/v, 0.20 ml) added. The pH of the solution was adjusted to 8.25 by the addtition of 1.0 ml of a solution containing tris-cacodylic acid (50 mmol/L) and diethylenetriaminepentaacetic acid (1 mmol/L), and the temperature maintained at 25°C. Finally, a pyrogallol solution (0.1 mmol/L, 0.20 ml) was added and immediately, the optical density was measured. Further measurements were made at appropriate time intervals. The optical densities of a blank solution without SOD, and of a standard SOD solution were measured at the same time as each specimen assay.

The difference between the optical densities of the SOD standard and the blank is represented by α, that between the patient group extract and the blank by β, and that between the normal group extract and the blank by ν. Then the ratios β/α and ν/α represent the relative activity measurement for the patient group and the normal group respectively. The bigger the relative activity value, the higher the activity of the SOD in the specimen, and the stronger its ability to catalyze the desappearance of O_2^-, thus the lower the amount of O_2^- present[4]. In other words, the smaller the relative activity value, the higher the amount of O_2^- present.

IV. Results and Discussion

The results are shown in Table 1.

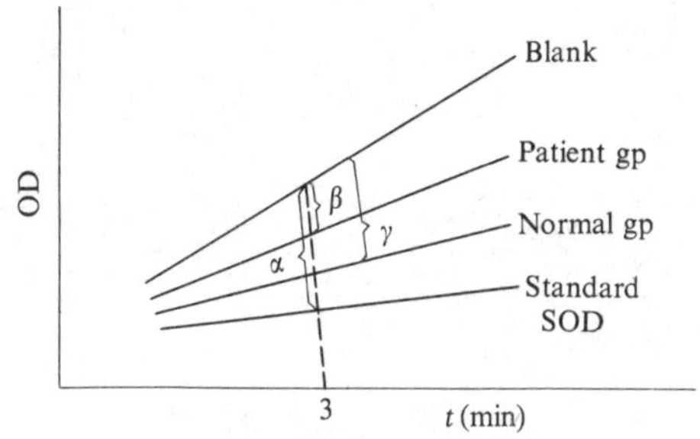

Fig. 2 SOD activity assay.

Table 1 Comparison of SOD Relative Activity Between G.C., E.C., C.G. Patient and Normal Groups

Group	n	Average Value±SD	P Value	O_2^- Level
G.C.	16	β/α: 0.307±0.164	$P<0.05$	high
E.C.	8	β/α: 0.250±0.090	$P<0.05$	high
C.G.	37	β/α: 0.361±0.159	$P>0.05$	low
Normal	19	γ/α: 0.439±0.208		low

In the patients with gastric cancer and esophageal cancer, the SOD activity is much lower than that in the normal group, i.e. the O_2^- level is much higher in these patients than in the normal people. The difference is statistically significant. In the patients with chronic gastritis, the result is different. The SOD activity is almost as high as that in the normal group, and the O_2^- level is not much higher than that in the normal group. There is no significant difference between them. This result is in agreement with that reported by Foyd[1] and Lohmann[2].

Slater[5] considered that free radicals, e.g. $Loo^{\cdot}$ and $L^{\cdot}$, could easily permeate and diffuse into the cell nucleus and attack the DNA or RNA to induce cancer. Since in gastric and esophageal cancer the O_2^- level is high, the level of its oxidation products will be also high, and thus there will be a higher chance for them to damage DNA and RNA and to induce the formation of cancer.

A low SOD activity level or a high O_2^- level may be used as an indicator in the supplementary diagnosis of gastric and esophageal cancer and to differentiate them from chronic gastritis.

References

1 Foyd, R.A., *Free Radicals and Cancer,* Marcel dekkey, Inc. NY, 1982, pp. 1-59.

2 Lohmann, W. *et al., Free Radical-Lipid Preoxidation and Cancer,* 1982.

3 Weng Qiliang *et al., Chin. J. Inorg. Chem.,* **2**(1986), 2: 99.

4 Weng Qiliang *et al., Chin. Prog. in Biochem. & Biophy.,* **69**(1986), 3: 51.

5 Slater, T. F., *Biochem. J.,* **222**(1984), 1: 1.

Effect of Rhodamine B on Transplanted Mouse Tumor*

HE Fengying,
(*Analysis and Testing Center of Gansu Province, Lanzhou 730000, PRC*)
WANG Liufang, YANG Zhengyin, LI Bingrui,
(*Department of chemistry, Lanzhou University, Lanzhou 730000, China*)
WANG Yumiao,
(*Louyang* No. 1 *Petroleum Cooperation, Fuzhou 350001, China*)
CHENG Guoguan and GUO Hongyun
(*Gansu Institute of New Medical and Pharmaccutical Science, Lanzhou 730000, China*)

Abstract In this paper, a study of the effects of HRhBCL on K_{562} and L_{1210} cells *in vitro* is reported. The inhibitory rates on K_{562} cells of concentrations of 100, 50, 10 and 5 μg/ml are 85, 84, 53 and 19% respectivrly while that on L_{1210} cells are 94, 92, 55 and 52% respectively.

The LD_{50} of HRhBCl i.p. in mice is 143.66±11.98 mg/kg.

In vivo, the growth of transplanted mouse tumors Hep and Ec has been inhibited, the rates being 38% and 68% respectively.

Further, abdominal injection of HRhBCl can increase markedly the weight of mouse spleen; this fact shows that HRhBCl has some stimulant function on the non-distinctive immunity system of the mouse.

I. Introduction

Rhodamine B ($C_{28}H_{31}O_3N_2Cl$ HRhBCl) has been used for the determination of Sb, Bi, Co, Nb, Au, Hg, Mo, Ta, Tl, and W[1]. Its aqueous and alcoholic solutions exhibit strong fluorescence and can stain bio-cells, so it has been used as a sensitive bio-dyeing agent[7]. However, no test for the antitumor pharmacology of either rhodamine or its derivatives has been reported. In this paper, the acute toxicity of HRhBCL by peritoneal injection in mice was tested, as well as its lethal effect on *in vitro* cultivated tumor cells K_{562} and L_{1210} and its inhibitory effect on the growth of transplanted mouse tumors Hep and Ec.

II. Experimental

1. *Materials*

(1) Rhodamine B, A.R. Beijing Chemical Factory.

* Project supported by the National Nutural Science foundation of China.

(2) Mice Healthy Kunming species, suppiled by Lanzhou Institute of Bioproducts.

(3) K_{562} human erythroleukemic cells and L_{1210} mouse leukaemia cells were received from Institute of Materia Medica, Chinese Academy of Sciences. Tumor Hep and Ec were supplied by Lanzhou Institute of Bioproducts.

2. *Lethal effect on K_{562} and L_{1210}*

The tumor cells were cultivated with cow serum RPMI 1640. A culture medium containing a 1×10^5/ml suspension of the cultivated tumor cells was prepared and used for testing by the micropore plate method. Into each cavity of the plate was put 0.2 ml of the cell suspension, then HRhBCl was added to give final concentrations of 100 μg/ml, 50 μg/ml, 10 μg/ml and 5 μg/ml. An equal volume of the corresponding solvent was used as a control. The plates were cultivated for 24 h under saturated humidity and 5% CO_2 atmosphere. The plates were then dyed with trypan-blue and the living cells counted under a microscope. The living cells of control group were taken as 100%, and the survival rate counted as follows:

$$\text{Survival rate} = \frac{\text{Average number of living cells of dosed group}}{\text{Number of living cells of control}} \times 100\%$$

3. *Acute Poison Test to Detemine LD*50

Healthy mice having a body weight of 20 ± 1 g were chosen.

These mice were injected peritoneally once with the required concentration of HRhBCL (0.1 ml/10 g), and they were observed for one week. The death rate was measured after 72 h.

4. *Effect of HRhBCl*

The effects of HRhBCl on the immune organs of mice transplanted with tumor colony Hep or EC are shown in Table 1.

Table 1 Effect of HRhBCl on the Growth of the Thymus Gland and Spleen of Mice

Tumor Colony	Dosage (mg/kg)	Thymus Gland ($X\pm$SD) (mg)		Spleen ($X\pm$SD) (mg)	
		Dosed	Control	Dosed	Control
Hep	10.0	38.1±12.74	37±9.44	107.9±20.55	102.9±27.39
	10.0	36.1±9.25	46.42±17.83	134.7±27.18	87.92±37.94
	15.0	35.3±9.81	31±9.44	124.5±31.54	102.9±27.39
	15.0	36.8±10.17	46.42±17.83	145.1±44.24	87.92±37.94
	30.0	35.44±6.89	46.42±17.83	149.55±36.7	87.92±37.94
EC	10.0	24.83±4.62	25.03±4.27	83.7±20.54	81.86±20.24
	30.0	19.66±8.6	25.03±4.27	12.76±28.79	81.86±20.24

From Table 1, it can be seen that HRhBCl has no apparent effect on the growth of the thymus gland of mice implanted with Hep or EC tumor colonies. However, HRhBCl has a positive effect on the growth of the spleen of the mice.

As seen from Fig. 1, HRhBCl has no apparent effect on the body weight of the mice. The body weight of the mice implanted with Hep or EC still increases with time.

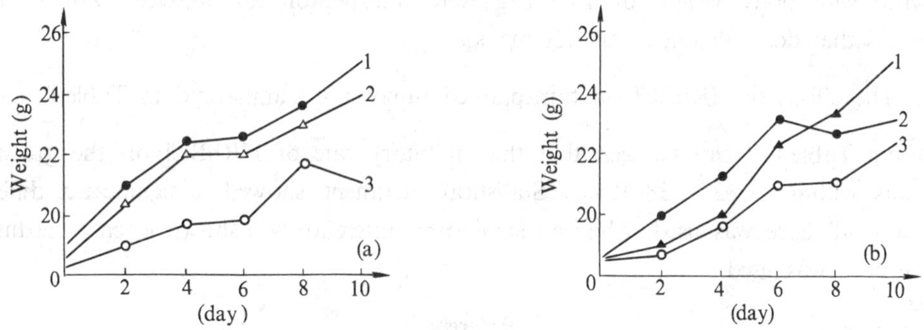

Fig. 1 Effect of HRhBCl on mice body weight.

(a) Mice implanted with Hep; (b) mice implanted with EC. (a) 1, Control; 2, 0.1% HRhBCl; 3, 0.3% HRhBCl. (b) 1, Control; 2, 0.1% HRhBCl; 3, 0.4% HRhBCl.

III. Conclusions

1. Lethal effects of HRhBCl on *in vitro* cultivated human erythroleukemic cellls K_{562} and leukaemia cells L_{1210} were observed. As much as 94% of L_{1210} and 85% of K_{562} could be killed. The lethal effect of HRhBCl was concentration-dependent.

2. When the mice were injected peritoneally once with HRhBCl, the LD_{50} was determined to be 143.66 ± 11.98 mg/kg.

3. HRhBCl has a certain inhibitory effect on the growth of transplanted HEP or EC tumor colonies. The sensitivities are different, the maximum inhibitory rates being 30% and 60% respectively.

4. HRhBCl has no apparent effect on the thymus gland weight but it can increase markedly the spleen weight of mice implanted with Hep or EC suggesting that it has a stimulating function on the nonspecific immune system of mice. Further HRhBCl has no apparent effect on the body weight of Hep or EC transplanted mice. This fact suggests that the dosage chosen was appropriate so that the toxic and side effects were rather small.

5. Because of its lethal effect on human erythroleukemic cells K_{562} and leukaemia cells L_{1210}, its inhibition of transplanted mice tumors Hep and EC, its acute toxicity and

influence on total body weight and spleen weight of mice transplanted with tumors, it can be concluded that HRhBCl has a definete inhibitory effect on tumor growth with low toxicity and few side effects so that it is worthy to study its pharmacology intensively.

IV. Results and Discussion

1. The result of acute toxicity test

Mice with body weight of 18—22g were intraperitoneally injected with HRhBCl. The half lethal dose obtained was 150 mg/kg.

2. The effects of HRhBCl on transplanted tumor are summarized in Table 1.

From Table 1 it can be seen that the inhibitory rate of HRhBCl on the growth of Hep was within 27.82— 38.45%. Statistical treatment showed a significanct difference when a small dose was used, while no significant difference was shown when a medium or a large dose was used.

References

1 Onishi, H. & Sandell, E. B., *Anal. Chim Acta,* 13(1955), 159.
2 Hesse, K. R., *Libre Bruexolles,* 1953.

A High-Yield New Synthesis Method of Benzo[k]fluoranthene

WANG Lihui, WANG Zhiqiang*, LI Yunxiang and DAI Qianhuan

(*Ctr. Chem, & Bioeng. of Cancer, Beijing Polytechnic Univ., Beijing* 100022)

Abstract Benzo[k]fluoranthene is a non-carcinogen, which would be a secure reference substance in the environmental analysis of carcinogens in polycylic aromatic hydrocarbon (PAH) fraction. Based upon the discussion of the stereo-chemistry of the corresponding reaction, a new method for the synthesis of benzo[k]-fluoranthene through bis-Wittig reaction by using the solid-liquid phase transfer catalysis technique with 40% overall yield, has been found in this laboratory, which is the most handy method with the highest overall yield compared with all the previous methods. A more precise analysis of MS ^{1}H- and ^{13}C-NMR spectra with purer sample than those in previous papers, is discussed in this paper.

Benzo[k]fluoranthene is widespread in the environment. It has been detected in the polycyclic aromatic hydrocarbon (PAH) fraction of the atmosphere or flue gas, gasoline and diesel machine exhaust from the combustion processes[1, 2]. In the chromatographic analysis with capillary column, it is eluted just after the peaks of two marked carcinogens, benzo[j]fluoranthene (+++) and benzo[b]fluoranthene (+++), and before the potent carcinogen, benzo[a]pyrene (++++)[3]. Although it has been reported with large dose i. p. administration on mice that benzo[k]fluoranthene shows slight carcinogenicity[4], all the other experiments including the skin painting test affirms that it is not a carcinogen[5] and the Ames test shows that it is not a mutagen either[6]. Obviously, it is appropriate that the American EPA classifies it as a non-carcinogen[7]. The above-mentioned three carcinogens are the main contents in PAH fraction of environmental sample, and have been detected with ppb degree in the samples of water, soil as well as in the smoked or non-smoked food. Therefore, the preparation of the reference substance of benzo[k]fluoranthene is important, because it has equal molecular weight with the above three carcinogens, and is useful as a nontoxic and secure standard in the analysis of polycylic aromatic hydrocarbons. This paper reports a new method for the preparation of benzo-[k]fluoranthene as well as for the measurement of its purification in order to obtain the standard substance of benzo[k]fluoranthene with gas chromatographic purity.

I. Synthesis Method of Benzo[k]fluoranthene

Now, there are four synthetic methods for benzo[k]fluoranthene. In 1964, a method with 7, 12-dicyanobenzo[k]fluoranthene was proposed by Moureu et al.[8] The overall yield was only 11—17% by this method. The decarboxylation of dicyano-BkF can be

* Present address: Shandong Institute of Chemistry, Jinan, Shandong Province, China.

proceeded directly by catalysis of phosphoric acid according to Vickery[9]. Then the overall yield of this preparation was increased to 13—18%.

A preparation with 1, 2′-binaphthyl was proposed by Orchin et al. in 1947[10]. The dehydration product of the alcohol formed from the reaction between tetralone and the Grignard reagent of α-bromonaphthene, was dehydrogenated by sulfur to yield 1, 2′-binaphthyl, and then the BkF was yielded by catalytic dehydrogenation with Cr_2O_3 at high temperature about 500°C. The overall yield was less than 9%.

The method of the first step by Friedel-Crafts reaction between fluoranthene and succinic anhydride was reported in 1954 by Bru-Hof et al. [11] The intermediate was reduced through Wolff-Kishner reduction, then transformed to acid chloride, and produced 8, 9, 10, 11-tetrahydro-BkF through the intramolecular Friedel-Crafts reaction and the following reduction (95%). BkF was obtained by dehydrogenation with selenium at 340°C. However, the overall yield was only 13%.

The common disadvantage of these methods is their having many steps. A handy synthetic method for BkF was reported in 1964 by Whitelock[12]. The BkF synthesis method consisted of the formation of bis-[diethyl methyleno phosphonate] through Arbuzov reaction between triethyl phosphite and α, α′-dibromoxylene and the condensation of the intermediate with acenaphthenone under the catalysis of sodium alcoholate.

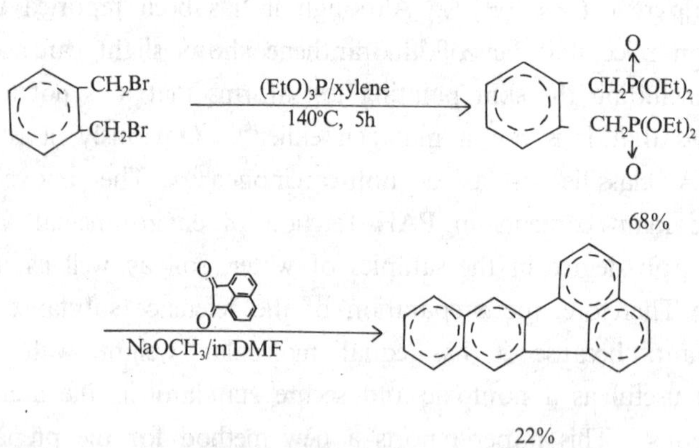

Fig. 1 Synthetic route of benzo[k]fluoranthene through bis-Wittig-Horner reaction.

Because of the rather low yield of the last step, the overall yield of this method from o-xylene, is only 7%, which is the method with the lowest yield among the above various routes. Therefore, in order to provide the standard substance for environmental analysis, a new handy method with high yield remains to be developed.

II. Bis-Wittig Synthesis of Benzo[k]fluoranthene

According to the published review[13], none of the yields of cyclic compound synthesized through bis-Wittig type reaction are high, and therefore this method has been used scarcely in the synthesis of six-member rings because of their easy formation, and often used in the syntheses of medium and large ring compounds which are difficult to gain through the routine methods. Most of the authors engaged in bis-Wittig type reaction often neglect the influence of stereo-chemistry in this reaction. In practice, the first step of bis-Wittig reaction before the cyclization reaction can offer two sorts of isomers, i.e. the Z isomer and E isomer; the former will be cyclized smoothly to form the target product. However, the latter cannot yield cyclic compound and form only the compound with higher molecular weight, which may be illustrated in Fig. 2.

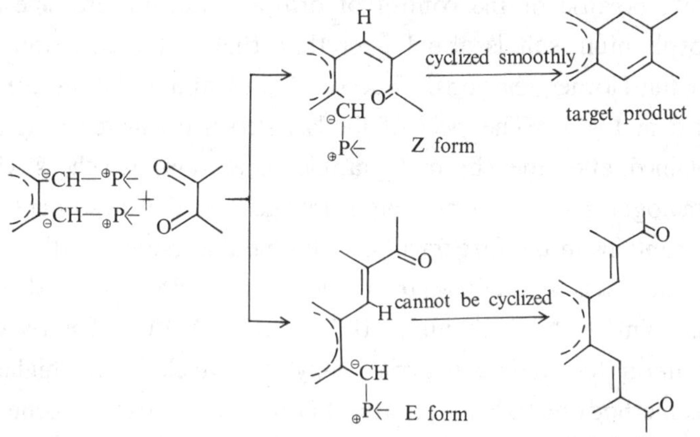

Fig. 2 Two distinct routes depend upon the stereo-direction of bis-Wittig type reaction.

The stereo-chemistry of Wittig reactions and Wittig-Horner reactions is a problem still under discussion[14]. Some work for this interesting task done in this laboratory will be published elsewhere. However, in practice, the stereo-chemistry of these reactions can be controlled semi-empirically based upon the experiential rules summarized through experiments. For example, the Wittig-Horner reactions always are stereo-specifically to yield the E isomers regardless of the variation of reaction condition; the anti-stereo-specificity of Wittig-Horner reactions is disadvantageous for the cyclization. It is more complex in Wittig reactions, for the unstable ylid. The one that is not connected with conjugate system, always gives the *cis* product stereo-specifically in non-polar or aprotic solvent, but for stable ylid, the one connected with conjugate system, often gives *trans* isomer as the main product. On the contrary, the protic solvent is advantageous for the ratio of *cis* product. The characteristics of metastable ylid is between the two conditions, in general, the reactions are non-stereospecificity, but the non-polar or aprotic solvent is advantageous for the increasing of *cis* product ratio[15].

In terms of the above discussion, obviously the Wittig-Horner reaction is difficult to offer high yield for the synthesis of aromatic compound. Therefore, in order to promote the formation of *cis* isomer intermediate from the metastable ylid, we adopt the Wittig reaction and use the aprotic solvent as reaction medium. It might be better to adopt the solid-liquid phase transfer catalysis technique instead of the routine method, which provides the reaction condition on solid intefacial surface to increase the possibility of cyclization. By using the potassium carbonate as the solid phase base, dioxane as the solvent and formamide as the conjugated acid of phase transfer base, the synthesis of benzo[k]fluoranthene through bis-Wittig reaction with 54% yield for high purity product has been achieved in this laboratory. Consistent with our expectation, the yield of BkF corresponds to 2.5 times of the analogous Wittig-Horner reaction. Additionally, the yield in the di-bromination of o-xylene, in the first step of BkF synthesis is higher than the report in literature[8], because of the control of dripping rate of bromine. The yield of bis-quaternary phosphonium salt is also higher than that of the corresponding bis-phosphonate ester in Wittig-Horner reactions. The conditions and yields in every step of this scheme are illustrated in Fig. 3. The yield of the last step is calculated in terms of the high purity product obtained after the chromatographic separation, which is yielded through the column chromatography by using the silica gel as the absorbent, and benzene as the eluate. BkF contains in the first fraction with blue fluorescene, and after concentration of the eluate, a golden yellow needle-shaped crystal is precipitated. After washing and drying, the melting point of this high purity BkF is 218—220°C. The overall yield comes up to 30% based upon the initiate material, o-xylene, which is the highest one among the present various methods of BkF preparation. Obviously, it has the general significance in the syntheses of polycyclic aromatic hydrocarbons because of the good yield achieved by this method in hand.

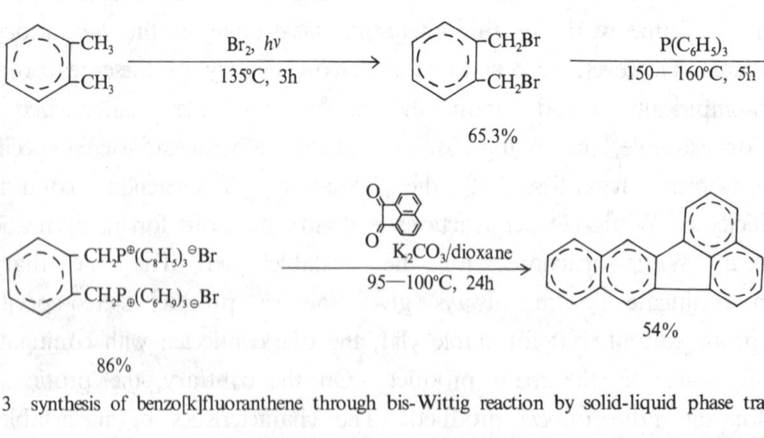

Fig. 3 synthesis of benzo[k]fluoranthene through bis-Wittig reaction by solid-liquid phase transfer catalysis.

III. Standard Substance Preparation and Spectral Properties of Benzo[k]fluoranthene

The yielded benzo[k]fluoranthene is recrystallized in 95% ethanol and then through the sublimation, the BkF of chromatographic purity is obtained. In HPLC with fluorescenc detector, during the signal of BkF amplified to 32 times, the impurity peak cannot be detected. Hence, the obtained benzo[k]fluoranthene is a standard substance with 100% purity by chromatographic verification.

The UV, IR, MS, ^{1}H- and ^{13}C-NMR of benzo[k]fluoranthene with 99.8% purity, have been reported by Karcher et al.[16] Owing to the higher purity of our sample and the development of the instruments at present with respect to those of 1983, the reports of the spectra of benzo[k]fluoranthene with modified discussions, are anew, but only MS, ^{1}H- and ^{13}C-NMR are recorded in the following paragraphs.

The electron impact MS spectrum of BkF in Fig. 4 is recorded with Varian MAT-232 instrument. The base peak is just the molecular ion peak (M/Z 225). In this peak cluster, in addition to the M+1 and M+2 isotope peaks, there are M−1, M−2, M−3 dehydrogenated peaks. The peak cluster of M/Z 226, 224 is the fragment ions eliminated HC≡CH from molecular ions accompanied by their dehydrogenated ions. The two clusters of M/Z 126 and 113 ion which both include the non-integer ions, are the double charge ions of the above two clusters.

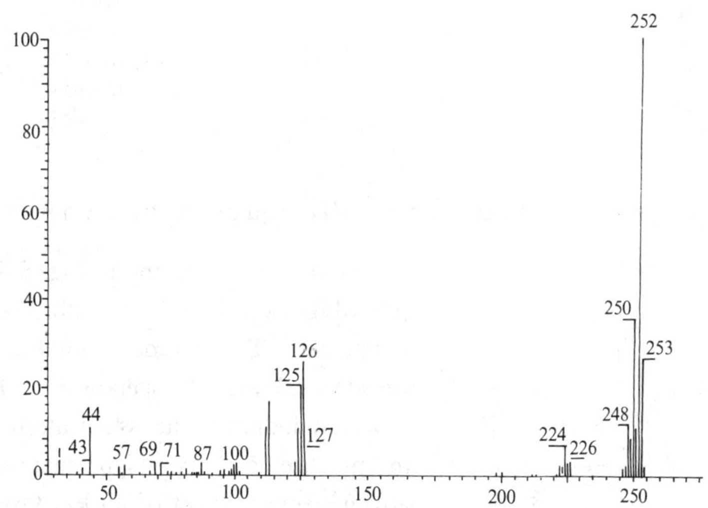

Fig. 4 Mass spectrum of benzo[k]fluoranthene.

^{1}H-NMR spectrum in Fig. 5 is recorded in $CDCl_3$ as solvent with Varian XL-300 type of 300 MHz instrument. All the peaks of proton in different environment are separated with each other in this 300 MHz spectrum, and their area ratios are 2:2:2:2:2:2. In terms of IUPAC nomenclature system, the classification of the peaks is indicated in the table. The high resolution spectrum in this paper makes the indication more exact

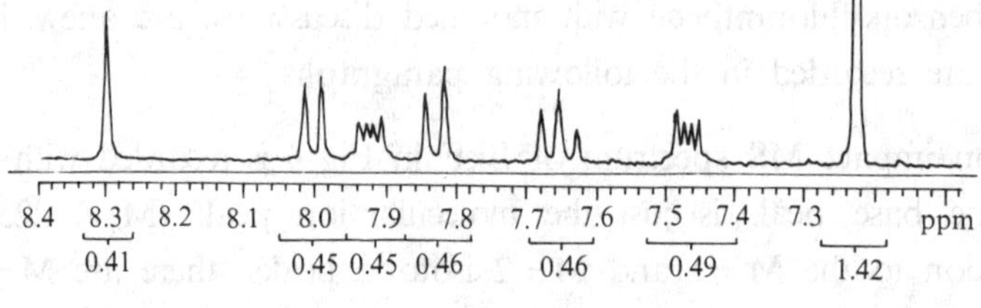

Fig. 5 ^{1}H-NMR spectrum of benzo[k]fluoranthene.

Proton No.	Chemical Shift (ppm)	Coupling Constant (Hz)
7 (12)	8.30	Undetected Coupling With Other Proton
1 (6)	8.00	$J_{1,2}=7.2$
8 (11)	7.93	$J_{8,9}=6.3$ $J_{8,10}=2.1$
3 (4)	7.84	$J_{3,2}=7.5$
2 (5)	7.66	$J_{2,1}=7.2$ $J_{2,3}=7.5$
9 (10)	7.49	$J_{9,8}=6.3$ $J_{9,11}=2.1$

than the complex spectrum recorded with 90 MHz equipment by previous authors[16].

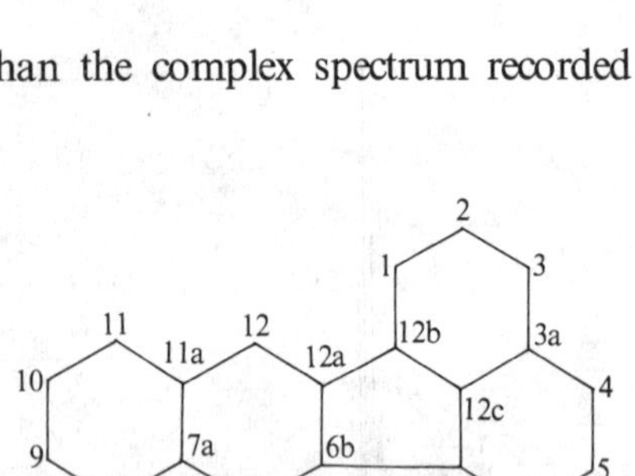

Fig. 5a Numbering of various positions on BkF according to IUPAC nomenclature.

^{13}C-NMR spectrum in Fig. 6 is recorded at 500 MHz field in $CDCl_3$ with Pruker AM 500 equipment. The recorded values of chemical shift are identical with the literature[16]. However, they have not indicated the issued atoms of the peaks. In practice on the high magnetic field, the obvious enhancement of nuclear Overhauser effects (NOE) on the peak intensity of tertiary carbon atoms bonded with proton causes distinct difference from the peak intensity of quaternary carbon atoms with only negligible NOE. The repulsion between the two hydrogen atoms on 1, 12-positions or 6, 7-positions, makes both corresponding carbon atoms on the highest upfield. The peaks of quarternary carbon atom reflect the much longer relaxation time, and keep roughly the relative intensities compatible with the corresponding number. The slight but notable higher intensities for 3a and 7a carbon atoms among other quarternary atoms, imply more α-protons neighbouring on them.

Carbon Atom No.	Chemical Shift (ppm)	Intensity	Note
1 (6)	119.1	0.88	strong NOE, push with 12H
7 (12)	120.2	0.87	strong NOE, push with 6H
2 (5)	126.0	1.00	strong NOE
3 (4)	126.2	0.95	strong NOE
9 (10)	128.2	0.89	strong NOE
8 (11)	128.8	0.84	strong NOE
3a	130.7	0.10	intensity≃1 with weak NOE
7a (11a)	133.6	0.18	intensity≃2 with weak NOE
12c	135.4	0.06	intensity≃1
6a (12b)	137.0	0.13	intensity≃2
6b (12a)	137.9	0.13	intensity≃2

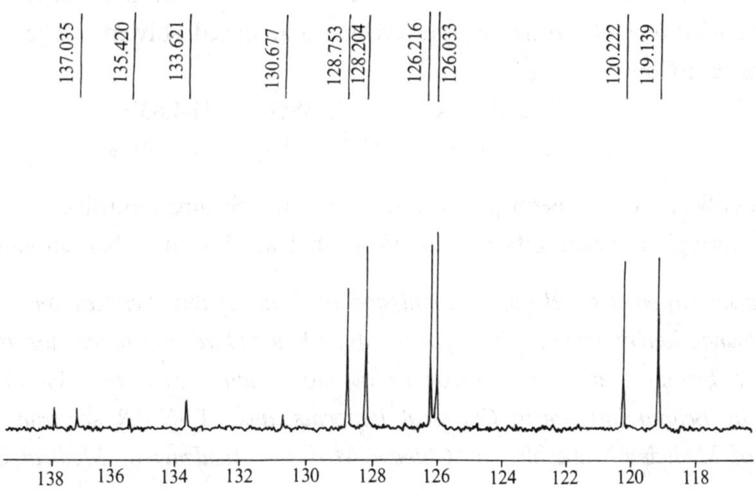

Fig. 6 ^{13}C-NMR spectrum of benzo [k] fluoranthene.

IV. Experiments

1. α, α′-dibromo-o-xylene: Under daylight lamp, at 135°C, stir the 10.6 g (0.1 mol) o-xylene for 2.5 h, when dropping 32.5 g (0.2 mole) bromide. After the dropping, the reaction keeps for another half hour. By addition of petroleum ether in the cooled reaction mixture, a greyish brown crystal was obtained. The product through filtration and

washing with petroleum ether is 17.3 g of 88% yield. By recrystallization with ethyl alcohol, it has m.p. 93—94°C[17]; UV, λ_{max} 219 nm; IR absorptions (strong absorptions only), 1491, 1454, 1432, 1233, 1217, 1038, 886, 838,765, 737, 606, 533, 476.

2. O-xylenyl-, bis-triphenylphosphonium dibromide: heat α, α′-dibromo-o-xylene 1.25 g (4.75 mmol) triphenylphosphine 2.5 g (9.5 mmol) and DMF 40 ml, at 150—160°C under reflux for about 5 h, then distill half volume of the solvent, filtrate the precipitated solid, wash with DMF, then with ethyl ether, the dried product is 3.2 g with 86% yield. m.p. 341—342°C. UV: λ_{max} 238.2 nm, IR (a part of the strong peaks): 3048, 3036, 3004, 2854, 2783, 1586, 1484, 1436, 1189, 1165, 1110, 997, 782, 752, 718, 690, 530, 510, 499, 456, 448.

3. Benzo[k]fluoranthene: Heat the above obtained bis-quarternary phosphonium salt 3.5 g (4.8 mmol), acenaphthacenone 0.73 g (4 mmol), anhydrous K_2CO_3 0.38 g (8 mmol), formamide 0.24 g (1.8 mmol) and 65 ml dry dioxane, at 100°C under reflux for 24 h, filtrate out the K_2CO_3, distill out the solvent and concentrate to dryness under vacuum. Collect the first fraction with blue fluorescence by chromatography on silica gel column through eluation with benzene. After distillation of the solvent, filtration and drying, the obtained high purity benzo[k]fluoranthene is 0.58 g corresponding to 54% yield, m.p. 218—220°C (literature 216—218°C)[12]. The melting point of the product has no change after the recrystallization with benzene and cyclohexane mixed solvent. The result of element analysis is as follows:

Found:	C 95.38%	H 4.83%
Calculation:	C 95.21%	H 4.79%

4. Purification of benzo[k]fluoranthene: the chromatographic purity product is obtained through recrystallization with 95% ethyl alcohol and then sublimation.

Financial supports by Beijing Commission of Municipality Services and National Natural Science Foundation of China. The purity of BkF standard substance has been checked and verified by Beijing Station of Environmental monitoring. MS and ¹*H-NMR spectra were prepared by Beijing Institute of Chemical Reagents, and* ¹³*C-NMR spectrum was prepared by Institute of Medicine Materials, the Chinese Medicine Academy of Medical Sciences.*

References

1 Dai Qianhuan, *Beijing Gongye Daxue Xuebao* (*Journal of Beijing Polytechnic University*), 1980, 1: 1—17.

2 Grimmer, G. et al., *Environmental Carcinogens, Polycyclic Aromatic Hydrocarbons*, CRC Press, 1983.

3 Lee, M. L., Novotny, M. V. and Bartle, K. D., *Analytical Chemistry of Polycyclic Aromatic Compounds*, Academic Press, 1981.

4 Bun-Hoi, N.P., *Cancer Res.*, **24**(1964), 1511.

5 Mohr, U., *Arch. Hyg*, **153**(1969), 495; Wynder, E.L. and Hoffmann, D., *Cancer*, **12**(1959), 1194.

6 Mossanda, K., Poncelet, F., Fouassin, A. and Moroier, M., *Food Cosmet Toxicol.*, **17**(1979), 141.

7 EPA, *Health Assessment for Polycyclic Organic Matter,* May, 1978.
8 Moureu, H., Chovin, P. and Rivoal, G., *Compt. Rend.,* **223**(1946), 951.
9 Vickery, E.H. and Eisenbracen, E.J., *Org. Prep. Proceed Int.,* **11**(1979), 259.
10 Orchin, M. and Reggel, L., *J. Am. Chem. Soc.,* **69**(1947), 505.
11 Bru-Hof, N.P., Lavit, D. and Lamy, I., *J. Chem. soc.,* 1959, p. 1845.
12 Whitelock, Jr. H.W., *J. Org. Chem.,* **29**(1964), 3129.
13 Vollhardt, K.P.C., *Synthesis,* 1975, p. 765.
14 cf. March, *J. Advanced Organic Chemistry,* 3rd Edition, 1985, p. 845.
15 cf. Anderson, R.J. and Henrick, C.A., *J. Am. Chem. Soc.,* **97**(1975), 4327.
16 Karcher, W., Fordham, R. J. et al., *Spectral Atlas of Polycyclic Aromatic Compounds,* D. Reidel Publishing Company, 1983.
17 Perkin, W.H., *J. Chem. Soc.,* **53**(1913), 5.

Studies on the Interaction of an Adriamycin-Calf Thymus DNA Complex With Nickel (II) Ions

YANG Pin, YANG Zuoyin and YANG Binsheng

(*Institute of Molecular Science, Shanxi University, Taiyuan, Shanxi 030006. China*)

Abstract Using visible absorption, fluorescence, CD and IR spectroscopy, as well as molecular mechanics and quantum chemistry calculations, the Ni (II) ion binding properties of adriamycin (ADM) in aqueous solution and the interaction of Ni (II) with the native and heat-denatured calf-thymus DNA complexes of adriamycin have been studied.

The CD spectra of ADM indicate that Ni (II) can bind to ADM and yield complexes of Ni (II) with ADM. Plots of absorbance at two wavelengths against equivalents of Ni (II) added show a clear break corresponding to a stoichiometry of 1: 1, Ni (ADM), and 1: 2, Ni $(ADM)_2$, within the pH range 7.2—8.0 and at pH8.4 respectively. Fluorescence quenching of ADM by Ni (II) give the same results. The IR spectrum of the solid complex, Ni (II)-ADM, shows that the binding site is coincident with that calculated from theory.

Of the two complexes, ADM-denatured DNA and ADM-native DNA, the Ni (II) ion affected the former much more than the latter. At pH8.0 and $R_t = 50$, where R_t is the molar ratio of DNA phosphate to ADM, titration of Ni (II) produced a ternary complex, Ni (II)-ADM-dDNA. A reasonable configuration for the ternary complex is suggested.

I. Introduction

Adriamycin (ADM) is an antitumor antibiotic which is in wide clinical use for the treatment of a variety of neoplastic diseases.

Since the discovery of the antibiotic[1], the mechanism of how ADM exhibits antitumor activity has been actively researched. To date most of the studies have been concentrated on the interaction of the drug with DNA and have suggested that the drug receptor site should be on DNA. In an effort to gain further information about the binding mechanism, several investigators have studied the binding of metal ions to the anthracycline-DNA complex. Spinelli and Dabrowiak[2] demonstrated that Cu (II) interacts with the native and heat-denatured calf-thymus DNA complexes with daunomycin to form ternary complexes involving the aglycone portion of the antibiotic, Cu (II) and DNA. Moreover, recent *in vitro* studies[3, 4] have shown that the drugs are capable of degrading DNA and the degrading process is affected by transition metal ions. This observation must be combined with the recognition that metal ions are necessary for the stabilization of double helical DNA[5]. In this paper, we describe the interactions which occur between Ni (II), ADM and calf-thymus DNA.

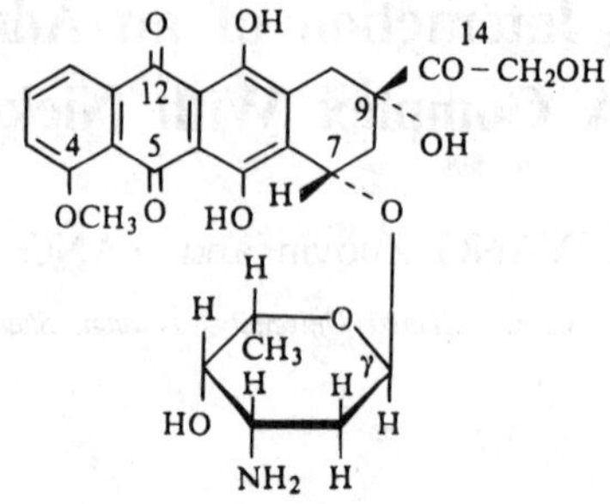

Adriamycin (ADM)

II. Materials and Methods

Adriamycin HCl was a generous gift of Professor Yang Zouzhong who works in the Drug Research Institute of Shanghai. Solutions of adriamycin were prepared by dissolving the drug in aqueous 5×10^{-3} mol/L NaCl solution immediately prior to use. ADM concentrations were measured using a molar extinction coefficient of 115 0 $(mol/L)^{-1}$ cm^{-1}[6]. $NiCl_2 \cdot H_2O$ used in the experiment was obtained from the Third Chemical Preparation Factory of Beijing. Calf thymus DNA (sigma) was prepared by dissolving the DNA (~ 2 mg/ml) in deionized water and exhaustively dialyzing, first against 0.1 mol/L EDTA and then against 5×10^{-3} mol/L NaCl. DNA concentrations are expressed as DNA phosphate (DNAp), and were determined optically at 260 nm using an extinction coefficient of 6600 $(mol/L)^{-1}cm^{-1}$. The DNA samples in 5×10^{-3} mol/L NaCl at pH=7.2 had an A_{260}/A_{280} ratio of ~ 1.9, indicating they were relatively protein free. Immediately prior to being titrated DNA was denatured by heating in a boiling water bath at 100°C for 15 min followed by rapidly soaking in ice water. The pH was adjusted using 0.1 mol/L NaOH or HCl.

All titrations were performed by adding microliter quantities of 0.1 mol/L Ni (II) to 1 ~ 9×10^{-5} mol/L solutions of the drug or to the ADM-DNA complex which had a molar ratio (ADM/DNAp) of 0.02. After each titration, the pH was adjusted and data were plotted at two wavelengths, after correcting for dilution.

The absorption spectra were obtained on a Shimadzu UV-365 spectrophotometer. The CD spectra were measured on a Jasco J-20 spectropolarimeter while the IR spectra of the ADM and the Ni (II)-ADM complex, which is a violet solid, were obtained on a Shimadzu IR-435 spectrometer. The fluorecence quenching data were obtained using a Hitachi RF-850 spectrometer. The spectra were measured using 1-cm cells. All of the spectroscopic work was carried out at ambient temperature.

Quantum chemistry calculations were performed on an MV/6000 computer. The programs for MMPM and CNDO were provided by Peking University.

III. Results and Discussion

Figure 1 shows the visible absorption spectrum of the titration of ADM with Ni (II). At both pH=7.2 and pH=8.4, there are two clear isobestic points, but they are not exactly the same, which shows that Ni (II) can bind to ADM and yield two different complexes. Plots of the absorbance at wavelengths of 480 and 560 nm against the equivalents of Ni(II) added indicate that the stoichiometry of the complexes are Ni (ADM) and $Ni(ADM)_2$ at pH=7.2 and pH=8.4 respectively (Fig. 2(a), Fig. 2(b)). The flourescence quenching curves (Fig. 3) correspond to the results from the visible absorption measurements.

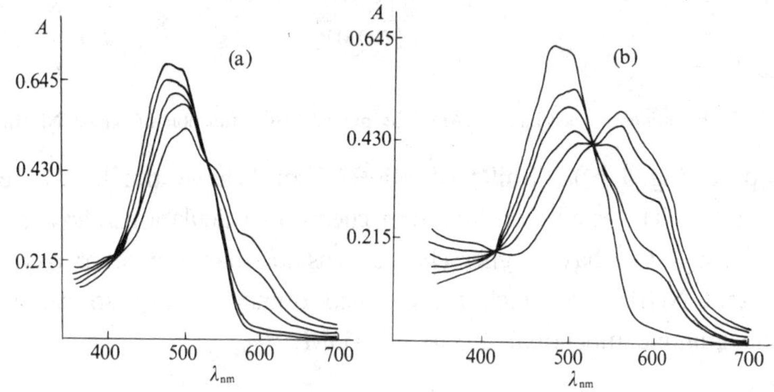

Fig. 1 Absorption spectra of ADM (5×10^{-3} mol/L NaCl) at pH=7.2 (left) and pH=8.4 (right) as a function of added Ni (II).

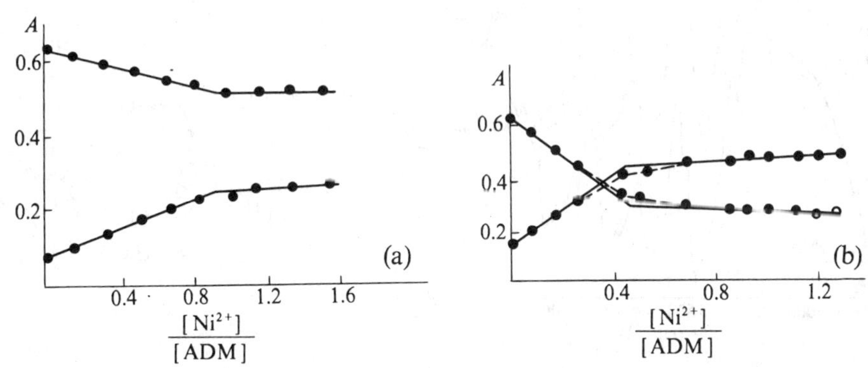

Fig. 2 Absorbance of ADM at pH=7.2(a) and pH=8.4(b) as a function of added Ni(II) at 480 nm and 560 nm.

The infrared spectrum of the solid complex of Ni (II) with ADM shows bands at 3440, 3000 and 1715 cm^{-1} due to the hydroxyl, amino and sidechain ketone respectively[7]. These bands are unaffected by the reaction, whereas the peaks at 1610 and 1580 cm^{-1} due to the quinone moiety in ADM (Fig. 4(a)) appear as a strong absorption at 1550 cm^{-1} in

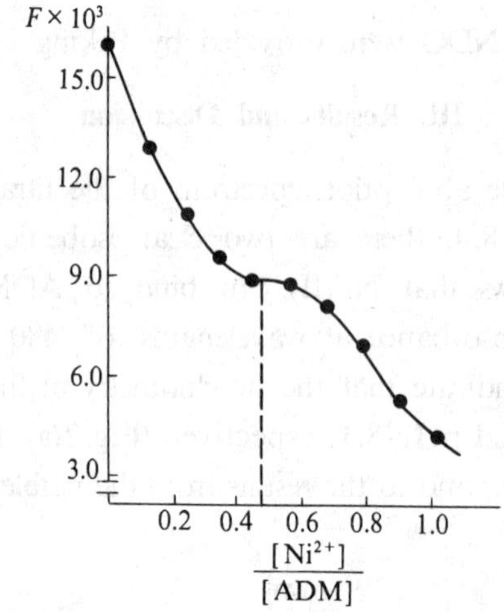

Fig. 3 Fluorescence quenching of ADM at pH=8.4 as a function of added Ni (II).

the nickel complex (Fig. 4 (b)). Shifts of 60— 85 cm^{-1} have previously been noted for chelated quinones[8, 9]. The results of quantum chemistry calculations show that the oxygen atoms on C_5, C_6, C_{11}, C_{12} have higher charge densities than the other oxygens in ADM, which indicates that Ni (II) can attack the chelated quinone easily, so we suggest that Ni (II) binds to the quinone functional group of ADM.

Since the complex is probably polymeric in nature, the structure shown in Fin. 5 has been assigned to the compound.

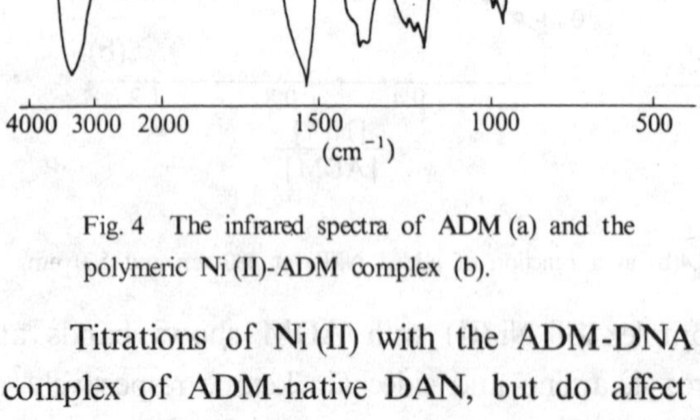

Fig. 4 The infrared spectra of ADM (a) and the polymeric Ni (II)-ADM complex (b).

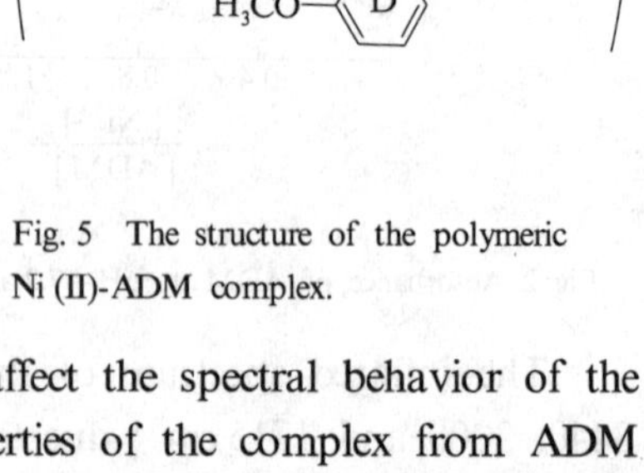

Fig. 5 The structure of the polymeric Ni (II)-ADM complex.

Titrations of Ni (II) with the ADM-DNA do not affect the spectral behavior of the complex of ADM-native DAN, but do affect the properties of the complex from ADM and denatured DNA. The latter is characterized by two isobestic points at 400 nm and 520 nm. At the end point of the titration, the system of Ni (II) / ADM / dDNA exhibits two well-definded absorption maxima at 560 nm and 590 nm, and the absorption bands associated with the hydroxyquinone chromophore of the drug become sharper and shift to lower energy (Fig. 6). In addition, the positive CD bands of the ADM-denatured DNA complex at 360 nm and 480 nm shift to 380 nm and 490 nm resp ctively (Fig. 7). In illustration, the bands of Ni(II)-ADM, ADM-dDNA and Ni(II)/ADM/DNA are collected in Table 1.

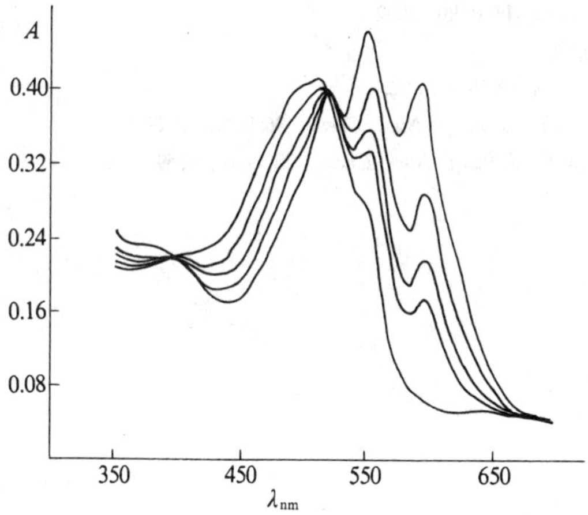

Fig. 6 The absorption spectrum of titrating Ni (II) to ADM-dDNA complex (pH=8.4).

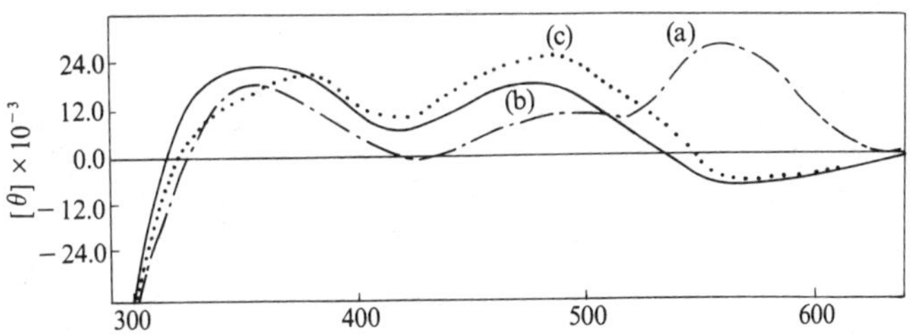

Fig. 7 The CD spectra of Ni/ADM (a), ADM/dDNA (b) and Ni/ADM/dDNA (c) (pH=8.4).

Table 1 The CD Bands of Ni/ADM, ADM/dDNA and Ni/ADM/dDNA (pH=8.4)

Band Position (nm)	350	360	380	480	490	560	570
Ni (II)-ADM	(+)				(+)	(+)	
ADM-dDNA		(+)		(+)			(−)
Ni (II) + ADM − dDNA			(+)		(+)		(−)

In summary, we suggest that Ni (II) ions be unable to react with the complex of ADM with nDNA, but can bind to the complex of ADM with dDNA to form a ternary complex which involves the intercalated aglyone. The reaction can be expressed as follows:

$$\text{Ni (II)} + \text{ADM} - \text{dDNA} = \text{Ni (II)} - \text{ADM} - \text{dDNA} + \text{Ni (II)} - \text{ADM}$$

References

1 Arcamone, F. *et al.*, *Biotechnol. Bioeng.*, **11**(1969), 1101.
2 Spinelli, M. and Dabrowiak, J.c., *Biochemistry,* **21**(1982), 2862.
3 Cown, J.W., Sim, S.K. *et al.*, *Biochem. Biophys. Res. Commun.*, **76**(1977), 705.
4 Someya, A. and Tanaka, N., *J. Antibiot.*, **32**(1979), 839.
5 Eichhorn, G.C., *Inorganic Biochemistry,* **2**(1973), 1210.
6 Gabbay, E.J. *et al.*, *Biochemistry,* **15**(1976), 2062.
7 Job, P., *Ann. Chem.*, **6**(1935), 97.
8 Dimarco, A., *Top. Antibiot, Chem.*, **2**(1978), 102.
9 Bottei, H.D. and Fangman, J.T., *J. Inorg. Nucl. Chem.*, **36**(1974), 1049.
10 Bottei, R.S. and Fangman. J.T., *J. Inorg. Nucl. Chem.*, **28**(1966), 1259.

QSAR Study on the Activity of Some Biological Fluorescent Agents Against ECa109*

LI Bingrui, WANG Liufang, PENG Zhouren

(Department of Chemistry, Lanzhou University, Lanzhou 730000, China)

and WANG Qi

(Lanzhou Institute of Chemical Physics, Academia Sinica, Lanzhou 730000, China)

I. Introduction

Fluorescein has been used for the fluorescence analysis of DNA and antibodies. In addition, we have studied the anti-tumor activity of its derivatives[1]. The results indicate the possibility of these compounds being useful medicines. Using Q-type stepwise informational cluster analysis, we have successfully carried out a QSAR (Quantitative Structure-Activity Relationships) study of the agents against ECa109.

In this paper, we describe the consequences and discuss their meaning.

II. Fundamentals of Mathematics

Q-type cluster analysis is a kind of non-supervision pattern recognition method. It enables us to classify a species without depending on any artificial standard. So it is important in quantitative medicine design research[2]. In the process of reducing a species for classification, some types of traditional cluster analysis generally arbitrarily delete species of smaller serial number. In this article, we report a method in which we reduce the species according to their relative information content, which we believe to be more reasonable. The principal steps are as follows:

(1) Construct the raw data matrix X with the P structure parameters of N species.

(2) Convert X into normalized data matrix X' by the formula:

$$X'_{ij} = \frac{X_{ij} - \overline{X}_i}{S_i} \qquad (i=1,2,\cdots,\ P; j=1,2,\cdots,\ N)\ ,$$

where $\overline{X}_i$ is the average of the variables, and the standard deviation S_i is defined in the usual manner as:

$$S_i = [\frac{1}{N-1} \sum_{j=1}^{N} (X_{ij} - \overline{X}_i)^2]^{1/2}$$

*Project supported by the National Natural Science Foundation of China.

(3) Calculate the real symmetric matrix Q of similarity coefficients. The matrix elements are,

$$q_{jk} \equiv \cos\theta_{jk} = \frac{\sum_{i=1}^{P} X'_{ij} \cdot X'_{ik}}{[\sum_{i=1}^{P} X'^2_{ij} \cdot \sum_{i=1}^{P} X'^2_{ik}]^{1/2}} \qquad (i, j = 1, 2, \cdots, N) .$$

(4) Select the largest matrix element $(\cos\theta_{jk})_{max}$ from the matrix Q, then calculate the information content corresponding to species j, k according to the Shannon equation,

$$I = -\sum_{i=1}^{m} \frac{S_l}{P} \log_2 \frac{S_l}{P} .$$

Here, P is the number of variables, m, the group number for calculating frequency distribution (in this paper, for example, $m=20$) and S_l, the emergence frequency of X'_{ij} in the lth group repectively.

(5) Compare I_j with I_k. If I_j is smaller, take the weighted sum of the jth and the kth column of X' for the new kth column and delete the jth column of X', and jth row and column of Q, then recalculate $\cos\theta_{ik}$, and *vice versa*. After completing this cycle, we return to step 4, and so on, until all elements of the matrix Q are chosen.

(6) Graph the dendrogram by the SAHN technique[3].

III. Data Processing

Crystal-structure analysis shows that the model of the fluorescein molecule has two almost mutually perpendicular planes. Fig. 1 shows the model with substituents located.

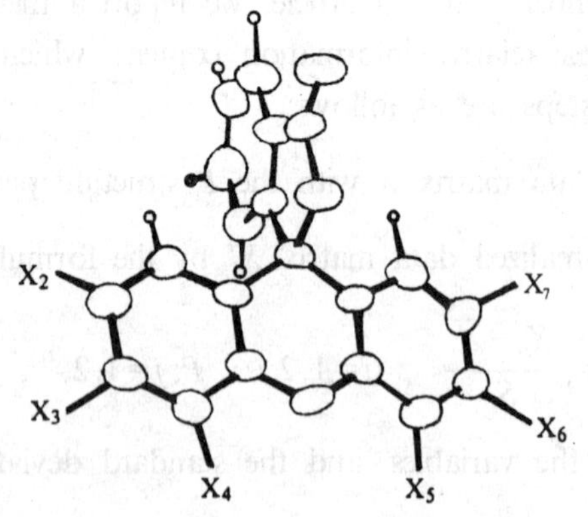

Fig. 1 Model of fluorescein with substituents located.

The series includes 16 derivatives symmetrically substituted: 1, Fluorescein diacetate; 2, fluorescein dipropionate; 3, fluorescein, disodium salt; 4, tetrabromofluorescein;

5, tetraiodofluorescein; 6, dibromodinitrofluorescein, disodium salt; 7, diiodofluorescein; 8, dibromofluorescein; 9, 2,7-dichlorofluorescein; 10, fluorescein dibutyrate; 11, dichlorofluorescein diacetate; 12, dibromofluorescein diacetate; 13, dibromodinitrofluorescein diacetate; 14,atetraiodofluorescein diacetate; 15, tetrabromofluorescein di cetate; 16, fluorescein.

The key to Q-type stepwise informational cluster analysis lies in selecting the structure parameters. We screened out two sets of parameters by combining this cluster analysis with stepwise regression:

$$\text{Set 1: } \sum \text{MR},\ F_2,$$
$$\text{Set 2: } \sum \text{MR},\ \sum \text{F},\ (\sum \pi)^2,$$

where MR is the molar refraction, F is the field inductive effect parameter, F_2 is the field inductive effect parameter of 2-substituent and π is the hydrophobic parameter of the substituents[4].

Table 1 lists the consequences of Q-type stepwise informational cluster analysis. Two correspondent dendrograms are shown in Fig. 2.

Table 1 The Consequences Clustered by (a) $[\sum \text{MR}, F_2]$ and (b) $[\sum \text{MR}, \sum \text{F}, (\sum \pi)^2]$

(a)

Species		Information Content		Similarity Coef.
j	k	I_j	I_k	$\cos\theta_{jk}$
3	16	0.5000	0.5000	1
6	11	1.0000	1.0000	0.9997
1	8	1.3750	1.3750	0.9920
5	15	1.6250	1.6250	0.9916
2	7	1.4982	1.7812	0.9911
12	13	1.7335	1.8750	0.9858
4	11	1.3725	1.8287	0.9835
14	15	1.6823	1.7390	0.9486
8	16	1.7810	1.8491	0.9359
13	15	2.3895	1.9236	0.8854
7	10	2.2384	1.6660	0.8356
7	16	1.5243	1.5489	0.7757
11	13	1.7915	2.2743	0.6914
9	16	1.9261	1.6984	0.2078
9	13	–	–	−0.9268

(b)

Species		Information Content		Similarity Coef.
j	k	I_j	I_k	$\cos\theta_{jk}$
3	16	0.5283	0.5283	1
8	9	0.8805	0.8805	0.9922
5	14	1.0566	1.0566	0.9656
1	16	1.0581	1.0581	0.9303
2	10	1.0651	1.1419	0.9036
11	12	0.7777	1.1400	0.8925
14	15	1.0193	1.1721	0.8837
6	13	1.1321	1.6345	0.8637
7	9	1.1698	1.1447	0.8287
7	16	0.8218	1.2327	0.8129
4	15	1.0664	1.7513	0.7554
12	13	1.1415	2.0501	0.5342
13	15	0.8120	1.8777	0.3527
10	16	1.0227	1.6414	0.3271
15	16	–	–	−0.9771

Pharmacological data are given in Table 2. The residual rate measured on given dosage (100 μg/ml)[1] has been transformed to lg[M/(residual rate × 100)] so as to examine the activity of a single molecule of the species. Here M is the molecular weight.

IV. Conclusions

(1) 16 species can be divided into two groups according to $[\sum MR, F_2]$ or $[\sum MR, \sum F, (\sum \pi)^2]$, see Table 3.

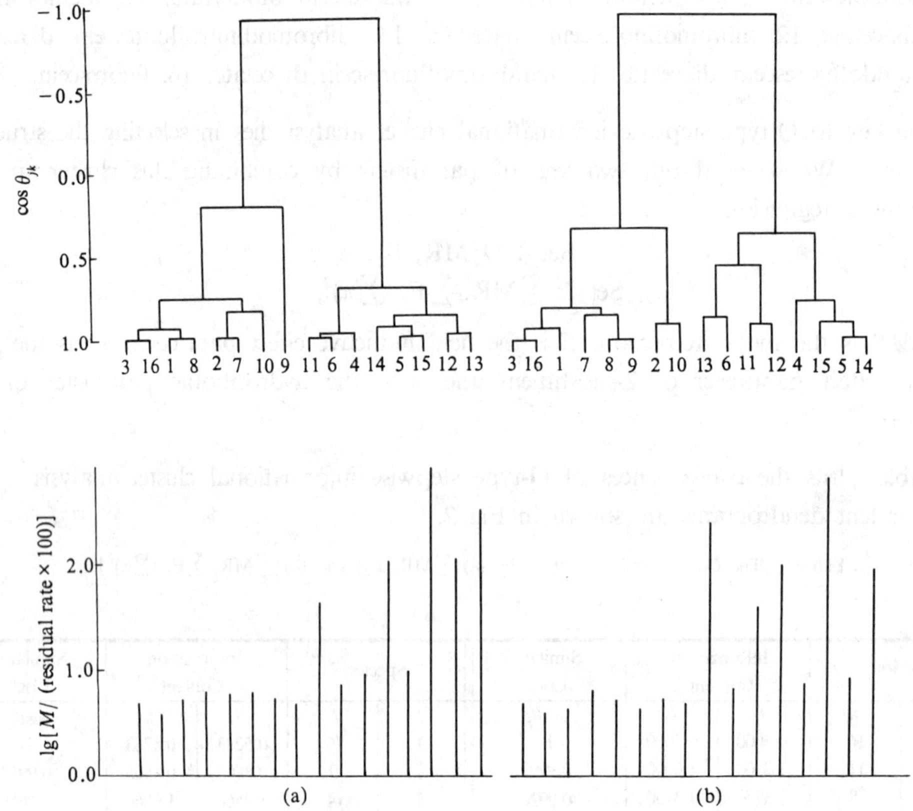

Fig. 2 The dendrogram and the activity against ECa109 of 16 species agglomerated by (a)[$\sum$MR, F_2] and (b)[$\sum$MR, $\sum$F, $(\sum\pi)^2$].

Table 2 Activity of Some Biological Fluorescent Agents Against ECa109 (Dosage: 100 μg/ml)

Species	Residual Rate × 100[a)]	lg[*M*/(Residual; rate × 100)]
1	82.5±6.3	0.703
2	83.0±11.3	0.729
3	69.0±15.5	0.683
4	86.0±9.5	0.877
5	93.0±9.9	0.954
6	81.5±10.6	0.852
7	86.5±2.1	0.829
8	94.5±4.9	0.715
9	85.5±11.3	0.674
10	94.0±4.2	0.701
11	11.6±10.0	1.621
12	5.6±5.5	2.011
13	2.3±2.0	2.461
14	9.0±1.3	2.010
15	1.0±1.0	2.864
16	88.7±9.3	0.573

a) Detemined 4h after dosing.

Table 3 Classification of Species and Their Activity

Higher activity group	species	15	13	12	14	11	5	4	6
	activity	2.864	2.461	2.011	2.010	1.621	0.954	0.877	0.852
Lower activity group	species	7	2	8	1	10	3	9	16
	activity	0.829	0.729	0.715	0.703	0.701	0.683	0.674	0.573

(2) Q-type cluster analysis shows that $\sum MR$ is a very important structure factor influencing the activity, and stepwise regression also shows that its variance-ratio $F(=1186)$ is much larger than the $F^{0.1}_{1,14}$ $(=3.10)$. This is meaningful both theoretically and practically. Since the determination of molar refraction has the advantage of being simple, rapid, accurate, needing only small amount of compound and the data are additive, it can be expected that molar refraction could be used as a valuable index in drug design and activity estimation.

(3) $\sum F$ is another very useful parameter for classification whereas $\sum R$ is not. This suggests that the field inductive effect is much more important than the field conjugative effect.

(4) F_2, the field inductive effect parameter of substituents in the 2-position is more closely related to activity than that of the other substituents. This fact may provide some valuable clues for researching Drug-Receptor interactions. The species may combine with a receptor only through their xanthane moiety, since the steric hindrance at position 2 is larger. Hence species substituted in the 2-position would be less able to interact with the receptor due to steric hindrance. One other possibility is that bond-breaking occurs between the spiro C atom and the O atom, then both the xanthane and isobenzofuran moieties combine with the receptor. In this case, substituents in the 2-position are in a favorable orientation.

The authors are indebted to professor A. B. Dai for suggesting and supporting the study.

References

1 Jin Danian, Zhang Peiyan and Wang Liufang, *journal of Lanzhou Medical College,* 1(1988), 19.

2 Martin, Y.C., *Quantitative Drug Design*, Marcel Rekkev, 1978.

3 Varmuza, K., *Pattern Recognition in Chemistry*, Springer, Berlin, 1980, p. 93.

4 Hansch C., and Leo, A., *Substituent Constants for Correlation Analysis is Chemistry and Biology*, Wiley, New York, 1979.

Sections E and F

Chemical Factor in Environment and Etiology of Cancer, Chemical Protection Against Cancer
Antitumor Agents, Structrue-Activity Relationship in Cancer Chemotherapy

Disposal Methods for Some Known or Suspect Chemical Carcinogens

Margaret-Ann Armour

(*Department of Chemistry, University of Alberta, Edmonton, Canada T6G 2G2*)

I. Introduction

Several groups of workers handle chemicals which are either known or suspect carcinogens in their daily work. These include researchers engaged in cancer research, laboratory technicians, hospital pharmacists, physicians, nurses and operators of some small businesses using chemical dyes or other reagents. In the interests of the health of these workers, and also to prevent these substances from being discarded into the sewer so that they may contaminate drinking water or in other ways harm the environment, it is desirable to have practical and reliable methods for the disposal of waste and surplus quantities of potentially carcinogenic materials. Frequently, the recommended method for disposal is incineration at temperatures above 1000°C. Many users of the chemicals do not have access to such facilities. Thus, it would be very desirable to be able to dispose of the materials on site, thus avoiding the need to transport them to a disposal site.

Since 1982, we have been collecting, developing and testing in the laboratory, chemical methods for converting these materials to non-physiologically active products. We began by searching the chemical and related literature for reactions which might be used to de-activate compounds such as aromatic amines, urethane and ethionine, ethidium bromide, azo dyes and chemotherapeutic drugs. When promising specific reactions had been identified, these were tested in the laboratory. The rate of disappearance of the suspect carcinogen was followed using an appropriate chromatographic technique. As far as possible, the products of the reaction were identified. This could be achieved in the case of relatively simple chemicals and when we were using reactions whose mechanisms were known so that the likely products could be predicted. In the case of large molecules with many functional groups, identification of all of the products was not always possible. This was especially true in the case of several chemotherapeutic drugs when drastic oxidation destruction was used. A large number of fragments were present in the reaction mixture. In these cases, the product mixture was subjected to an Ames test to determine whether the products showed excess mutagenicity over standards.

For a disposal method to be acceptable, several criteria had to be met. At least

99% of the suspect carcinogen had to be destroyed in a reasonable length of time, the products had to be identified as non-carcinogenic, often by using the Ames test, and it had to be possible for workers having minimal chemical background to perform the method safely and reproducibly.

Several of the methods developed for the destruction of chemotherapeutic agents were developed and tested collaboratively with the International Agency for Research on Cancer in Lyons, France. We have been particularly concerned with devising practical and safe ways of treating spills of these compounds or their solutions, especially when a spill occurs in a hospital corridor or patient treatment area.

II. Specific Disposal Methods

Details of a variety of the disposal methods which we have developed are presented here.

1. *Disposal of aromatic amines*

Many aromatic amines have been shown to cause cancer in rodents and are confirmed or suspect human carcinogens. They can be rendered physiologically inactive by removal of the amino group. For example, 4-aminobiphenyl **1** is converted to biphenyl **2** by treatment with sodium nitrite and then hypophosphorous acid. Thus, to

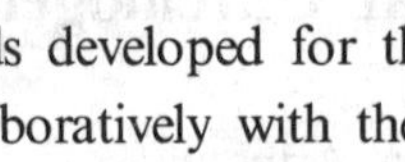

1

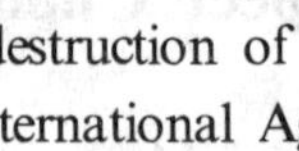

2

1.0 g of 4-aminobiphenyl in a 125 mL. Erlenmeyer flask, is added a mixture of 0.8 mL of water and 2.5 mL of concentrated hydrochloric acid. The mixture is stirred for 10—15 minutes until a homogeneous slurry is formed. The slurry is cooled to 0°C in an ice-salt bath and dropwise, a solution of 1.0 g of sodium nitrite in 2.5 mL of water is added at such a rate that the temperature of the mixture does not rise above 5°C. After stirring for 1 hour, 13 mL of ice-cold 50% hypophosphorus acid is added slowly. Some foaming may occur. After addition of the acid is complete the mixture is stirred for 18 hours at room temperature. The solid is collected by filtration, the filtrate washed into the drain with a large volume of water, and the solid (biphenyl) discarded with normal refuse or disposed of by burning.

Other aromatic amines such as **2**-aminofluorene **3** can be made harmless by a similar reaction which results in the product fluorene, **4**.

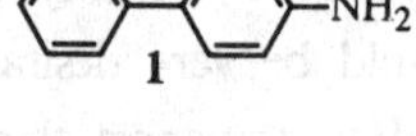

3

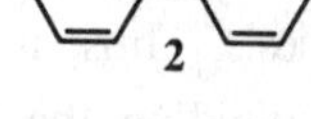

4

The acetyl group of 2-acetylaminofluorene **5** is first removed by acid hydrolysis then the resulting amino group is removed by nitrosation and reduction to again yield fluorene **4**. These reactions can be performed sequentially in the same flask. Details of the

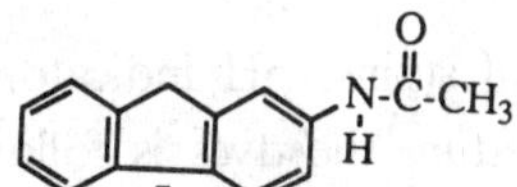

5

reaction are as follows. To 0.25 g of 2-acetylaminofluorene in a 50 mL round-bottomed flask is added 10 mL of 3.6 mol/L hydrochloric acid. The flask is fitted with a condenser and heated at reflux for at least 10 hours when all trace of yellow should have disappeared. The contents of the flask are cooled to 0°C in an ice-salt bath and over a period of 5 minutes, a solution of 0.13 g of sodium nitrite in 0.3 mL of water is added dropwise. The mixture is stirred for 30 minutes, then 2.7 mL of ice-cold 50% hypophosphorus acid are slowly added. After stirring at room temperature for 16 hours, the mixture is filtered, the filtrate washed into the drain and the solid (fluorene) discarded with normal refuse or disposed of by burning.

2. *Disposal of urethane* **6**

$$NH_2\overset{O}{\overset{\|}{C}}OCH_2CH_3$$

6

Also known as ethyl carbamate, this compound is a cancer suspect agent. It can be hydrolyzed in base at room temperature. To urethane (2 g) contained in a 125 mL Erlenmeyer flask equipped with a magnetic stirrer is added 45 mL of 10% aqueous sodium hydroxide solution. After stirring at room temperature for 6 hours or heating under reflux for 10 minutes, no urethane remains and the liquid can be washed into the drain.

3. *Disposal of ethionine* **7**

$$CH_3CH_2SCH_2CH_2\overset{NH_2}{\overset{|}{C}}HCOOH \qquad CH_3SCH_2CH_2\overset{NH_2}{\overset{|}{C}}HCOOH$$

7 **8**

The amino acid ethionine is a cancer suspect agent. All of its physiological effects can be prevented and reversed by the essential amino acid methionine **8**. Ethionine is oxidized and split into fragments by household bleach. The progress of the reaction has been followed by infrared spectroscopy. Ethionine (1 g) is dissolved in 50 mL of water in a 250 mL Erlenmeyer flask and, with stirring, 60 mL of household bleach (5% sodium hypochlorite is added). Stirring is continued at room temperature for 2 hours, then the liquid can be washed into the drain.

4. *Disposal of azodyes*

Azo dyes are used as biological stains, pH indicators and textile dyes. A description of the general method used to denature the dyes is followed by a table giving the weight of each azo dye which can be decomposed by the quantities of reagents given in the general method. The azo dye is dissolved in 10 mL of 6 mol/L hydrochloric acid (5 mL of concentrated hydrochloric acid added to 5 mL of water). To the solution is added 0.5 g of tin powder, and the mixture stirred at room temperature for 2 hours. The excess tin can be removed by filtration, or the mixture allowed to stand until the solid has settled to the bottom of the container and the clear liquid decanted. The tin can be washed with dilute hydrochloric acid and reused. To the clear solution is added 100 mL of 2 mol/L sulfuric acid (11.1 mL of concentrated sulfuric acid carefully added to 90 mL of water) and 100 mL of freshly prepared 0.2 mol/L potassium permanganate solution (5.7 g of potassium permanganate in 100 mL of water). The mixture is stirred for 24 hours and solid sodium bisulfite is added until the liquid is clear and colourless. It is then neutralized by the addition either of sodium bicarbonate or of 5% sodium hydroxide solution and poured into the drain.

Azo Dye	Wt. of Dye to be Used in General Procedure
o-Aminoazotoluene	0.3 g
Benzopurpurin	0.5 g
Congo Reg	0.4 g
Methyl Orange	0.4 g
Methyl Red	0.35 g
Oil Red XO	0.35 g
Sudan IV	0.3 g

5. *Disposal of ethidium bromide* **9**

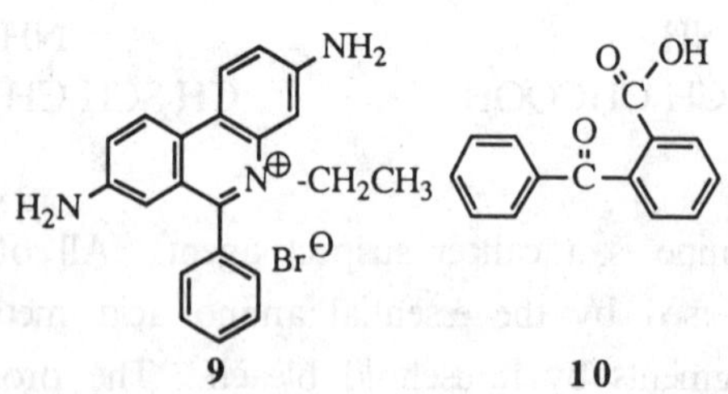

9 **10**

Ethidium bromide is a compound frequently used in genetic testing since it intercalates double stranded DNA and RNA. It is known to be mutagenic and therefore must be handled with care. It is normally used in very dilute solution, and we have found that it can be destroyed in these solutions by treatment with household bleach. When a solution of 34 mg of ethidium bromide in 100 mL of water is stirred at room temperature with 300 mL of household bleach for 2 hours, the ethidium bromide is converted to the physiologically inactive product 2-carboxybenzo-phenone **10**. The p oduct solution does not show excess mutagenicity over standards in the Ames test.

6. *Disposal of chemotherapeutic drugs*

Disposal methods for a variety of chemotherapeutic drugs are described. For each method is included a table listing the drugs which can be destroyed, and including reagent quantities and reaction conditions, and a description of how to treat solid residues, solutions of the drug and glassware contaminated with the drug.

(i) Treatment with acidic potassium permanganate Acidic potassium permanganate is a powerful oxidizing medium and can often be used to break a molecule into non-toxic and non-mutagenic products which can be washed into the drain. Table 1

Table 1

Drug and Quantity	Volume of Water	Volume of Concentrated Sulfuric Acid	Weight of Potassium Permanganate	Time Mixture Stirred at Room Temperature
Chlorambucil				
50 mg (25 tablets)	10 mL	2 mL	1.8 g	4 hours
Daunorubicin				
30 mg	10 mL	2 mL	1.0 g	2 hours
30 mg in 10 mL solution	0	3 mL	1.0 g	2 hours
Doxorubicin				
30 mg	10 mL	2 mL	1.0 g	2 hours
30 mg in 10 mL solution	0	3 ml	1.0 g	2 hours
Dichloromethotrexate				
10 mg	10 mL	2 mL	0.5 g	1 hour
10 mg in 10 mL solution	0	2 mL	0.5 g	1 hour
Methotrexate				
50 mg	10 mL	2 mL	0.5 g	1 hour
50 mg in 10 mL solution	0	2 mL	0.5 g	1 hour
6-Mercaptopurine				
18 mg	17 mL	3 mL	0.13 g	12 hours
9 mg in 10 ml solution	0	3 mL	0.13 g	12 hours
6-Thioguanine				
18 mg	17 mL	3 mL	0.13 g	12 hours
9 mg in 10 mL solution	0	3 mL	0.13 g	12 hours
Streptozotocin				
48 mg	10 mL	2 mL	2 g	12 hours
48 mg in 10 mL solution	0	2 mL	2 g	12 hours
Vincristine sulfate				
10 mg	10 mL	2 mL	0.5 g	2 hours
10 mg in 10 mL solution	0	3 mL	0.65 g	2 hours
Vinblastine Sulfate				
10 mg	10 mL	2 mL	0.5 g	2 hours
10 mg in 10 mLsolution	0	3 mL	0.65 g	2 hours

lists the drugs which are made harmless by treatment with this reagent, the quantities of potassium permanganate and concentrated sulfuric acid required to deactivate a given quantity of the drug, and the time for which the solutions should be allowed to stand. Conditions are given for both solid material and reconstituted aqueous solutions. Solid material is dissolved in the water and the sulfuric acid added. Sulfuric acid is added to the reconstituted solutions. In both cases, solid potassium permanganate is slowly added to the stirred mixture. Should the purple colour fade before reaction time is complete, more potassium permanganate should be added. When the reaction is complete the mixture is neutralized with 10% sodium hydroxide then sodium bisulfite is added until a colourless solution is formed. This solution is washed into the drain.

Glassware including vials containing residues of the drugs is immersed in a solution prepared by dissolving 4.7g of potassium permanganate in 83 mL of water and 17 mL of concentrated sulfuric acid. After standing overnight the glassware is rinsed thoroughly with water and discarded or reused. The permanganate solution is neutralized by the careful addition of 10% sodium hydroxide, then sodium bisulfite is stirred into the mixture until a colourless solution is formed. This solution is washed into the drain.

As a safety precaution when using potassium permanganate wear gloves, goggles and a laboratory coat. As far as possible work in a fume hood. Concentrated sulfuric acid is extremely corrosive and should be handled with care. Immediately, wash spills on the skin with cold running water for 20 minutes. Always add sulfuric acid to water, never the other way round. Heat is produced during the neutralization of the acidic solution with 10% sodium hydroxide. When sodium bisulfite is added, some sulfur dioxide may be produced; therefore this addition should be made in a fume hood or in a well ventilated area.

(ii) Treatment with household bleach (5% sodium hypochlorite) or calcium hypochlorite solution Household bleach and calciun hypochlorite solution, although not as powerful oxidizing agents as acidic potassium permanganate, can be used to decompose several hazardous pharmaceuticals. Conditions for the effective denaturation of these materials are listed in Table 2. Calcium hypochlorite solution is prepared by stirring 10 g of calcium hypochlorite with 100 mL of water for 2 hours, then removing the undissolved material by decantation or filtration. The bleach or calcium hypochlorite solution is added to the solid or solution. When reaction is complete, the solution is washed into the drain.

Glassware including vials containing residues of the drugs is immersed in bleach and allowed to stand overnight. It is rinsed thoroughly with water and reused or discarded. When reaction is complete, the mixture is washed into the drain.

As a safety precaution when using bleach wear gloves, goggles and a laboratory coat.

Table 2

Drug and Quantity	Volume of Bleach or Calcium Hypochlorite Solution	Time Mixture to Stir at Room Temperature
Amsacrine 10 mg	100 mL bleach	30 minutes
Dactinomycin 10 mg soild or 10 mg in 20 mL solution	200 mL bleach	1 hour
Methotrexate 20 mg solid or 20 mg in 10 mL solution	25 mL bleach	30 minutes
Fluorouracil 500 mg in 10 mL solution	40 mL calcium hypochlorite solution	30 minutes
Procarbazine Hydrochloride 500 mg in 30 mL solution	60 mL calcium hypochlorite solution	12 hours
Mercaptopurine 3.2 mg in 1 mL solution	25 mL bleach	90 minutes
Thioguanine 3.2 mg in 1 mL solution	25 mL bleach	90 minutes

As far as possible, work in the fume hood. Bleach solution is corrosive. Immediately wash spills on the skin with cold running water for 15 minutes. Avoid breathing the vapors from bleach.

(iii) Base hydrolysis Hydrolysis in base denatures mytomycin C, thiotepa, cyclophosphamide, and ifosphamide. The conditions of hydrolysis are listed in Table 3.

Table 3

Drug and Quantity	Base Concentrations and Volume	Time and Conditions of Reaction
Mitomycin C 5 mg solid or 5 mg in 10 ml solution	50 mL of 10% sodium hydroxide	12 hours
Thiotepa 20 mg solid or 20 mg in 20 mL solution	20 mL of 4% sodium hydroxide	Heat under reflux for 1 hour
Cyclophosphamide 500 mg solid or 500 mg in 25 mL water	50 mL of 12% sodium hydroxide and 100 ml of dimethylformamide	Heat under reflux for 4 hours
Ifosphamide 100 mg solid or 100 mg in 25 mL water	10 mL of 12% sodium hydroxide and 20 mL of dimethylformamide	Heat under reflux for 4 hours
DETERGENT SOLUTION		
Lomustine 100 mg solid or 100 mg in 25 mL water	20 mL of detergent solution	Heat at 55°C for 30 minutes
Carmutine 100 mg solid or 100 mg in 25 mL water	20 mL of detergent solution	Heat at 55°C for 90 minutes

The base is added to the solid drug or its solution. When reaction is complete, the solution is neutralized by careful addition of 2 mol/L hydrochloric acid (10 mL of concentrated hydrochloric acid added to 50 mL of water), and washed into the drain.

Lomustine and carmustine are decomposed in basic synthetic detergent solution. The solution (100 mL) is prepared by dissolving 4.8 g of sodium pyrophosphate in 100-mL of water and adding 1 mL of Triton X100. When 100 mg of either drug is added to 20 mL of the detergent solution and heated at 55°C for 90 minutes, non-toxic and non-carcinogenic products are formed. The solution is washed into the drain.

Glassware including vials containing residues of mitomycin C and thiotepa is immersed in 10% aqueous sodium hydroxide, allowed to stand overnight and washed thoroughly with water before reusing or discarding. Glassware containing residues of cyclophosphamide and ifosphamide is rinsed thoroughly with dimethylformamide. The rinses are added to one half their volume of 10% sodium hydroxide solution and the mixture heated under reflux for 4 hours. The cooled solution is neutralized by careful addition of 2 mol/L hydrochloric acid (10 mL of concentrated hydrochloric acid added to 50 mL of water) and washed into the drain. Glassware containing residues of carmustine and lomustine is decontaminated by immersing in synthetic detergent solution at 55°C for 2 hours. The glassware is rinsed thoroughly or reused. The solution is washed into the drain.

As a safety precaution when using base, wear gloves, goggles and a laboratory coat. As far as possible, work in the fume hood. Basic solutions are corrosive especially when hot. Should a spill occur on the skin, immediately wash with cold running water for 15 minutes. Avoid breathing vapor of dimethylformamide and skin contact. Should skin contact occur, wash immediately with soap and water.

(iv) Treatment with diethyldithiocarbamate Diethyldithiocarbamate complexes with platinum so this reagent is used to denature cisplatin and carboplatin. A solution containing 1 g of diethyldithiocarbamate in 100 mL of 0.1 mol/L sodium hydroxide is prepared. For each 10 mg of cisplatin or carboplatin is added 3 mL of the diethyldithiocarbamate solution and 3 mL of a saturated solution of sodium nitrate. After mixing thoroughly, the solution is discarded into the drain.

Glassware containing residues of cisplatin or carboplatin is immersed in a 1: 1 diethyldithiocarbamate solution and saturated sodium nitrate solution. After standing overnight it is rinsed thoroughly with water and reused or discarded. The solution is discarded into the drain.

As a safety precaution when using diethyldithiocarbamate, wear gloves, goggles and a laboratory coat. And possible work should be done in the fume hood.

(v) Treatment of spills Before handling a hazardous pharmaceutical, be ready to take appropriate action, should a spill occur. This requires both knowing what to do, and having appropriate materials and reagents available.

Isolate the area of the spill and wear protective clothing including gloves and eye protection. In general, spills of solid or solutions are deactivated using the reagents and conditions which destroy surplus quantities as described. However, the initial treatment of the spill depends upon the danger to health which the spilled compound presents, thus solid spills of less hazardous compounds are scooped into a container, then treated with the appropriate reagent, and spills or solutions of these compounds are absorbed on suitable material and similarly treated. The area of the spill is washed thoroughly with a strong soap solution.

On the other hand, the appropriate deactivating solution such as bleach, acidified potassium permanganate or other reagent is poured directly onto spills of compounds which are particularly hazardous to handle. The liquid is absorbed onto suitable material, the material covered with deactivating solution and allowed to stand overnight. If the deactivating solution is acidic potassium permanganate, the solution is carefully neutralized with 10% aqueous sodium hydroxide, decolourized by the slow addition with stirring of solid sodium bisulfite and washed into the drain; bleach solution is washed into the drain; hydrochloric or sulfuric acids are carefully neutralized with 10% aqueous sodium hydroxide and washed into the drain; sodium hydroxide solutions are carefully neutralized with 2 mol/L hydrochloric acid (1 volume of concentrated hydrohloric acid to 5 volumes of water) and washed into the drain; solutions of diethyldithiocarbamate and sodium nitrate are washed into the drain. The area of the spill is washed thoroughly with strong soap solution. The material used to absorb the spill may be paper towels, gauze or a chemical spill absorbent. We have found a 1: 1: 1 mixture of soda ash, clay cat litter (bentonite) and sand to be very effective. After denaturing the spill, the liquid is washed into the drain, and the solid residue from whatever absorbing material was used discarded as normal refuse.

Solutions of potassium permanganate for treating spills are prepared by dissolving 4.7 g of potassium permanganate in 100 mL of 3 mol/L sulfuric acid (17 mL concentrated sulfuric acid added to 83 mL of water). This solution should be freshly prepared daily. If the pink colour fades during treatment of the spill leaving a brown mixture, more potassium permanganate should be added.

Previously unopened containers of bleach should be used.

Compounds which are particularly hazardous to handle so that deactivating solution should be poured directly onto spills of them include lomustine, streptozotocin, chlorozotocin, cisplatin, cyclophosphamide, ifosphamide, 6-thioguanine, 6-mercaptopurine and ethidium bromide, mitomycin C, procarbazine, chlorambucil and thiotepa. Compounds not included in this list must also be handled with care.

The author is grateful to the agencies who provided funds for this work, the Alberta Environmental Research Trust, the Alberta Heritage Foundation for Medical Research, the Heritage Grant Program of Alberta Occupational Health and Safety, to the collaborators in th project, Dr. Lois Browne and Ms. Rosemary Bacovsky, and to the researchers involved in the project, Katherine Ayer, Patricia McKenzie, Carmen Miller, Roger Klemm and Donna Renecker.

Much of the work described was part of a collaborative study with IARC, the International Agency for Research on Cancer. A book[1] *describing this work has been published. Our group has produced two manuals*[2] *which detail, for individual chemicals, many of the disposal methods which we have tested. The second edition of Potentially Carcinogenic Chemicals Information and Disposal Guide is in preparation.*

References

1 Castegnaro, M., Adams, j., Armour, M. A. *et al.,* Laboratory decontamination and destruction of carcinogens in laboratory wastes: some antineoplastic agents, *IARC Scientific Publications,* No. 73, 1986.

2 a) Armour, M. A., Bacovsky, R. A., browne, L. M. *et al., Potentially Carcinogenic Chemicals Information and Disposal Guide,* University of Alberta, Department of Chemistry, 1986.

b) Armour, M. A., *Hazardous Laboratory Chemicals Disposal Guide,* CRC Press, Boca Raton, FL, 1991.

Carcinogenicity of Dinitrobenzo(a)pyrenes and Dinitrofluoranthenes in F344 Rats

Kazumi Horikawa, Nobuyuki Sera, Koichi Murakami,
Takeshi Otofuji, Hiroshi Tokiwa,

(*Department of Health Science, Fukuoka Environmental Research Center,* 39 *Mukaisano, Dazaifu, Fukuoka* 818-01, *Japan*)

Keisuke Izumi and Hisashi Otsuka

(*Second Department of Pathology, School of Medicine, The University of Tokushima, Kuramoto-Cho* 3-18-15, *Tokushima* 770, *Japan*)

Abstract: In general, dinitroarenes are more mutagenic than the othe nitrated aromatic compounds. Dinitropyrenes (DNPs), dinitrofluoranthenes (DNFs), and dinitrobenzo (a) pyrenes (DNBPs) are extraordinary mutagens, inducing revertants at a level of 10^5 for *Salmonella typhimurium* strain TA 98. In addition, the 1, 3, 1, 6-and 1, 8-isomers of DNPs are well known to be potent carcinogens in rats and mice, 3, 9- and 3, 7-DNFs were tested for tumorigenicity by implantation into the lungs of rats, and their risk for human carcinogenesis was determined. 3, 6-DNBP, a new mutagen, was detected in airborne particulates. This compound also induced 137, 000 revertants in strain TA98 per nmol. The related compounds including 1, 6-DNBP, were found to be activated by acetyltransferase but not nitroreductase. It is important to know whether or not the ability to reduce activation is associated with the bioligical activity. In this study, the major mutagens 3, 6-and 1, 6-DNBP were tested for carcinogenicity in F344 rats, and the correlation with their mutagenicity was investigated. The incidence of lung cancer induced by 3, 9-DNF was twice as high as that of BaP when tumorigenicity was compared at approximately equivalent dose levels of 0. 34 μmol 3, 9-DNF and 0.39 μmol BaP. Tumorigenicity of 3, 7-DNF was lower than 3, 9-DNF when compared with a dose level of 0.68 μmole per rat. Most tumors induced by 3, 9-DNF at a higher doses were identified as squamous cell carcinomas. 3, 6-DNBP was a tumorigenic compound in rats whereas 1, 6-DNBP did not induce any tumors up to 45 weeks after inoculation with the chemical.

I. Introduction

In general, dinitroarenes are more mutagenic than the other nitrated aromatic compounds. Dinitropyrenes (DNPs), dinitrofluoranthenes (DNFs), and dinitrobenzo (a) pyrenes (DNBPs) are extraordinary mutagens, inducing revertants at the magnitude of 10^5 for *Salmonella typhimurium* strain TA98[1, 2, 3]. In addition, 1, 3, 1, 6- and 1, 8-isomers are well known to be potent carcinogens in rats and mice[4, 5]. 3, 9-and 3, 7-DNFs were tested for tumorigenicity by implantation into the lungs of rats, and their risk for human carcinogenesis was determined.

3, 6-DNBP, a new mutagen, was detected in airborne particulates[6]. This compound also induced 137,000 revertants of strain TA98 per nmole. The related compounds including 1, 6-DNBP, were found to be activated by acetyltransferase but not nitroreductase. It is important to know whether or not the ability to reduce activation is associated with the biological activity.

In this stud , the major mutagens 3, 6- and 1, 6-DNBP were tested for carcinogenicity in F344 rats, and the correlation with their mutagenicity was investigated.

II. Materials and Methods

1. *Chemicals*

3-Nitrofluoranthene (3-NF) was purchased from R. K. Chemical Co. Ltd., USA, and purified to 99.9% purity by high-performance liquid chromatography (HPLC). 3, 7- and 3, 9-DNF were synthesized by nitration of fluoranthene in the presence of fuming nitric acid, fractionated on an alumina column and finally purified on a column of Unisile C18 (Gasukuro Kogyo Inc., Tokyo, Japan) by HPLC[1]. The purity of the two compounds was 99.9 and 99.98%, respectively. 1, 6- and 3, 6-DNBP were synthesized by nitration of 3, 4-benzo(a)pyrene (Wako Pure Chemical Industries, Ltd., Osaka, Japan) in the presence of fuming nitric acid, fractionated on an alumina column and finally purified on a column of Unisile C18 for HPLC[3]. The purity of the compounds was 99.53 and 99.46% respectively. Benzo(a)pyrene (BaP), used as a positive control, was obtained from Aldrich Chemical Co., Inc., Milwaukee, WI, USA.

2. *Mutagenicity test*

Mutagenicity was tested by the *Salmonella* microsome assay system[7]. Strains used in this study were *Salmonella typhimurium* TA98, TA98NR (a nitroreductase-deficient mutant), and TA98/1, 8-DNP$_6$ (an acetyltransferase-deficient mutant)[2].

3. *Animals*

Six-week-old male F344/DuCrj rats used in the two experiments were purchased from Charles River Japan Inc., Atsugi, Japan. The rats were housed in stainless steel cages containing sterilized granulated wood bedding and given a commercial pellet diet (Oriental MF; Oriental Yeast Co. Ltd., Tokyo) and tap water *ad libitum*.

4. *Pulmonary imlantatin of* 3, 7*-and* 3, 9*-DNA*, 3*-NF and BaP*

The rats were treated with chemicals when they were 11 weeks old, at which time their body weight had reached 250g. The chemicals were implanted by the method of Stanton *et al.*[8] as a suspension in a mixture of equal volumes of beeswax (Nakarai Chemicals, Kyoto, Japan) and tricaprylin(Sigma Chemical Co., St. Louis, MO, USA). The doses were

100 μg for 3-NF, 200 μg for 3, 7-DNF, and 200, 100 and 50 μg for 3, 9-DNF and BaP. Control rats were given only the beeswax-tricaprylin mixture. The rats were anesthetized by i. m. injection of ketamine hydrochloride (100 mg/kg body weight; Sankyo Zoki Co. Ltd, Tokyo), a left lateral thoracotomy was performed, and 50 μl of beeswax-tricaprylin containing the test chemical was injected directly into the lower third of the left lung. After injection, the mixture formed a solid, defined pellet in the lung. No rats died within one week after this injection. All rats were observed for up to 100 weeks after injection.

5. *Subcutaneous injection of* 1, 6-*and* 3, 6-*DNBP and BaP*

Rats were inoculated in the back s.c. with 50μl of a mixture of equal volumes of beeswax and tricaprylin. The doses of 1, 6- and 3, 6-DNBP and BaP were 8, 40, 200 and 1000μg. Some of the rats given these chemicals are still under study. Rates that died or were killed because they became moribund due to the occurrence of tumors during this period were autopsied, and survivors were killed for autopsy after 100 weeks. The lungs, liver, spleen, heart and kidneys were weighed. All organs were fixed in 10% neutralized formalin solution. Grossly apparent lesions and tissues from all major viscera were studied histologically. Sections were routinely stained with hematoxylin and cosin, and some sections were stained by the periodic acidSchiff reaction, alcian blue at pH 2.5 or by silver impregnation for reticulin.

III. Results

1. *Lung tumors induced by a single injection of* 3-*NF, and* 3, 7- *and* 3, 9-*DNF*

Table 1 shows the incidence of lung tumors caused by 3-NF, 3, 7-and, 3, 9-DNF and BaP. These results were obtained by the 100th week after injection of the chemicals into the lungs of rats. The first tumor found in rats given 200 μg of 3, 9-DNF was seen on day 257 after injection of the chemical, and most of the rats (90.5%) developed lung tumors within 27 weeks after the first tumor appeared. In the rats treated with 100 μg of 3, 9-DNF, the first tumor was seen on day 371 after injection, and 70% of the rats developed lung tumors within 29 weeks after the first tumor appeared. Only one rat treated with 50 μg of 3, 9-DNF developed a tumor, indicating that this is the minimum dose for tumor induction. In the rats given 200 μg of 3, 7-DNF, the first tumor was seen on day 351 after injection, and 12 (54.5%) of the 22 rats developed lung tumors within 73 weeks after injection. In the 3-NF-treated rats, a tumor developed in only one (5.0%) of the 20 rats during 100 weeks of observation.

Macroscopically, the tumors were grayish-white, solid and hard, with irregular foci of hemorrhage and necrosis. Most tumors showed expansive growth, but secondary involvement of the adjacent organs, e. g. the diaphragm, heart, ribs and vertebrae, was usually observed. In many cases the esophagus was compressed by the tumor mass.

Table 1 Lung Lesions Isduced by Intrapulmonary Implantation of the Chemicals

Chemical	Dose (nmol / rat)	Initial No. of Rats	Effective No. of Rats	No. of Rats With Lung Lesion					Total With Tumors (%)
				Granulo-matous lesions	Squamous metaplasia	Squamous cell carcinoma	Adeno-squamous carcinoma	Undiffer-entiated neoplasm	
3, 9-DNF	200	22	21	0	1	18	1	0	19 (90.5)
	100	10	10	1	0	5	1	1	7 (70.0)
	50	10	10	4	0	0	0	1	1 (10.0)
BaP	200	9	9	0	0	3	0	1	4 (44.4)
	100	10	10	6	1	2	1	0	3 (30.0)
	50	10	10	3	1	0	0	0	0 (0.0)
3, 7-DNF	200	22	22	2	3	11	0	1	12 (54.5)
3-NF	1000	20	20	14	0	1	0	0	1 (5.0)
Control	—	20	19	15	0	0	0	0	0 (0.0)

Histologically, the lung lesions induced by 3, 9-and, 3, 7-DNF, 3-NF and BaP were classified as simple granulomatous lesions, keratinizing squamous metaplasias, squamous cell carcinoma, adenosquamous carcinoma and undifferentiated neoplasms. Most tumors induced by 3, 9-DNF were squamous cell carcinomas, and the others were adenosquamous cell carcinomas and undifferentiated neoplasms. Squamous cell carcinomas were found in rats given higher doses of 3, 9-DNF (Fig 1). The tumors induced by BaP also were mostly squamous cell carcinomas, and only one adenosquamous cell carcinoma and one undifferentiated neoplasm were observed. Poorly differentiated squamous cell carcinomas, which were squamous cell carcinomas with sarcomatoue components, were found in 5 rats treated with 200 μg of 3, 9-DNF and one rat treated with 3, 7-DNF.

As shown in Table 1, 3, 9-DNF induced a higher incidence of lung cancer than the equivalent doses of BaP; with doses of 200 μg (3, 9-DNF and BaP equivalent to 0.68 and 0.79 μmole respectively), the incidence was 90.5 and 44.4%; and with doses of 100 μg (3, 9-DNF and BaP equivalent to 0.34 and 0.4 μmole, respectively), it was 70 and 30%, respectively. The tumorigenic potency of 3, 9-DNF was approximately twofold that of BaP (Fig. 2).

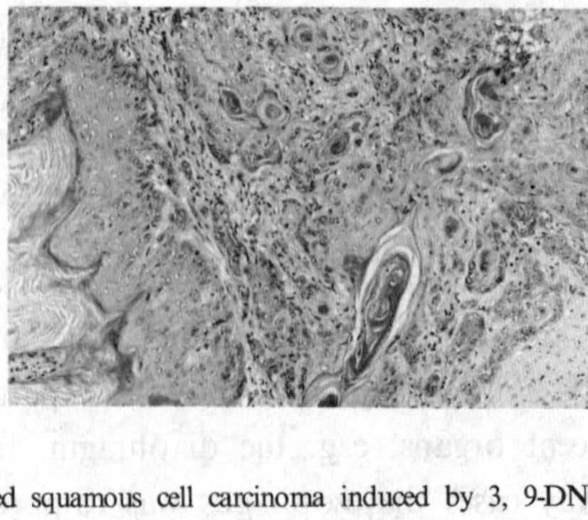

Fig. 1 Well-differentiated squamous cell carcinoma induced by 3, 9-DNF (H&E, ×50)

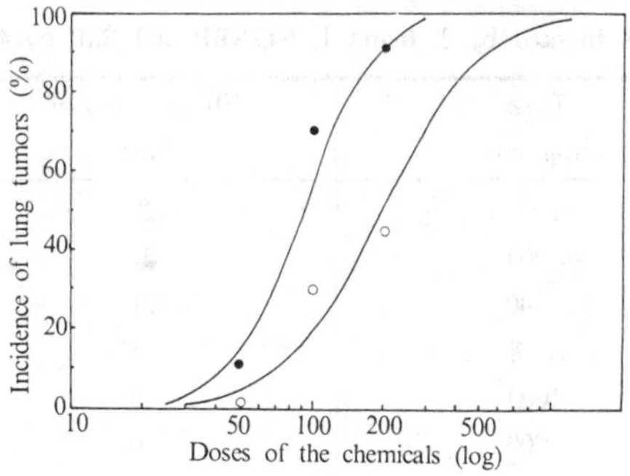

Fig. 2 Dose-response curves of the incidence of lung tumors induced by 3, 9-DNF (●—●) and BaP (○—○).

Table 2 Mutagenicity of 1, 6- and 3, 6-DNBP in the *Salmonella* Test Microsome System

Chemical	Revertants per ng for *Salmonella* His-strains (-S9)		
	TA98	TA98NR	TA98/1, 8-DNP$_6$
1, 6-DNBP	4.4	0.9	0.1
3, 6-DNBP	400	256	3.8

Dose-response relationships of tumors induced by 3, 9-DNF and BaP were examined statistically by the probit method. Sigmoid curves were obtained with both 3, 9-DNF and BaP at P values of 0.01 and 0.05, respectively, and fitted very well the data of this experiment, when the incidence of lung tumors was plotted against the logarithms of the doses of the two chemicals.

2. *Mutagenicity of* 1, 6- *and* 3, 6-*DNBP for strain TA98, TA98NR and TA98/*1, 8-*DNP*$_6$

Fig. 3 shows the chemical structure of 1, 6-and 3, 6-DNBP. For strain TA98, 1, 6- and 3, 6-DNBP induced 4.4 and 400 revertants, respectively, per ng of the chemical (Table 2). The mutagenic potency of 3, 6-DNBP corresponded to 100 times that of 1, 6-DNBP. In addition, the mutagenicity of 3, 6-DNBP was greatly reduced for the acetyltransferase-deficient strain TA98/1, 8-DNP$_6$, compared with that for the parent strain TA98. This result indicates that 3, 6-DNBP was activated by acetyltranferase but not nitroreductase. The activation was associated with the substituted position of nitro function in the chemical structure; nitro function substituted at the 3-position was reducible to amino derivatives (data not shown).

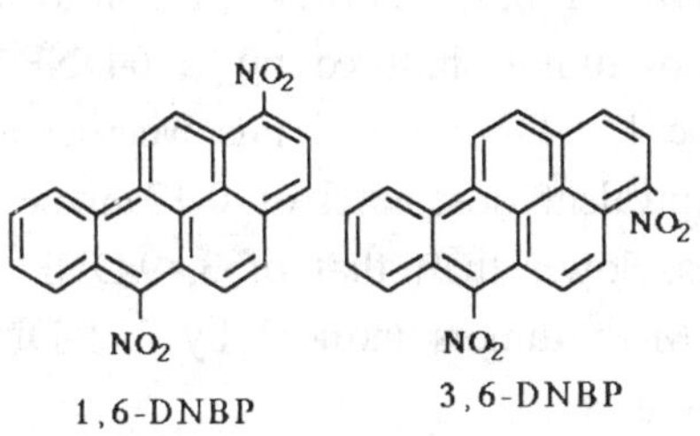

Fig. 3 Structure of Dinitrobenzo(a)pyrenes.

3. *Subcutaneous tumors induced by a single injection of* 1, 6- *and* 3, 6-*DNBP and BaP*

In rats given 1000 μg of 3, 6-DNBP, the first tumors were found on day 183 after

Table 3 Incidence of Tumors Induced by 3, 6-and 1, 6-DNBP and BaP by 45 Weeks After Inoculation

Chemical	Dose (μg/rat)	Effective No. of Rats	No, of Rats With s.c. Tumor (%)
3, 6-DNBP	1000	20	11 (55)
	200	21	4 (19)
	40	21	1 (5)
	8	21	0
1, 6-DNBP	1000	10	
	200	10	
	40	10	
	8	11	
BaP	1000	11	8 (73)
	200	11	4 (36)
	40	11	2 (18)
	8	11	0
Control	-	20	0

inoculation of the chemical, and 11 (55%) of the 20 rats developed subcutaneous tumors within 40 weeks after the inoculation. Of the 21 rats treated with 100 μg of the chemical, 4 (19%) developed tumors at the inoculation site. No tumors were induced by 1, 6-DNBP up to 40 weeks after inoculation (Table 3). Of the 11 rats given 1000 μg of BaP, 8 (73%) developed tumors after the first inoculation, and 4 (36%) of the 11 rats given 200 μg of BaP developed tumors at the inoculation site. Histologically, tumors induced by 3, 6-DNBP were malignant fibrous histiocytomas.

IV. Discussion

The incidence of lung tumors induced by 3, 9-DNF and BaP was dose-dependent. The incidence of lung cancer induced by 3, 9-DNF was twice as high as that induced by BaP when tumorigenicity was compared at the approximately equivalent dose levels of 0.34 μmole of 3, 9-DNF and 0.39 μmole of BaP. However, the incidence of tumors induced by 3, 9-DNF was lower than that of tumors induced by 1, 6-DNP[9]; the incidence of tumors was approximately 50% for the 1, 6-DNP-treated rats whereas it was only 10% for the 3, 9-DNF-treated rats at the equivalent dose level of 0.17 μmole. On the other hand, the tumorigenicity of 3, 7-DNF was lower than that of 3, 9-DNF when compared at a dose level of 0.68 μmole per rat. Most tumors induced by 3, 9-DNF at higher doses were identified as squamous cell carcinomas.

On the other hand, both dinitrobenzo (a) pyrenes mutated *Salmonella* tester strain TA98, and the mutagenic activity of the 3, 6-isomer corresponded to 100 times that of the 1, 6-isomer; the activation of these chemicals was due to the formation of an amino derivative through a nitros derivative at the 3-position of the chemical structure. In this study, 3, 6-DNBP was also tumorigenic in rats whereas 1, 6-DNBP did not induce any tumors up to 45 weeks after inoculation. It is suggested that the poor carcinogenicity of 1, 6-DNBP at the dose levels used may be due to the lack of metabolic activation at the 1- or 6-position of the chemical structure.

References

1 Nakagawa, R., Horikawa, K., Sera, N. *et al.*, *Mutation Res.*, **191**(1987), 85.
2 Rosenkranz, H. S. and Mermelstein, R., *Mutation Res.*, **114**(1983), 212.
3 Fukuhara, K., Miyata, N., Matsui, M. *et al.*, *Chem. Pharm. Bull.* (in press).
4 Tokiwa, H., Otofuji, T., Horikawa, K. *et al.*, *Carcinogenesis,* **8**(1987), 1919.
5 Ohgaki, H., Negishi, C., Wakabayashi, K. *et al.*, *Carcinogenesis,* **5**(1984), 583.
6 Sera, N., Kai, M., Horikawa, K. *et al.*, *Mutation Res.*, **263**(1991), 2.
7 Maron, D. M. and Ames, B.N., *Mutation Res.*, **113**(1983), 173.
8 Stanton, M. F., Miller, E., Wrench, C. *et al.*, *J. Natl. Cancer Inst.*, **49**(1972), 867.
9 Iwagawa, M., Maeda, T., Izumi, K. *et al.*, *Caoinogenesis,* **10**(1989), 1285.

Quantum Chemical Study of Antitumor Agents—Lycobetaine and Its Derivatives*

Quantum Chemical Indexes and Molecular Electrostatic Potentials

GAN Ling, CHEN Kaixian, WU Ji'an and JI Ruyun

(*Laboratory of New Drug Research, Shanghai Institute of Materia Medica, Academia Sinica, Shanghai* 200031, *China*)

Abstract: In this paper are reported the results of employing MNDO and CNDOEP programs to calculate the quantum chemical indexes and the molecular electrostatic potentials of a new kind of antitumor agent— lycobetaine and its analogues. Results show that the absence of steric hindrance, and the formation of two strong positive electrostatic potential areas and one negative area are factors which are necessary for the antitumor activity of these compounds.

I. Introduction

Lycobetaine (Ungeremine, AT-1840, I), developed by our institute, is a new antitumor agent which is partially synthesized from *Lycorine*[1]. It inhibits the growth of many experimental tumor systems: Ehrlich ascites carcinoma, leukemia L1210, P388, Lewis lung carcinoma, Yoshida sarcoma and sarcoma 180. It is attractive in that it shows only low inhibition of the hemopoietic system and leads to no other severe harmful side reactions[2]. Early examinations of the structure activity relationship of lycobetaine gave the following results[3-5]. Firstly, the potential betaine and the methylendioxy group in this compound are critical to its exhibiting antitumor activity. Secondly, fission of the five—membered ring of lycobetaine does not affect its antitumor activity. Thirdly, changes in the distance of the betaine in lycobetaine obviously influence its antitumor activity.

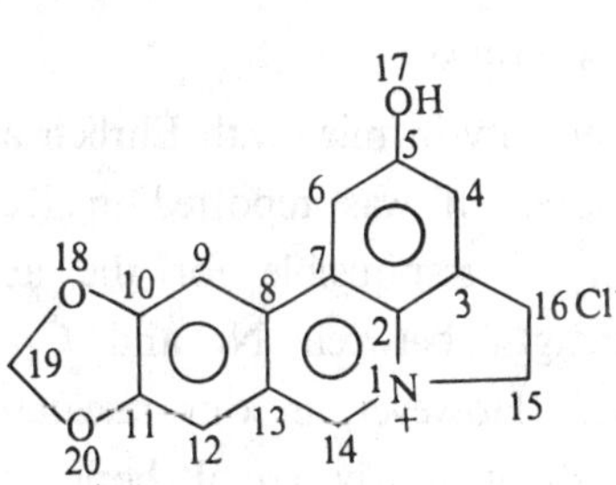

I

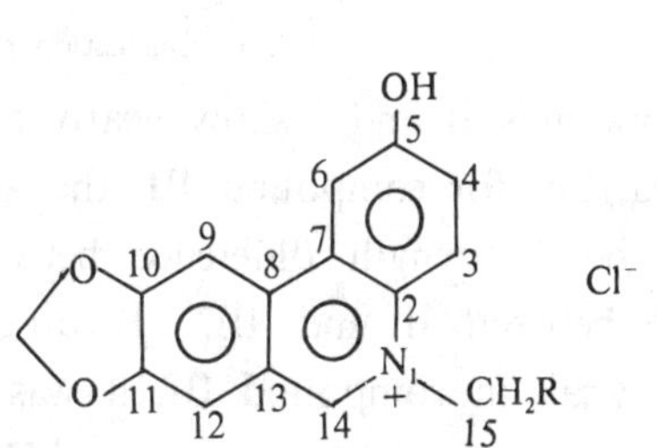

II. R = H   III. R = CH_3

In order to understand the antitumor mechanism of lycobetaine and discover more

* Project supported by the National Natural Science Foundation of China.

active antitumor agents of this type of compound, the quantum chemical calculation method has been employed to study the structural character, electrostatics of lycobetaine and its derivatives.

II. Methods and Calculations

An MNDO[6] program was used to optimize the chemical structure of AT-1840 and some of its derivatives on a VAX/11/780 computer. A number of analogous compounds were then calculated by using the CNDOEP[7] program so that molecular electrostatic potential (MEP) maps were obtained.

III. Results and Discussion

The net charge distribution and the bond orders of AT-1840 are shown in Fig. 1. The eigenvalues of the frontier orbitals are $E_{\mathrm{HOMO}} = -12.3919\,\mathrm{eV}$ and $E_{\mathrm{LUMO}} = -5.2783\,\mathrm{eV}$, and the LUMO consisted mostly of electrons from C_{14} and N_1. It is suggested that the N_1-C_{14} double bond plays an important role in its antitumor activity because most antitumor agents are electrophilic. A tentative conclusion can be made that any steric hindrance to the C_{14}-N_1 double bond would affect its electrophilic reaction and reduce its antitumor activity. The results of pharmacological experiments[4] are consistent with our conclusion.

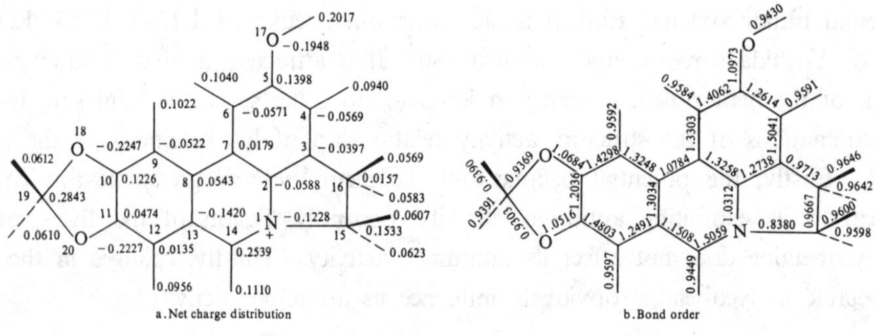

Fig. 1 Calculation results of the cation of AT-1840.

Compounds II and I show nearly equal antitumor activity in mice with Ehrlich ascites carcinoma, but for compound III, the activity is very low. It was reported in Ref. [4] that the bond strength difference between N_1 and C_{15} is responsible for the activity difference between II and III. Because the bond strength between N_1 and C_{15} was relatively weak in compound III, it was not very active. However, in our research, the results obtained by employing the MNDO program show nearly equal bond orders between N_1 and C_{15} for compound II and III,

$$\text{Bond order } (N_1 - C_{15},\ \text{II}) = 0.8513,$$

$$\text{Bond order } (N_1 - C_{15},\ \text{III}) = 0.8431.$$

Further, both of them are slightly higher than in the case of AT-1840 (0.8380). It can be considered that there is no difference in the bond strength between these three compounds. Therefore, in our opinion, the reason for the great difference in antitumor activity seems to be the steric hindrance to the N_1-C_{14} double bond which is caused by the N_1 side chain rotating along the N_1-C_{15} bond. The larger the steric hindrance to the N_1-C_{14} double bond, the lower the antitumor activity. It is obvious that the steric hindrance caused by the ethyl group (in compound III) is larger than that caused by the methyl group (in compound II). In compound I, the formation of a five-membered planar nitrogen heterocycle ensures that there is no steric hindrance by the side chain on N_1.

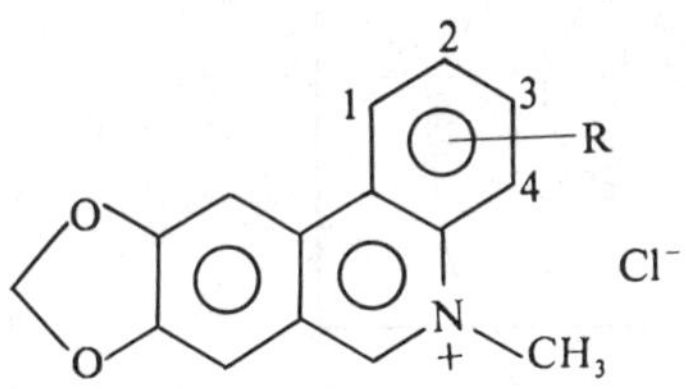

IV. R=1−OH

V. R=3−OH

VI. R=4−OH

X. $R=2-OCH(CH_3)_2$

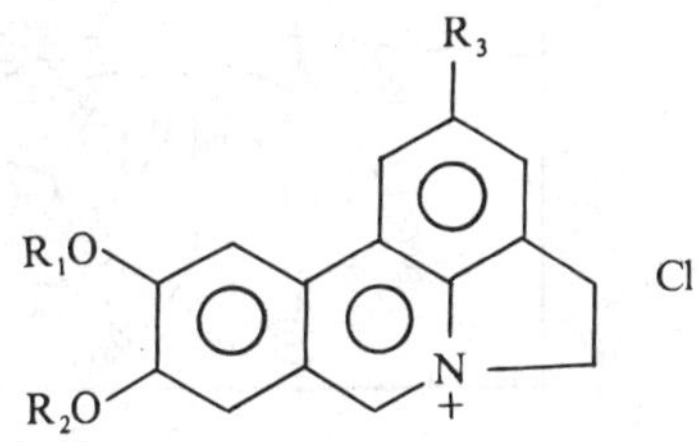

VII. $R_1=CH_3$ $R_2=CH_3$, $R_3=OH$

VIII. $R_1=H$ $R_2=CH_3$, $R_3=OH$

IX. $R_1'R_2=-CH_2-$, $R_3=H$

In order to understand why only a betaine can be a potential antitumor agent and what kind of betaine can be such an agent, ten compounds were selected for further research. These included eight betaines (I-VIII) and two cations (IX, X). The CNDOEP calculations were performed by using the coordinate parameters taken from the MNDO optimized AT-1840 skeleton and standard bond parameters. The molecular electrostatic potential of these betaines and cations were obtained.

Fig. 2 to Fig. 9 show the molecular electrostatic potential contour maps in a special plane which is 1.5 Å above and parallel to the molecular plane. For compounds I and II, which are relatively more active, the maps are clearly divided into two regions of different potential, positive and negative. There are two intense positive potential regions in the MEP map separated by a distance of nearly 9 Å (one is created by the nitrogen and the carbons around it, and the other is formed by the methylendiox group), and one negative potential region created by the phenolic betaine. The values of these three intense potentials are nearly equal (Fig. 2, Fig. 3). When the phenolic group moves closer to the nitrogen atom (VI), the value of the positive potential around the nitrogen is reduced (Fig. 4), and the antitumor activity becomes low. If the methylendioxy bond is broken (VII), the electrostatic potential around it changes from positive to negative (Fig. 5), and no antitumor activity is observed. Compound VIII has two types of betaine (a, b). The MEPs (Fig. 6, Fig. 7) of both betaines are quite different from those of compounds I and

II, in that both VIIIa and VIIIb have only one intense positive potential region. And for compounds IX and X, which have no negative potential areas in the maps (Fig. 8,

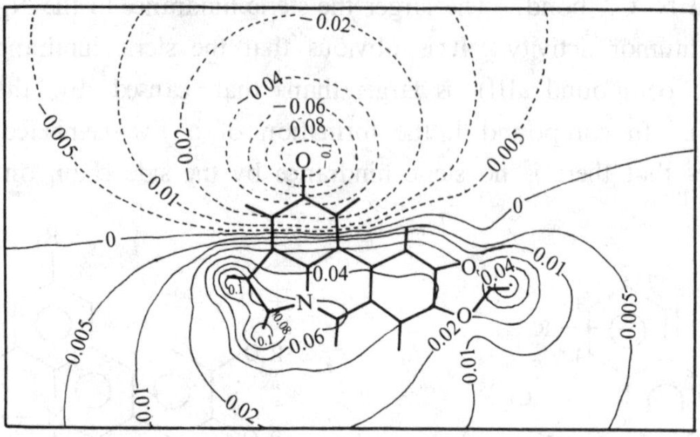

Fig. 2 MEP map of I.

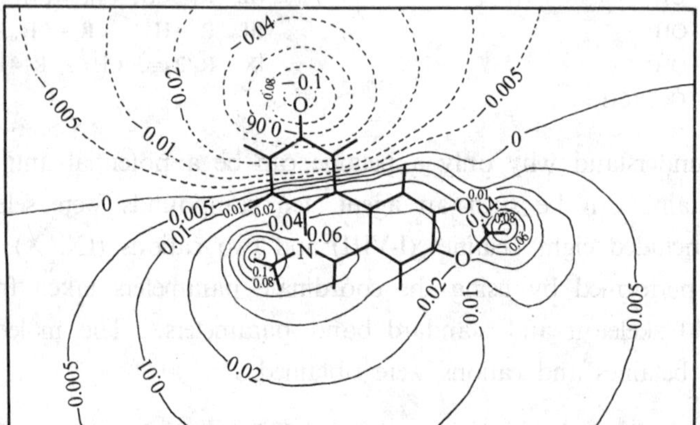

Fig. 3 MEP map of II.

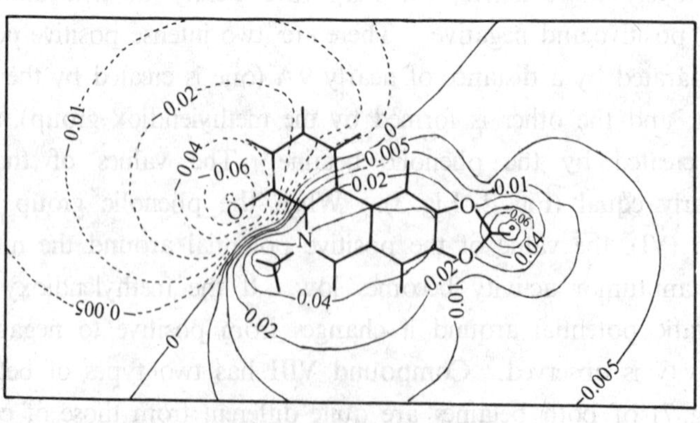

Fig. 4 MEP map of VI.

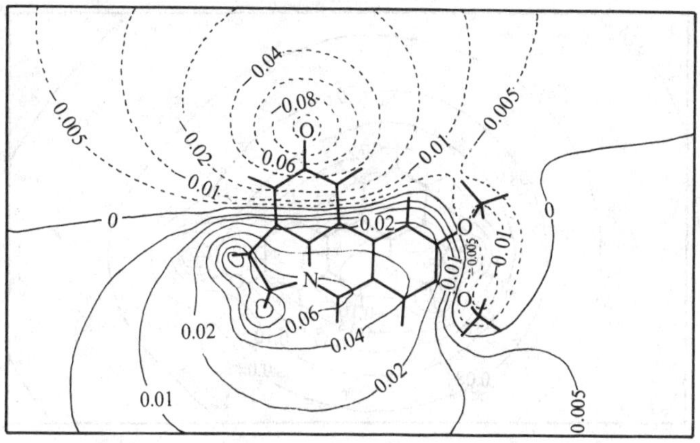

Fig. 5 MEP map of VII.

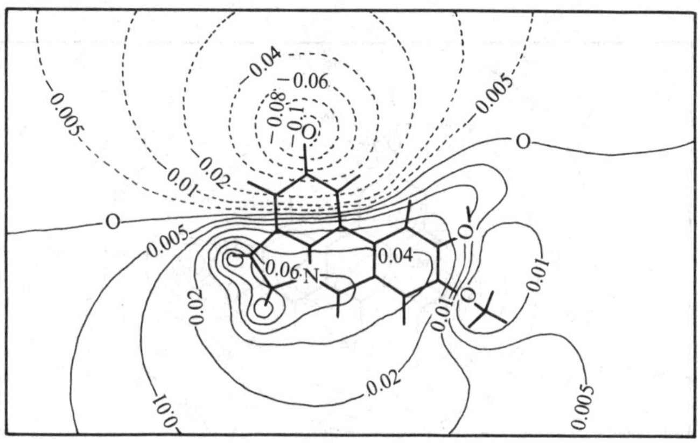

Fig. 6 MEP map of VIIIa.

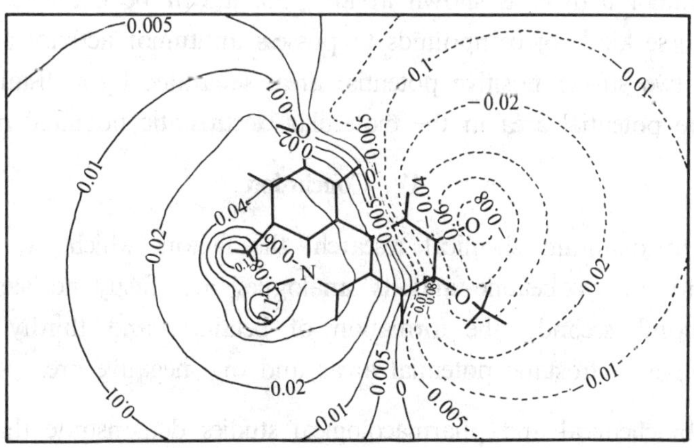

Fig. 7 MEP map of VIIIb.

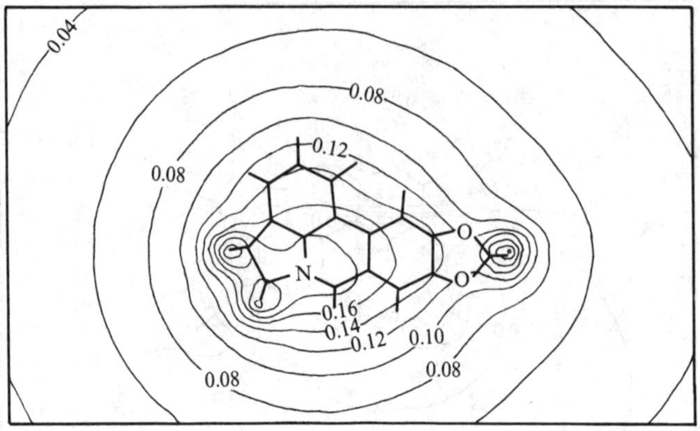

Fig. 8 MEP map of IX cation.

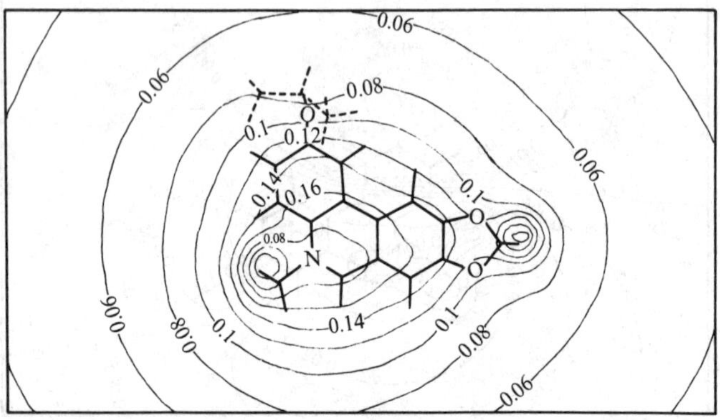

Fig. 9 MEP map of X cation.

Fig. 9), no antitumor activity is shown at all. So, it can be deduced that the necessary conditions for these kinds of compounds to possess antitumor activity are those in which there should be two strong positive potential areas separated by a distance of about 9 Å, and one negative potential area in the molecular electrostatic potential map.

IV. Conclusion

According to quantum chemical research, the factors which are necessary for the antitumor activity of lycobetaine and its analogues are firstly no steric hindrance on C=N double bond, secondly the formation of betaines, and thirdly the formation of two strong positive electrostatic potential areas and one negative area.

The latest biochemical and pharmacological studies demonstrate that lycobetaine is a good DNA intercalator[8]. Further theoretical research on the interaction of these kinds of compounds and DNA is being carried out in our institute.

References

1 Weng Zun-yao et al., *K'o Hsueh T'ung Pao,* **21**(1976), 285.
2 Zhang Su-yin et al., *Acta Pharmacol Sin.*, **2**(1981), 1: 41.
3 Weng Zun-yao et al., *Acta Pharmaceutica Sin.,* **17**(1982), 10: 744.
4 Weng Zun-yao & Zhant Guang-rong, *Acta Pharmaceutica Sin.,* **19**(1984), 1: 28.
5 He Hu-ming et al., *Acta Pharmaceutica Sin.,* **24**(1989), 4: 302.
6 Provided by Prof. Li Shu-sen.
7 Wu Ji-an et al., *W C J. PS* (China)., **1**(1986), 2: 71.
8 Liu Jie et al., *Acta Pharmacol. Sin.,* **10**(1989), 5: 437.

Synthesis and Antitumor Activity of 4-Methyl-6-carbazoyl-pyridazinone- 3*

WANG Liufang**, CHEN Xingguo, PENG Zhouren, LI Bingrui, WANG Qiguang,

(Department of Chemistry, Lanzhou University, Lanzhou 730000, China)

CHEN Guoquen

(Gansu Institute of New Medicine and Pharmaceutical Science. Lanzhou 730050, China)

and WANG Qi

(Lanzhou Institute of Chemical Physics, Academia Sinica, Lanzhou 730000, China)

Some hydrazine derivatives possess certain bio-activity[1, 2] and anti-ozonization ability[3]. The pyridazine and pyridazone compounds which contain a hydrazine group on the ring show pharmaceutical activity other than common bio-activity[4, 5]; therefore, many workers have been interested in studying these compounds. In 1984, J. Mayrargue *et al.* condensed ethyl pyruvate with a nucleophilic reagent, acetylenic magnesium bromide, and isolated a lactone, 2-hydroxy-5-carbethoxy-5-methyl-5H furanone. On reacting this lactone with hydrazine they obtained a new hydrazine, the title compound(MCP), in 25% yield based on ethyl pyruvate[5]. We now report a new route to synthesize the title compound. Its crystals were obtained from alcohol. By means of a four-circle diffractometer its structure was suggested to be:

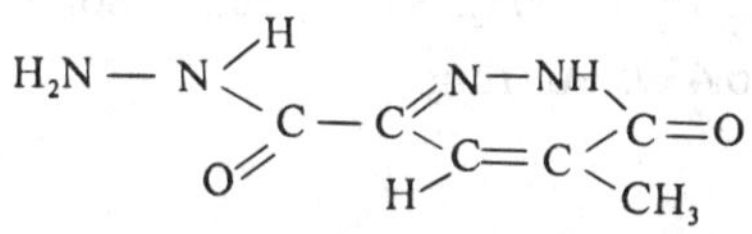

A test of the antitumor activity of MCP on transplanted mouse tumor EC showed that MCP has a definite inhibition effect on the growth of EC with an inhibitory rate of 41%. The acute toxicity was also tested.

I. Experimental

1. *Preparation of La-pyruvate*[6]

Freshly prepared La-carbonate was dissolved in excess pyruvic acid, the mixture was warmed up to remove the CO_2 formed and then filtered under vacuum while hot. Ether was added to the filtrate and the mixture was stirred under reflux for 2 h. The La(Pyr)$_3$

* Project supported by the National Natural Science Foundation of China.

* To whom correspondence should be addressed.

formed was filtered and washed several times with ether then dried in a vacuum desicator.

2. *Synthesis of the title compound*

The La-pyruvate was added to aqueous hydrazine hydrate to give a pH value of about 10. The mixture was then stirred under reflux for 30 min. Pyruvic acid was added to the clear solution until the precipitate dissolved completely and the pH was between 6 and 7. An equal volume of absolute alcohol was added, and the mixture was heated under reflux for a further 4 h. After cooling ether was added and a large amount of precipitate was obtained. The precipitate was filtered with suction and washed with water several times. The elemental analysis of the precipitate gave C% 42.90, N% 32.79, H% 4.71; calcd (title compound, $C_6H_8N_4O_2$): C% 42.86, N% 33.33, H% 4.76.

3. *Crystal formation of the title compound and its diffraction data*

When an alcoholic solution of the precipitate was allowed to evaporate, after a few days well-formed single crystals of the title compound were obtained.

The diffraction data were collected using a CDA 4K diffractometer with CuK_α radiation ($\lambda = 1.5418$ Å). The unit cell parameters were: $a = 7.386$ Å, $b = 10.290$ Å, $c = 10.037$ Å, $\alpha = \gamma = 90.00°$, $\beta = 101.27°$, $V = 748.1$ Å^3, $d_c = 1.493$ g/cm^3. The space group was $P/21\ c$ and $Z = 4$.

4. *IR study*

The main peaks in the IR spectrum (Fig. 1) could be assigned empirically as: 3301.284 vs, NH_2, asym.; 3200.215 w, NH_2, sym.; 1658.886, C=0, side chain; 1621.332, ring C=0[8]; 1600.618 and 1556.439, Ar ring.

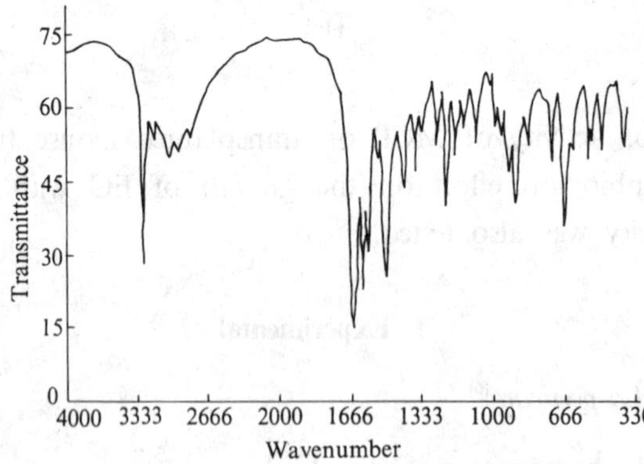

Fig. 1 IR spectrum of title compound.

5. *The Antitumor test*

A suspension of MCP and Tween-80 was prepared for the antitumor test, and a suspension of Tween-80 was used as a control.

Tumor species EC was obtained from Beijing Pharmaceutical Institute and it was cultivated by the Gansu Tumor Institute. Mice species with body weight of 18—22 g were obtained from Kunming. Mice of the same sex were used. These mice were abdominally transplanted with tumor species EC.

The transplanted mice were randomly divided into groups, each treated group contained 10 mice and each control group contained 15 mice. The weight difference of the mice was less than 1 g. The drug (MCP) was given 24 hours after transplanting, one dose each day. The dosage was continued for 10 days. On the 11 th day, the weight of the mice bodies and tumors were measured.

II. Results and Discussion

The M.P. of the title compound was 235°C and the MS gave m/e: 168, 137, 109, 81, 68(weak) and 54. Its molecular structure is shown in Fig. 2 and bond lengths are listed in Table 1.

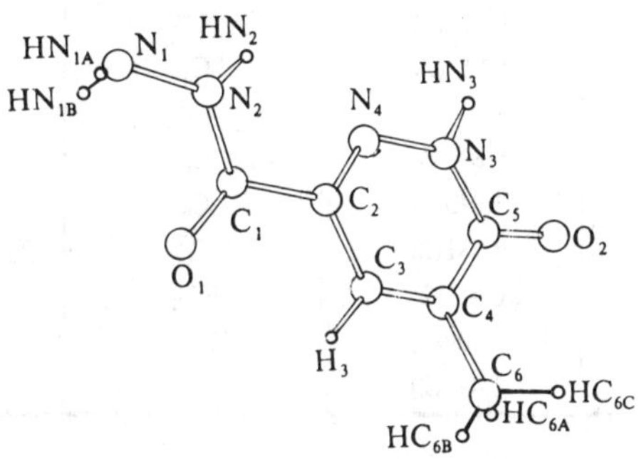

Fig. 2 Molecular structure and labelling sequence of atoms.

The bond lengths of C_1-O_1(1.232 Å) C_5-O_2(1.299 Å) and the weak OH peak in the IR spectrum indicated that some of the title compound exists in the enolic form when it is a non-crystalline. But the result of X-ray diffractometry suggested that it exists in the keto form when it is a crystalline, i.e. the following tautomerism probably exists:

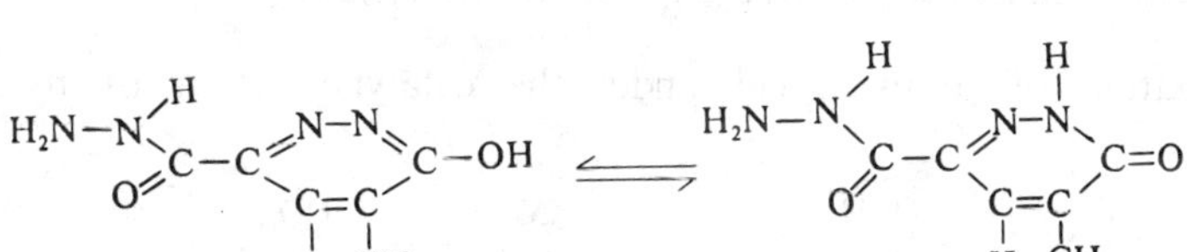

(enol form) (keto form)

From the bond lengths in Table 1, it can be seen that the six-membered ring is a strongly conjugated system. This can also be ascertained by the presence of the two aromatic peaks (1600.108 and 1556.439 cm^{-1}) and the C=O peak (1621.332 cm^{-1}) in the IR spectrum. The atoms of this six-membered ring exist fundamentally in a plane (Table 2). The C=O group outside the ring is not conjugated with the six-membered ring and the bond length of C_1-C_2 becomes even longer than that of C_4-C_6 due to the repulsive force between the electron-rich C=O groups outside the ring and in the ring system itself. Further, the carbazoyl group shows some tendency to enolize which causes the bond length C_1-N_2 to be shorter than C_5-N_3 and the bond length C_1-O_1 to be longer than C_5-O_2, and lowers the energy of the whole system thus stabilizing the compound.

Table 1 Bond Distances in Å

Atom 1	Atom 2	Distance	Atom 1	Atom 2	Distance
O_1	C_1	1.232(2)	C_2	C_3	1.421(2)
O_2	C_5	1.229(2)	C_3	C_4	1.352(3)
N_1	N_2	1.410(2)	C_3	H_3	0.96 (2)
N_1	HN_{1A}	0.91 (2)	C_4	C_5	1.453(3)
N_1	HN_{1B}	0.85 (2)	C_4	C_6	1.492(3)
N_2	C_1	1.334(2)	C_6	HC_{6A}	0.94 (2)
N_2	HN_2	0.83 (2)	C_6	HC_{6B}	0.91 (2)
N_3	N_4	1.343(2)	C_6	HC_{6C}	1.03 (2)
N_3	C_5	1.381(2)	HC_{6A}	HC_{6B}	1.54 (3)
N_3	HN_3	0.93 (2)	HC_{6B}	HC_{6C}	1.53 (3)
N_4	C_2	1.302(2)	HN_{1A}	HN_{1B}	1.46 (3)
C_1	C_2	1.495(2)			

Table 2 Least Square Plane and Displacement of Atoms From the Plane (P)

Plane $0.8827x+0.4251y-0.2001z-0.2251=0$						
Atoms	C_2	C_3	C_4	C_5	N_4	N_3
P(Å)	−0.009	0.014	−0.005	−0.010	−0.007	−0.017

We found that it is easy to prepare the title compound in good yield and high purity by reacting pyruvic acid-RE complex with hydrazine hydrate, and the reaction time is short. The reaction mechanism is suggested to be as follows:

(1) Dimerization of pyruvic acid under the catalytic action of hydrazine hydrate (base)[6]:

$$2\ CH_3-\overset{\overset{O}{\|}}{C}-\overset{\overset{O}{\|}}{C}-O^- \rightleftharpoons CH_3-\overset{\overset{CO_2^-}{|}}{C}(OH)-CH_2-\overset{\overset{CO_2^-}{|}}{C}=O$$

(2) Condensation of pyruvic acid dimer with hydrazine[7]:

$$CH_3-\overset{\overset{CO_2^-}{|}}{C}(OH)-CH_2-\overset{\overset{CO_2^-}{|}}{C}=O \overset{N_2H_4}{\rightleftharpoons} CH_3-\overset{\overset{CO_2^-}{|}}{C}(OH)-CH_2-\overset{\overset{CO_2^-}{|}}{C}=NH_2$$

(3) Complexation of the condensation product with La^{3+}: The complex has the following structure:

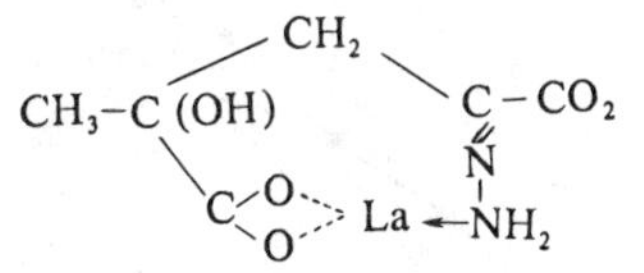

(4) As the reaction temperature is increased, the La−N bond begins to break and N(b) attacks the nearby C(a) to cause decomposition of the complex, and allow cyclization to occur. One molecule of water is lost, lowering the energy content of the whole system and stabilizing it.

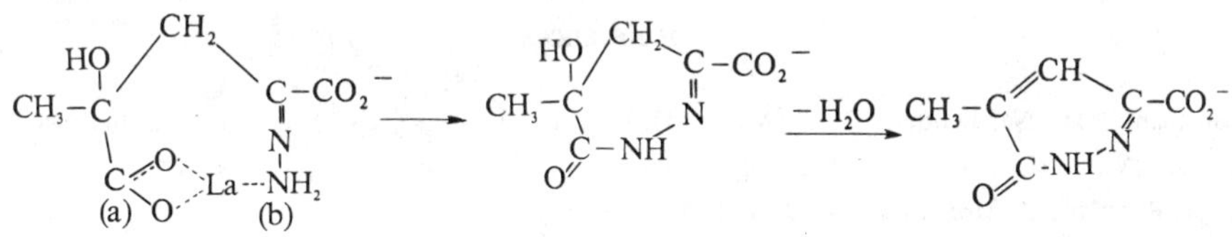

(5) Finally, at the reflux temperature, the carbonyl group outside the ring reacts with hydrazine to form the title compound:

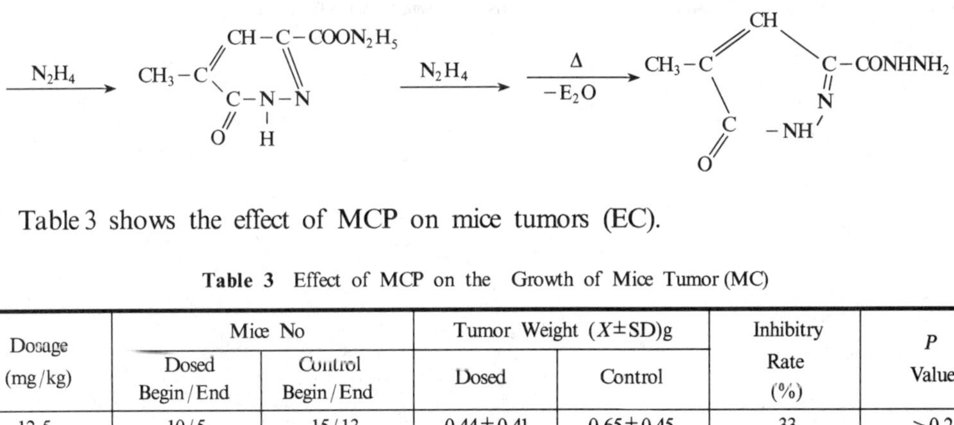

Table 3 shows the effect of MCP on mice tumors (EC).

Table 3 Effect of MCP on the Growth of Mice Tumor (MC)

Dosage (mg/kg)	Mice No		Tumor Weight ($X\pm SD$)g		Inhibitry Rate (%)	*P* Value
	Dosed Begin/End	Control Begin/End	Dosed	Control		
12.5	10/5	15/13	0.44±0.41	0.65±0.45	33	>0.2
25	10/6	15/13	0.38±0.26	0.65±0.45	41	>0.1

From Table 3, it can be seen that MCP has a definite effect on inhibiting the growth of the tumor EC. But no such effect was observed for a liver abdominal cancer species (Hep).

The average body weight of mice which were treated steadily increased as shown in Fig. 3 and there was no abnormal change of their hair color. The treated mice were all healthy and energetic. The acute toxicity test showed that $LD_{50}=250$ mg/kg.

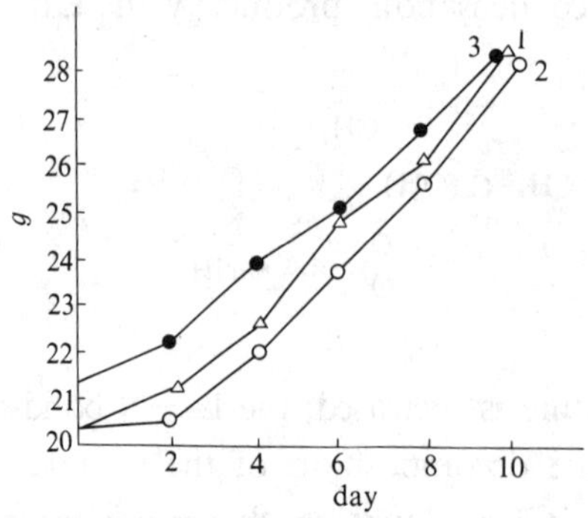

Fig. 3 Effect of MCP on transplated mice body weight.

References

1 Ramanathan, J. D., Namboothiri, D. G., Mehta, H. J. *et al.*, *J. India Chem. Soc.*, **55**(1978), 10: 1036.

2 Albert, A., *Nature* (London), 1953, 172, 201.

3 Ecluarol, R. *et al.*, *J. Med. Chem.*, **8**(1963), 1: 29.

4 Guo, H. Y., Sun, L. Y., Tang, Y. *et al.*, *Acta Pharmaceutica Sinica*, **23**(1988), 8: 566 (CH).

5 Mayrargue, J., Avril, J. L. and Miocque, M., *Bull. Soc. Chim.*, France, 1984, part 2, (3-4), 129.

6 Senasing, D. D. *et al.*, *J. Am. Chem. Soc.*, 1964, 8: 2805.

7 Pino, T. and Cordes, E. H., *J. Org. Chem.*, **86**(1971), 12: 1068.

8 Kaji, K., Nagashima, H., Ohhata, Y. *et al.*, *J. Heterocycl. Chem.*, **22**(1983), 1: 161.

Inhibition of Benzo(a)pyrene Binding to DNA by Ellagic Acid

K.L. Khanduja and S. Majid

(Department of Biophysics, Postgraduate Institute of Medical Education and Research, Chandigarh - 160012, India)

Abstract Ellagic acid has been found to inhibit the binding of ^{3}H-benzo(a)pyrene (^{3}H-BaP) to DNA *in vitro* and *in vivo*. In *in vitro* systems the carcinogen was activated by NADPH, ascorbic acid, and hematin. This study describes the mechanism of action of EA in inhibiting the carcinogen-DNA adduct formation.

A number of polycyclic aromatic hydrocarbons (PAH) widely distributed in our surroundings[1,2] are known to induce cancer in man and animals. PAH are metabolized into reactive electrophiles by mixed function oxidases, and these reactive metabolites known as ultimate carcinogens interact with cellular macromolecules like DNA, RNA and proteins[3,4] to elicit cell transformation, mutagenic and carcinogenic activities. The susceptibilities of certain tissues to PAH-induced cancer correlate well with their ability to bind with DNA[5]. This binding is catalyzed by the cytochrome P-450 dependent mixed function oxidase system (MFO) and may also via the peroxidative cooxidation by the prostaglandin synthetase and by the lipid peroxidation. Diet is important in modulating the carcinogenic risk from the chemicals. Ellagic acid (EA), a naturally occurring plant polyphenol, has been found to inhibit the carcinogen-DNA binding[6,7] and the tumorigenesis induced by PAH's[8,9]. In the present study we report that EA was capable of inhibiting the carcinogen-DNA binding *in vivo*, and *in vitro* mediated through different modes.

In vitro ^{3}H-BaP-DNA binding studies were conducted by activating the carcinogen in three ways. (i) The enzymatic activation was done by using the post-mitochondrial supernatant (PMS) of NMRI mouse lungs. The reaction mixture in final volume of 3 ml contained 50 μmol of sodium phosphate pH 7.4; 10 μmol EDTA, 0.5 mg NADPH, 2 mg calf thymus DNA, 100 mg tissue equivalent PMS and varying concentrations (0 — 500 μmol/L) of EA. The reaction at 37 °C was initiated by adding 40 μmol of ^{3}H-BaP, sp. act. 5000 mCi/mmol, in 25 μl of acetone. The reaction was stopped after 30 min. (ii) Ascorbate-dependent lipid peroxidation-mediated activation was done with microsomes separated by calcium aggregation. The reaction mixture in a final volume of 3 ml contained 0.15 mmol Tris-HCL, pH 7.4, 3 nmol ascorbic acid, 6 nmol $FeSO_4$, 2 mg DNA,

1 mg hepatic microsomal protein and varying concentrations of EA. The reaction at 37 °C was stopped 20 min after adding 40 nmol of ^{3}H-BaP. (iii) Activation by peroxidation of linoleic acid was done with hematin. The reaction mixture in a final volume of 1 ml contained 50 μmol Tris-HCl, pH 7.4, 5 nmol hematin, 1 μmol linoleic acid in 10 μl of ethyl alcohal, 2 mg DNA and EA (0— 500 μmol). The binding was initiated by adding 40 nmol ^{3}H-BaP (500 mCi/nmol) in the reaction mixture incubated at 37 °C for 20 min. The reactions in three cases were stopped by adding 3.0 ml of stopping reagent (2% SDS, 0.03 *N* NaCl and 0.003 *N* sodium citrate, pH 7.0). DNA was isolated as described by us earlier[10].

For *in vivo* studies, mice on plain drinking water or EA (12 μg EA/ml drinking water) for 8 weeks were i.p. injected 200 μCi of ^{3}H-BaP/100 gm body weight (sp. act. 5.3 Ci/mmol). Animals were killed after 8 and 12 h. Pulmonary DNA was extracted by Marmur's method[11]. A ratio of A260/A280 1.9 was taken as an index for DNA purity to be 98%. The DNA-carcinogen adduct formation was estimated by liquid scintillation counting.

The effect of EA on *in vitro* carcinogen-DNA binding triggered by three modes is shown in Table 1. The maximum inhibition in carcinogen-DNA adduct formation was 43— 47% in all the cases. But the concentration of EA required to produce maximum inhibition was different. For example in NADPH mediated binding this was 500μmol/L, whereas in case of binding mediated by lipid peroxidation triggered by ascorbic acid or hematin it was 125 μmol/L. The basal levels of carcinogen-DNA adduct formation in hematin-, ascorbic acid- and NADPH-mediated binding were 8250±415, 145±9.0 and 173±9.7 fmol/mg respectively. Effect of EA feeding at a dose of 12 μg/ml for 8 weeks on ^{3}H-BaP binding to mouse pulmonary DAN is depicted in Fig. 1. The maximum binding of the carcinogen (2057±317 fmol/mg DNA in the control animals was observed at 12h which was significantly more than at 8h (1306±240). It was found that binding of the carcinogen in EA pretreated animals at 8 h (962±86 fmol/mg) and 12 h (1048±76 fmol/mg) was significantly less than the values in control animals at these timings. Furthermore, in EA-pretreated mice the level of carcinogen-DNA adduct formation at 12h was not significantly different from the level at 8h.

Table 1 Effect of Ellagic Acid on ^{3}H-benzo(a)pyrene-DNA Binding Mediated by NADPH, Ascorbic Acid and Hematin. Mean±SD Values Are in fmol/mg DNA/min

	Ellagic Acid Concentration (μmol/L)			
	0	125	250	500
NADPH	173±9.7	136±3.67	124±32.6	97.7±13.6
Ascobic acid	145±9.0	74.5±18	88±4.5	68±9.5
Hematin	8250±415	4740±535	4300±304	5100±495

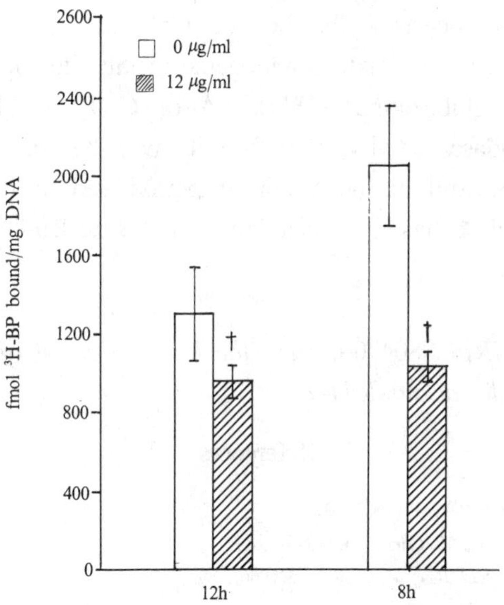

Fig. 1 Effect of EA on ^{3}H-BP binding with pulmonary DNA *in vivo*. +, $P<0.05$.

The difference in EA requirement to produce maximum inhibition in three *in vitro* carcinogen-DNA adduct studies could be ascribed to the differences in the modes of activation of BaP. In NADPH-dependent system, the initial st p in carcinogen activation is carried out by cytochrome P-450 dependent oxidation, and the metabolites formed may be further activated to ultimate reactive forms either chiefly by the MFO system and/or by peroxidative mechanisms. Whereas, during the activation of carcinogens by peroxidative mechanisms, the activation is wholly carried out by the free radicals. As the saturation effect of EA in inhibiting the BP-adduct formation, mediated by peroxidative mechanisms, is achieved at 125 μmol/L, we feel that there may be some radicals which EA is not able to quench directly or indirectly. This may be because they are somehow trapped in the lipid millieu and EA is not able to reach them, and before they are quenched they react with the carcinogen, starting a self-propagating chain of reactions. Thus, this nearly fixed ratio of free radicals, which are not accessible to EA for a particular *in vitro* system at least, remains the same.

Though the activation of procarcinogens to reactive metabolic forms can be carried out by non-enzymatic processes, *in vivo* the activation is carried out chiefly by cytochrome P-450 dependent MFO localized mainly in the microsomal fraction of the liver. The reactive metabolites either bind covalently with macromolecules or are detoxified by the drug detoxifying enzymes including glutathione-S-transferase (GST). The inhibition in carcinogen-DNA adduct formation by EA *in vivo* reflects that despite quenching free radicals responsible for activation of the carcinogen, EA may promote the system responsible for detoxification of reactive metabolities of the carcinogen. We have already reported that EA feeding increased the hepatic GST activity and reduced glutathione levels[12, 13]. GST conjugates the ultimate carcinogenic metabolites of BaP, i.e. baP-7, 8-diol-9, 10-epoxide with reduced glutathione (GSH). Also, GST has been observed to have Se-dependent GSH-peroxidase activity; therefore it may be an important alternative in detoxifying lipid peroxides, and in the repair of peroxidized liver nuclear DNA since the Se-dependent GSH-peroxidase has low abundance in the nucleus[14].

The financial grant, IRIS 8804900, *from the Indian Council of Medical Research, New Delhi*-110029, *India is dully acknowledged.*

References

1 Boyland E., *Prog. Exp. Tumor Res.*, **11**(1967), 222.
2 Armstrong, B. and Doll, R., *Int. J. Cancer*, **15**(1975), 617.
3 Lawley, P.D., *Prog. Nucleic Acid Res. Mol. Biol.*, **5**(1966), 89.
4 Miller, J.A., *Cancer Res.*, **30**(1970), 557.
5 Eastman, A. and Bresnick, E., *Cancer Res.*, **39**(1979), 2400.
6 DelTito, B.J., Mukhtar, H. and Bickers, D.R., *Biochem. Biophys. Res. Commun.*, **114**(1983), 388.
7 Dixit, R., Teel, R.W., Daniel, F.B. *et al.*, *Cancer Res.*, **45**(1985), 2951.
8 Lesca, P., *Carcinogenesis*, **4**(1983), 1651.
9 Mukhtar, H., Das, M. and Bickers, D.R., *Cancer Res.*, **46**(1986), 2262.
10 Dogra, S.C., Khanduja, K.L., Gupta, M.P. *et al.*, *Indian J. Biochem. Biophys.*, **21**(1984), 117.
11 Marmur J.A., *Biophys. Mol. Biol.*, **3**(1961), 208.
12 Majid, S., Khanduja, K.L., Kapur, S. *et al.*, *J. Clin. Biochem. Nutr.*, **10**(1991), 127.
13 Majid, S., Khanduja, K.L., Kapur, S. *et al.*, *Biochem. Pharm.* (in press).
14 Kitterer, B. and Meyer, D.J., *Mutation Res.*, **214**(1989), 33.

Antitumor Activities of 5′-Iodo-indirubin

DU Deji, ZENG Qingtian, SI Xiaofeng,
RAN Changqing and WANG Xiaoping

(Sichuan Institute of Chinese Materia Medica, Chongqing 630065, China)

Abstract Comparative experiments of 5′-I-ind, one of the derivatives of indirubin (ind), with ind for toxicities, antitumor activities and ^{3}H-isotope precursor incorporations were reported in this paper. The results showed that 5′-I-ind was more potential against experimental transplantable tumours than ind.

I. Introduction

Indirubin, isolated originally from QINGDAI, a Chinese traditional medicine in 1975, is an anticancer drug for the treatment of chronic granulocytic leukemia[1]. We have been investigating the structure activity relationships of indirubin derivatives for ten years in order to find more active anticancer drugs which are less toxic than indirubin[2]. Among the derivatives that we have synthesized, 5′-Iodoindirubin (5′-I-ind) was found to be one of the active derivatives against W256, L7212 and so on[3]. The results of pharmacological studies on 5′-I-ind are reported herein.

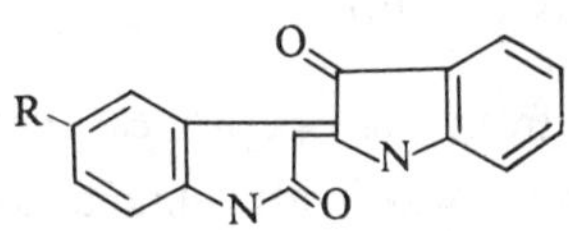

Fig. 1 Structure formula of indirubin and 5′-indoindirubin.
(1) 5′-iodoindirubin R=I;
(2) indirubin R=H.

II. Materials and Methods

1. *Animals*

C57BL/6, DBA/2 and 615 inbreeding mice and Kunming hybrid strain mice, weighing 18— 22 g, and Wistar strain rats, weighing 60— 90 g, were used in our experiments. All animals were obtained from the Animal Laboratory in our institute (SICMM).

2. *Tumors*

Walker 256 carcinosarcoma in Wistar rats, Leukemia L7212, L7712, L759 in 615 mice, Leukemia P388 in DBA/2 mice, Hepatocarcinoma 22 and Ehrlich ascites carcinoma (ECA) in Kunming mice were all maintained in our laboratory.

3. *Reagents and drugs*

5′-I-ind (purity 96%) was kindly provided by Gu Y.C. in SICMM. Its impurities, indigotin and indigo brown, have no antitumor activity reported so far. Ind and other derivatives were also synthesized by the Chemical Lab. of SICMM. The purity of Ind was 97% with impurities of indigotin and indigobrown. Other chemotherapeutic drugs such as Myleran, Cyclophosphamide (CY), 6-Mercaptopurine (6-MP), 5-Fluorouracil (5-FU), Mitomycin C (MMC) and Vincristine (VCR) were purchased from market.

(Methyl-^{3}H) thymidine (^{3}H-TdR), ^{3}H-uridine (^{3}H-UR), ^{3}H-Leucine (^{3}H-Leu) were all purchased from Chinese Academy of Atomic Energy Science. Their purities were not less than 95%.

4. *Antitumor tests*

The antitumor assay was carried out according to the screening protocol *in vivo*[5]. Drugs were given po or ip to tumor-bearing animals once a day for seven days after tumor transplantation. The inhibition rate of tumor growth in solid tumor models was calculated by the formula $TW_c\text{-}TW_t/TW_c \times 100\%$, where TW_c and TW_t represented the mean tumor weights of the control group and the test group respectively. The prolongation rate of animal survival time in ascites tumors or leukemia models was calculated by $LS_t\text{-}LS_c/LS_c \times 100\%$, where the LS_t and LS_c represented the mean life spans of the test group and the control group respectively.

5. *Incorporation of* ^{3}H-*isotope precursors into tumor cells in vitro*

P388 cells, H22 cells or ECA cells were harvested from the peritoneal cavity of tumor-bearing mice 6 or 7 days after transplantation, washed twice with saline and diluted with RPMI1640 to a concentration of 4×10^3/ml. Serial concentrations of test drugs or vehicle PEG 600 in triplicate were added into glass tubes in which there was 0.1 ml of the described cell suspension and 0.9 ml of RPMI1640. The mixtures were incubated at 37 ℃ for 1 h; then 1 Bg of isotope precursors (^{3}H-TdR, ^{3}H-UR or ^{3}H-Leu) was added into the tubes, which were finally incubated for 1 h more. DNA, RNA, or protein fractions were extracted from the incubated cells and the CPM was measured in a Beckman Liquid Scintillation Counter according to our previous method[6].

III. Results

1. *Acute toxicity of 5′-I-ind to mice and rats*

The LD50 of 5′-I-ind could not be estimated since oral administration of the largest volume (1 ml) of suspension (200 mg/ml) to mice resulted in diarrhea but not death. The same toxic response to the agent was observed in rats administered the drug orally with 5 g/kg of 5′-I-ind dose.

2. *Antitumor activities on W256 Carcinosarcoma-bearing rats and other solid tumour-bearing mice*

Compared with ind, 5′-I-ind was more effective either at 800 mg/kg (at the same weight of the two agents per kg of animals) or at 2 mmol/L (namely at the same gram molecule of the two agents per kg of animals). The inhibition rate of 5′-I-ind was 59—72%, significantly differing from the 30—34% of ind as shown in Table 1. The ID50 of 5′-I-ind was estimated to be 490±2.9 mg/kg by diagram assay.

Table 1 The Antitumor Effect of 5′-Iodo-indirubin on Walker 256 Carcinosarcoma in Rats

Drugs	Dose mg/(kg · d)	Days of ig. adm	No. of Rats	Mean Wt. (g) of Tumor $\overline{x}\pm SD$	Inhibition (%)	"*P*" Compared With Control
Control	—	7	18	5.3±1.4		
5′-I-ind	776 (2 mmol/L)	7	8	1.5±1.4	72	<0.01
Ind.	524 (2 mmol/L)	7	8	3.5±1.5	34	>0.05
Control	—	7	15	5.4±1.1		
5′-I-ind	500	7	8	2.3±0.4	57	<0.01
Control	—	6	14	6.2±1.9		
5′-I-ind	800	6	10	2.1±0.4	66	<0.01
Ind.	800	6	10	4.3±1.2	30	<0.06
Control	—	6	30	5.5±1.9		
5′-I-ind	800	6	10	2.3±1.1	59	<0.01
Ind.	800	6	10	4.6±1.5	16	>0.05
Myleran	40	1	10	0.2±0.1	97	<0.01

Oral administration of 1000 mg/kg of 5′-I-ind for 8—10 days to mice bearing Lewis lung carcinoma inhibited tumor growth by 48%, whereas when given to mice bearing ECS and S180 it did not inhibit tumor growth.

3. *Experimental therapeutic effects of 5′-I-ind on L7212 and other leukemia models*

The comparative experiment with 5′-I-ind to ind, N′-alkylind, or other chemotherapy drugs were carried out on L7212 leukemia-bearing mice. The results showed that the mean survival time of 5′-I-ind, ind, N′-methylind, N′-ethylind group were prolonged by 63, 18, 25, and 37% at 1000 mg/(kg · day) for 8—9 days, respectively, and 5′-I-ind appeared to have almost the same effect as 6-MP, 5FU and MMC at the MTD dosage (see Table 2).

Table 2 The Therapeutic Effect of 5′-Iodo-indirubin and Other Antitumor Agents on L7212 in 615 Mice

Drug	Dose mg/(kg.d)	Days of ig.	No. of Tumor Cell ($\times 10^4$)	No. of Mice	Survival Time (days) ($\bar{x}\pm$SD)	ILS (%)	Significance P
Control	—	6	420	10	7.3±0.4		
5′-I-ind	1000	9	420	5	12.7±1.4	73	<0.01
Control	—	6	220	12	7.4±0.4		
5′-I-ind	1000	9	220	6	12.4±1.5	68	<0.01
Control	—	6	340	14	6.9±1.1		
5′-I-ind	1000	6	340	7	9.7±1.2	41	<0.01
Control	—	6	204	20	8.6±1.1		
5′-I-ind	1000	6	204	6	12.6±2.6	47	<0.01
5′-I-ind	500	6	204	6	11.2±1.9	30	<0.01
Control	—	7	460	27	8.3±1.9		
5′-I-ind	1000	9	460	7	13.5±2.0	63	<0.01
Ind	1000	8	460	7	9.9±2.4	18	>0.05
N′-M-Ind	1000	8	460	7	10.4±2.7	25	<0.01
N′-E-Ind	1000	9	460	7	11.4±1.1	37	<0.01
Myleran	10	6	460	7	9.1±1.6	9	
CY	50	5	460	7	11.3±2.1	36	<0.01
6-MP	30	6	460	7	12.2±1.0	47	<0.01
5-FU	20	6 (ip)	460	7	12.2±2.3	47	<0.01
Mitomycin-C	1.5	6 (ip)	460	7	12.9±2.5	55	<0.01
VCR	1.0	6 (ip)	460	7	7.7±1.0	−7	>0.05

5′-I-ind was also active against L759 and L7712 as the increase in life span was 37 and 42% respectively; however, it had no activity against L615 and P388 leukemia. (cf. Table 3).

4. *Influence of 5′-I-ind on the Incorporation of* ^{3}*H-precursors into Tumor Cells*

The ^{3}H-TdR incorporation experiment carried out on H22 hepatocarcinoma cells and P388 cells demonstrated that 5′-I-ind was much more effective than ind as shown in Fig. 2 and Table 4. The IC50 of 5′-I-ind and ind were 6.4 and 17.0 μg/ml respectively. But both of the agents had a similar effect on ECA cells. In the ^{3}H-UR incorporation experiment on ECA cells, 10μg/ml of 5′-I-ind was shown to inhibit the incorporation of ^{3}H-UR into tumor cells by 32%, while ind was not. The inhibition effect of ^{3}H-Leu incorporation was not observed either in 5′-I-ind or in the ind group when compared with PEG the control group.

IV. Discussion

Comparative experiments of 5′ -I-ind to ind on toxicities, antitumor activities and ^{3}H-isotope precursor incorporations were reported in this paper. Although low toxicities were observed on both of them, in view of the maximum inhibition rate of

Table 3 The Effect of 5′-Iodo-indirubin on Other Leukemias and Solid Tumors in Mice

Tumor	Drug	Dose mg/(kg.d)	Route	Days of Adm.	Mean Wt. Tumor (g) ($\bar{x}$ ±SD)	Inhibition (%)	"*P*" Value
L759	control	—	ig	8	1.7±0.4	37	<0.01
	5′-I-ind	1000	ig	8	1.1±0.3	37	<0.01
	Ind	1000	ig	8	1.1±0.6		
ECS	control	—	ig	7	2.5±0.6		
	5′-I-ind	1000	ig	7	2.3±0.9	9	
S180	control	—	ig	7	2.3±1.0		
	5′-I-ind	1000	ig	7	2.9±0.7	9	
Lewis	control	—	ig	9	3.0±0.8		
	5′-I-ind	1000	ig	9	1.6±0.7	47	<0.01
	control	—	ig	10	2.1±0.9		
	5′-I-ind	1000	ig	10	1.1±0.3	48	<0.01
	control	—	ig	9	1.6±0.7		
	5′-I-ind	1000	ig	9	0.9±0.4	46	<0.01
	CY	50	ig	3	0.0	100	<0.01
					Days of Survival	ILS(%)	
P388	control	—	ig	10	11.6±0.5		
	5′-I-ind	1000	ig	10	11.4±0.5	0	
L7712	control	—	ig	8	9.2±0.8		
	5′-I-ind	1000	ig	8	13.1±3.9	42	<0.01

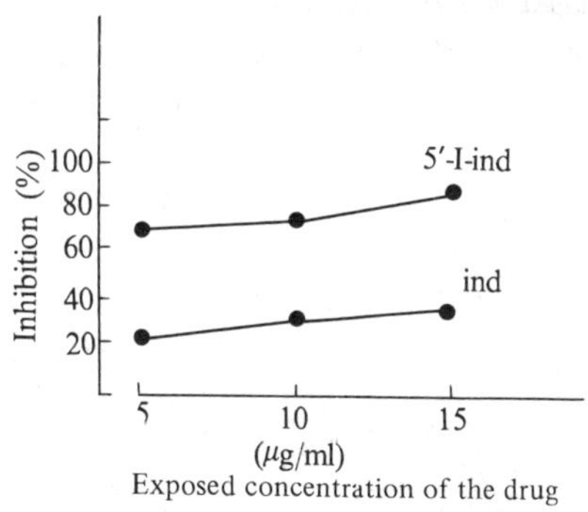

Fig. 2 The effect of 5′-iodo-indirubin on incorporation of ^{3}H-TdR into DNA of hepatoma$_{22}$ ascites carcinoma cell *in vitro*.

tumor growth 5′-I-ind was able to reach up to 73— 83%, which was almost the same as 6-MP, 5-FU and MMC, whereas ind was only able to reach less than 50%, indicating that 5′-I-ind was more potential against experimental transplantable tumors. The results suggest that the substitution of iodine for the H atom of 5′ position on the benzene ring enhances antitumor activities. In addition, the antitumor mechanism of ind has been reported to be of partial interference with biosynthesis of DNA in tumor tissue[6, 7]. The result of the incorporation experiments of ^{3}H-isotope precursors indicated that 5′-I-ind

Table 4 The Effect of 5′-Iodo-indirubin and Indirubin of ^{3}H-TdR Into DNA of Leukemia P388 Tumor Cell *in vitro*

Drugs	5′-I-Ind		Ind	
Concentration (μg/ml)	dpm ($\bar{x}\pm$SD)	Inhibition (%)	dpm ($\bar{x}\pm$SD)	Inhibition (%)
1	71649.25±5624.32	16		
5	43215.61±10782.26	49	78151.55±9298.16	8
10	40270.93±4135.45	53	62840.05±6791.43	26
20	22976.69±6679.30	73	37597.12±4901.86	56
30			18516.11±3894.53	78
Control (PEG 600 20μl/ml)	85120.62±8292.36		85120.62±8292.36	
IC50	6.4μg/ml		17.0μg/ml	
IC10	0.72μg/ml		6.2μg/ml	
b	1.349		2.922	

could also interfere with biosynthesis of DNA and sequential biosynthesis of RNA in tumor tissue.

References

1 Clinical study Group of Indirubin, *Chinese Journal of Hematology,* **1**(1980), 3: 132.
2 Zheng, Q.T. *et al., Chinese Traditional and Herb Drugs,* **13**(1982), 1: 24.
3 Gu, Y.C. *et al., Acta Pharmaceutica Sinica,* **24**(1989), 8: 629.
4 Zheng, Q.T. *et al., Chinese Traditional and Herb Drugs Bulletin,* **10**(1979), 11: 35.
5 Pen, X.G., in *Pharmacological Experimental Methodology* (Ed. Xue, S.Y.), People Health Press, 1982, pp.1115–1146.
6 Du, D.J. *et al., Chinese Traditional and Herb Drugs,* **12**(1981), 9: 22.
7 Wu, K.Y. *et al., Chinese Medical Journal,* **60**(1980), 451.

Binding Between Beta-elemene and Nucleic Acids

LI Deshan, QIN Liya,

(*Dalian Institute of Medical and Pharmaceutical Sciences, Dalian* 116013, *China*)

CUI Xiuyun

(*Dalian Medical College, Dalian* 116024, *China*)

and SHI Shouheng

(*Dalian Institute of Light Industry, Dalian* 116024, *China*)

Abstract In this paper, the binding between beta-elemene and calf thymus DNA *in vitro* has been verified by thermal denaturation measurements and fluorimetry analysis. Thermal denaturation measurements showed that beta-elemene caused a reduction in T_m of about 2 °C and this value was reproducible. After incubation of calf thymus DNA (30 μg/ml) with beta-elemene (20 μg/ml), the fluorescence intensity at *Ex* 304 nm and *Em*358 nm increased to 0. 315 compared with 0. 020 for the control solurtion of DNA (30 μg/ml). A similar increase in fluorescence intensity was demonstrated in the incubation of beta-elemene with yeast t-RNA. The mechanism of the antitumor activity of beta-elemene was explored by quantum chemistry using the CNDO/2 method. The frontier orbital energy level ELUMO for beta-elemene is −0.0168 a. u. and the EHOMO is −0. 3239 a. u. For quanine the ELUMO is 0. 1629 a. u. and the EHOMO is −0.2596 a.u.: for thymine, the ELUMO is 0.1324 a.u. and the EHOMO is −0.3550 a.u.; for uracil, the ELUMO is 0.0888 a.u. and the EHOMO is −0.3940 a.u. One of the methyl groups in beta-elemene results in a more positive net charge. This suggests that there could be an interaction between beta-elemene and the nucleic acid bases with a selective interaction between the methyl group and the nitrogen atoms of the bases.

I. Introduction

Beta-elemene was isolated from the traditional Chinese medicine, the essential oil of curcuma wenyujin, and it was found to be effective in the treatment of tumors a few years ago. Previous work showed that beta-elemene reduced the level of DNA and RNA in ascites cancer cells, suggesting that there was an interaction between beta-elemene and the DNA template. The work reported here shows the binding between beta-elemene and calf thymus DNA *in vitro* by fluorescence analysis and by DNA thermal denaturation measurements. Also explored is the binding function between beta-elemene and DNA using the quantum chemical CNDO/2 method.

II. Materials and Methods

1. *Reagents*

Beta-elemene was provided by the Dalian Institute of Medical and Pharmaceutical

Science; calf thymus DNA was obtained from the Reagent Factory of Institute of Biophysics under the Chinese Academy of Sciences. The DNA solution was prepared in a buffer of 0. 15 mol/L NaCl and 0. 015 mol/L sodium citrate. Beta-elemene does not dissolve in water, but a solution in water can be prepared using tween −80. The control solution contained the same concentration of tween −80. Yeast t-RNA was obtained from the Institute of Biophysics, Chinese Academy of Sciences. All reagents used were of analytical grade.

2. *Fluorimetry study of the binding between beta-elemene and DAN/t-RNA*

Reactions were carried out in sodium citrate buffer at room temperature. The fluorescence spectra of beta-elemene after reaction with DNA or t-RNA were measured with a Hitachi 650 −60 fluorescence spectrophotometer. The wavelength of excitation was 304 nm and the wavelength of emission was 358 nm. The concentration of the calf thymus DNA solution was 30 μg/ml; the concentrations of the solution of beta-elemene were 0 μg/ml, 20 μg/ml, 60 μg/ml, 120 μg/ml and 200 μg/ml respectively.

3. *Thermal denaturation measurements of DNA*

Sodium citrate buffer was used as the reaction medium. The optical density at 260 nm was recorded using a Shimadzu UV −240 spectrophotometer and used the optical density values to determine the changes of T_m.

4. *Molecular orbital calculations for beta-elemene*

A molecular model was constructed using a published CNDO/2 molecular calculation. The standard parameters of Pople. Lide and Geiser were used. There are three double bonds in beta-elemene, two of which have sterically hindered rotation. One can rotate by 360°, and this one has been considered in our calculations.

III. Results

1. *Binding between beta-elemene and DNA*

The intensity of fluorescence of the solution of calf thymus DNA at a concentration of 30 μg/ml was low. When the solution reacted with beta-elemene solution, the fluorescent intensity increased (Tables 1 and 2). Similar results were observed with yeast t-RNA.

2. *Effect of beta-elemene on T_m of DNA*

The T_m value of calf thymus DNA in the presence of tween −80 was 93.3 ℃, while that of the beta-elemene DNA complex in the presence of tween −80 was 91.4 ℃. Thus the addition of beta-elemene to DNA solution resulted in a reduction of about 2 ℃ in the value of T_m which was reproducible. When the reaction medium was tris-HCI-cellosolve buffer (2: 1, v: v) the result was similar, the reduction in T_m being 2.5 ℃ .

Table 1 Effect of Beta-elemene Contained Tween −80 on DNA Fluorescent Intensity

DNA (μg/ml)	Beta-elemene (μg/ml)	Tween −80 (μg / ml)	Intensity
30	0	0	0.024
30	20	200	0.70
30	60	600	1.53
30	120	1200	2.40
30	200	2000	3.15

Table 2 Effect of Tween −80 on DNA Fluorescent Intensity

DNA (μg/ml)	Tween −80 (μg/ml)	Fluorescent intensity
30	200	0.33
30	600	0.73
30	1200	1.24
30	2000	1.85

3. *Results of calculation*

Table 3 Energy of All Conformation of Beta-elemene (a. u.)

a(°)	0	30	60	90
Totae energy (a.u)	−124.4799	−124.4735	−124.4692	−124.4675
a(°)	120	150	180	210
Total energy (a.u)	−124.4763	−124.4769	−124.4768	−124.4775
a(°)	240	270	300	330
Total energy (a.u)	−124.4766	−124.4656	−124.4678	−124.4726

Table 4 Energy of Frontier Orbital of Beta-elemene (a.u)

a(°)	0	30	90	180	210	270	330
ELUMO	−0.0168	−0.0166	−0.0152	−0.0156	−0.0157	−0.0153	−0.0166
EHOMO	−0.0239	−0.3240	−0.3266	−0.3228	−0.3231	−0.3226	−0.3240

Table 5 Energy of Frontier Orbital of Nucleic Acid Bases (a.u)

	Guanine	Adenine	Cytosine	Thymine	Uracil
ELUMO (a.u)	0.1629	0.1366	0.1459	0.1324	0.0888
EHOMO (a.u)	−0.2596	−0.3695	−0.3342	−0.3550	−0.3940

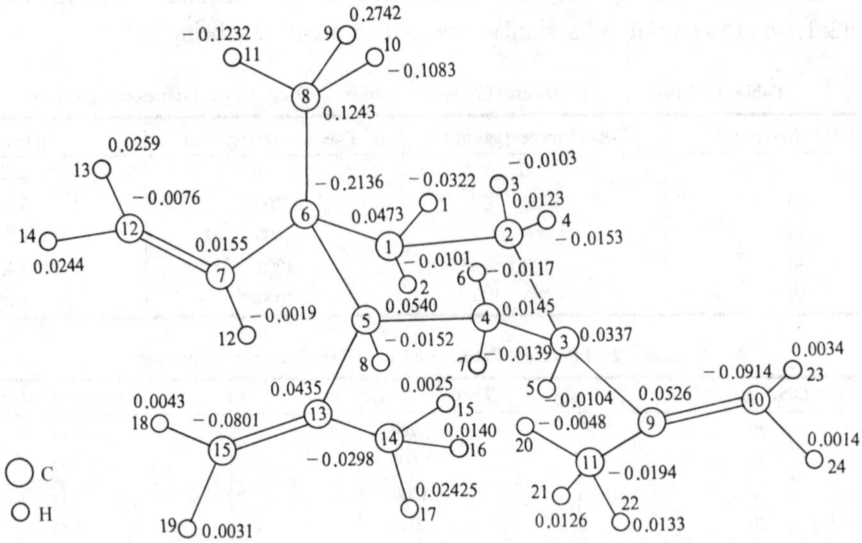

Fig. 1 Net charge configuration of beta-elemene when the double bond was at a = 0 °C .

IV. Discussion

Fluorescence analysis method was used to prove the binding of drug to DNA, The higher fluorescent intensity showed that there could be an interaction between beta-elemene and DNA. The complex of beta-elemene and DNA was produced. Changes in T_m was often used as a criterion of DNA binding with drug. Addition of beta-elemene to DNA solution resulted in a reduction of T_m, though the change was not marked and this value was reproducible. This suggested that the binding of DNA with beta-elemene reduced stability of DNA. And the binding between beta-elemene and DNA was weak because the reduction of T_m was only near 2 °C, but it could affect the function of DNA template and the function of t-RNA as well. Beta-elemene is a compound which belongs to the sesquiterpense. It does not contain any atoms of oxygen or nitrogen which possess larger electric negativity, and it is not capable of forming hydrogen bonds with DNA and t-RNA, but a methyl group in beta-elemene results in more positive net charge. This suggests that there could be an interaction between beta-elemene and the nucleic acid bases and riboses with a selective interaction between the methyl group and the nitrogen atoms of bases and the oxygen atoms of riboses. On the other hand, comparing the energy level of frontier orbit of beta-elemene with nucleic acid bases, this suggests that there could be an interaction between frontier orbit of beta-elemene and nucleic acid bases. π electron of beta-elemene could be excited onto the LUMO of some nucleic acid bases and the molecular complex of beta-elemene with DNA or RNA could be formed; functions of DNA and RNA would be affected by beta-elemene.

References

1 Shi Jihui, *Zhong Yao Tong Bao* (in Chinese), **32**(1981), No. 6.

2 Fu Naiwu *et al., Zhong Yao Tong Bao* (in Chinese), **35**(1984), No. 2.

3 Glasby, J. S., *Encyclopaedia of the Terpenoids,* p. 877.

4 Lide, D. R. *et al., J. Chem. Phys.,* **35**(1961), 1374.

5 Geise, H. J. *et al., J. Mol. Struct.,* **13**(1972), 211.

References

The Effect of Chemotherapy on the Activity of NK Cells and T Cells in Peripheral Blood of Cancer Patients

ZHOU Lizhong, WEN Fugang, LU Jinfang
(*Anshan No.* 4 *Hospital Anshan,* 114033, *China*)

LI Shiqing
(*Anshan Central Hospital, Anshan* 114001, *China*)

This paper is based on observation and study of the activity of NK cells and differences in T cells in peripheral blood before and after chemotherapy. Although there have been some reports about this in the past few years, the results differ greatly.

I. Patients and Method

From July 1990 to Feb. 1991, 33 patients, who were being treated with chemotherapy, and volunteered to allow examination of NK cells activity and of T cells in peripheral blood. All were suffering from malignant tumors as confirmed by pathological and cytopathological diagnosis; 12 patients had stage III and IV lung cancer; 4 patients had stage IV breast cancer and 5 patients were in postoperative accessory chemotherapy; 4 patients had advanced gastric carcinoma; 2 patients were suffering from postoperative carcinoma of the colon and had stage IV of malignant lymphoma, respectively. Four patients had other tumours. The average age was 49 years (ranging between 24 and 70 years). They consisted of 16 men and 17 women.

Only one patient smoked like a chimney. Another six were light smokers who had stopped three months before.

The chemotherapy medicines were CTX, ADM, DDP, Vp-16, 5Fu, MTX and Carboplatin. The combination chemotherapy fell into five groups: CAP, PEF, CAF, CEF and CMF. The number of patients in each group was 8, 8, 6, 6 and 5 respectively.

One day before chemotherapy, NK, T3, T4 and T8 were tested for the first time and tests were repeated before and after each treatment. When two cycles of chemotherapy had been completed, we had obtained five sets of data using a Flow Cytometry Analyzer.

The patients had not received any therapy for at least one month before the first examination.

II. Result

The NK cells activity and the T cells in peripheral blood of normal adults and of cancer patients before and after chemotherapy were compared (see Table 1).

Table 1 Comparison of NK Activity and T Cells Between Normal Adult and Cancer Patients Before and After Chemotherapy

	Normal	First	Second	Third	Fourth	Fifth
NK	39±12	40.53±2.74	44.8±3.59	45.6±3.9	44.63±3.14	53.44±4.47
P		>0.05	>0.05	>0.05	>0.05	<0.01
T3	60.47±5	64.95±1.76	64.6±1.99	66.19±1.8	69.66±2.5	67.54±2.32
P		<0.05	−0.05	<0.01	<0.01	<0.05
T4	36.74±2	39.66±1.55	39.76±1.61	41.34±1.63	43.72±1.68	43.04±2.13
P		>0.05	>0.05	<0.01	<0.01	<0.02
T8	20.33±1	25.31±1.16	24.84±0.84	25.05±0.97	25.98±1.18	24.12±1.05
P		<0.01	<0.01	<0.01	<0.01	<0.01
T4/8	1.89±0.2	1.67±0.099	1.62±0.07	1.72±0.098	1.71±0.0068	1.82±0.119
P		<0.025	<0.005	<0.05	<0.01	>0.1

III. Discussion

It has been shown by numerous experiments that natural killer cells (NK cells) are able to kill tumor cells directly and to cause T cells to regain their sensitivity so that they are activated to strike the cancer cells. Our results show that the activity of the NK cells of normal adults and of cancer patients before chemotherapy was similar ($P>0.05$). It has been reported that lower NK activity is found only in advance and metastasis patients[1] Eremin *et al.*[2] have suggested that there is no difference between breast cancer patients and normal adults. In the study reported here, the fact that the NK activity values for the 33 patients and the normal adults were very close may result from the number of breast cancer and stable stage patients.

After the combination chemotherapy the NK activity gradually rose. When the second cycle of therapy was completed, the NK activities were found to be markedly higher than those after the first cycle and the normal values ($P<0.02$, $P<0.01$). This differs from the report of Tentori[3] and Xia Yanxing[4] that NK activity was strikingly reduced after chemotherapy. Müler[5] and Sun Weiming[6] observed that single doses of chemotherapeutic drugs did not affect the activity of the NK cells in peripheral blood. Our research indicates that the activity of the NK cells was increased after combination chemotherapy. Masumiotoko and Hosogawa suggested that ADM and DDP increase the activity of NK cells. In our study, 22 patients were treated with ADM and DDP and 6 patients were treated with carboplatin which has the same mode of action as DDP. We have no results to report to date as to whether the two drugs affect the activity of NK cells.

The T cell value is one of the signs of the body's immune state. Generally, the T4 subgroup functions as helpers and inductors (TH/Ti) and the T8 as suppressors and cytotoxins (Ts/Tc)[8]. In our research, the patients had higher than normal values of T_3 and T_8 ($P<0.05$, $P<0.01$) while that of T4 was the same as in normal adults. However, the T4/8 value was lower ($P<0.025$). Taku and Watanabe[9] reported that Th/Ts drops strikingly when a malignant tumor advances. We obtained similar results. It may be noted that T4/8 is higher than that of AIDS patients[10]. After combination chemotherapy, T3 and T8 were still similar to the first values measured. However T4 was higher than the normal ($P<0.02$) and T4/8 was also increased compared with the normal ($P>0.1$). Mizushima *et al.*[11] report that some chemotherapy drugs, by selectively inhibiting Ts cells, may cause Th cells to increase rapidly, thus resulting in an excessive cell immunity reaction. Masumiotoko and Hosogawa[7] suggested that some anti-cancer drugs should strengthen the immune response in three ways, i. e. by removing negative tropism immunity, by increasing positive tropism immunity, and by adding immunity sensitivity. ADM, DDP and CTX can raise positive immunity to Tc, TH and MΦ. ADM and CTX serve to remove negative tropism immunity to Ts. Taku and Watanabe[9] reported a decrease in T cells after chemotherapy, resulting in low values of Th/i and Ts/c, especially of Th/i. In contrast, our results show a rise in T4 and no change in T8. Shinichro and Yamamoto[12] treated HCC with PEIT and found an increase in T4/8 which was due to a decrease in T8. They also found a decrease in the activity of NK cells. However, our research shows a rise in T4/8 due to an increase in T_4. Therefore this immunization state is different from that after PEIT therapy. Barbara *et al.*[19] pointed out that the activity of NK cells and Th/s in heavy smokers were notably reduced. In our study, only one patient was a heavy smoker so the various values were not affected.

In summary, the study reported here indicates that combination chemotherapy with a predetermined mixture, can serve to excite the body's natural resistance to cancer and activate the T cells' immunological reaction to killing tumor cells.

References

1 Wang Changan, *Medicine Immunology Abroad*, **8**(1985), 6: 288.

2 Eremin, O. *et al.*, *Int. J. Cancer*, 1978, 21: 35.

3 Tentori, L. *et al.*, *Cancer Immunol. Immunother.*, **24**(1987), 1: 86.

4 Xia Yanxing *et al.*, *Tumour*, **6**(1986), 2: 81.

5 Müller, C., *Clin. Immunol. Immunopathol.*, 1987, 44: 12.

6 Sun Weimin *et al.*, *Chinese Journal of Microbiology and Immunology*, **8**(1988), 2: 92.

7 Hosogawa, M., *Biotherapy,* **4**(1990), 7: 1229.
8 Reinherz, E.L. *et al.*, *Cell*, 1980, 19: 821.
9 Watanabe, T., *Medical Immunology,* **10**(1985), 4: 471.
10 Geber, H.M., *New Eng. J. Med.*, **316**(1987), 2: 113.
11 Mizushima, Y. *et al.*, *J. Natl. Cancer Ints.*, 1981, 66: 659.
12 Yamamoto, S., *Liver,* **30**(1989), 1: 142.
13 Barbara, P. *et al.*, *Cancer,* **56**(1985), 12: 2789.

Design and Synthesis of Antineoplastic Agents Based on a Natural Blueprint

Hsing-Jang Liu, Milan Ralitsch and Shu Yuan Yu

(*Department of Chemistry, University of Alberta, Edmonton, Alberta, Canada T6G2G2*)

Abstract Based on the natural blueprint of terrecyclic acid **2**, several simple analogs have been prepared, and their biological activity has been examined.

(-)-Quadrone **1**[1,2] and (+)-terrecyclic acid A **2**[3,4] are sesquiterpene metabolites isolated in small quantities from *Aspergillus terreus.* Both of these Compounds exhibit high antineoplastic activity, the former against KB cells *in vitro*[1] and the latter against lymphocytic leukemia P-388 in mice[3]. The interesting cytotoxic properties and the challenging structural features of these novel sesquiterpenoids have elicited extensive synthetic activity, culminating in several total syntheses[5-16] including the one developed in our laboratory[16]. Due to the structural complexity of the target molecules, these synthetic routes, however efficient, are impractical to produce the final products in large quantities.

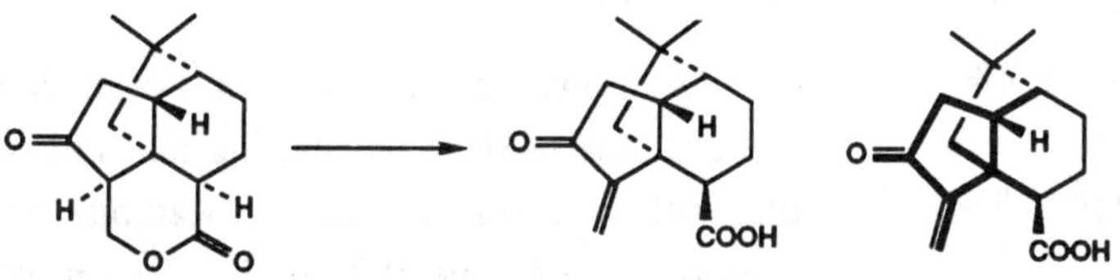

1 (–)-Quadrone **2** (+)-Terrecyclic Acid A

Scheme 1

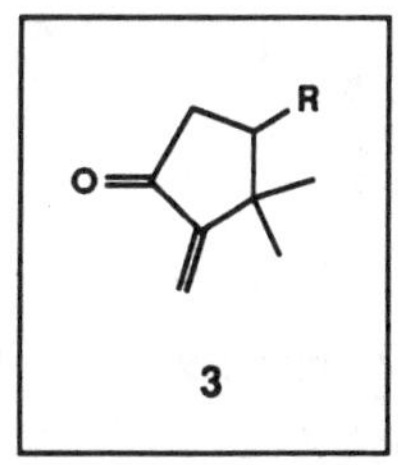

Fig. 1

The antineoplastic activity observed for quadrone and terrecyclic acid A is believed to be due to the presence of the α-methylenecyclopentanone moiety, which is an excellent Michael acceptor, in the latter compound, and the ability to liberate such a moiety in the case of the former compound (Scheme 1). A further examination of the structure of **2** reveals the presence of a quaternary *β*-carbon, which could stabilize the otherwise labile α-methylene ketone functionality, and a highly polar carboxyl group which, along with a hydrocarbon spacer, forms an appendage of the cyclopentanone ring. Under these considerations, it is highly conceivable that simple analogs with the stripped-down structural features shown in general formula 3 (Fig. 1) might still retain the desired biological activity of the natural blueprint.

Rcently, we have embarked on a project directed towards the synthesis of compounds of general type **3** with the ultimate goal being to develop useful therapeutic agents for cancer treatment. During the course of these studies, two general synthetic routes have been developed, each making use of a readily available chiral starting material. As well, several compounds were prepared and tested.

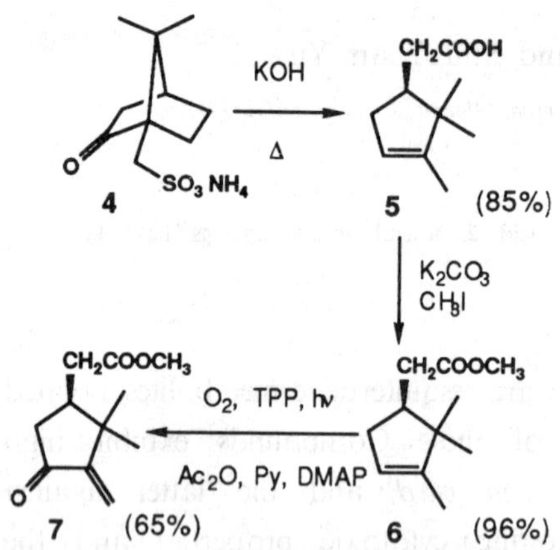

Scheme 2

In one route, the ammonium salt of (-)-10-camphorsulfonic acid **4** was heated with potassium hydroxide to give (-)-α-campholenic acid **5**[17, 18]. This acid was esterified with potassium carbonate and methyl iodide in refluxing acetone. The corresponding methyl ester **6** thus obtained was subjected to photooxidation. Irradiation (tungsten lamp) of a solution of **6** in methylene chloride in the presence of oxygen, acetic anhydride, pyridine and 4-dimethylaminopyridine using 5, 10, 15, 20-tetraphenyl-21*H*, 23*H*-porphine as a photosensitizer[19] gave rise to the desired α-methylenecylopentanone derivative 7. These results are outlined in Scheme 2.

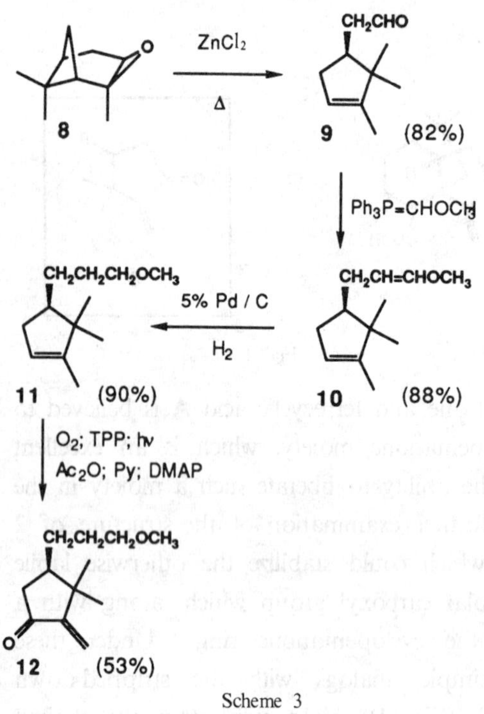

Scheme 3

As shown in Scheme 3, (-)-α-pinene oxide **8** was used as the starting material in the other synthetic route leading to compounds of general type **3**. Treatment of (-)-α-pinene oxide **8** with zinc chloride resulted in its skeletal rearrangement to give (-)-α-campholenic aldehyde **9**[20, 21]. This compound was subjected to Wittig reaction using (methoxymethyl) triphenylphosphonium chloride and potassium hydride in a solution of dimethyl sulfoxide and benzene at room temperature. Catalytic hydrogenation of the resulting enol ether **10** with 5% palladium on carbon, in the presence of potassium carbonate in ethyl acetate at room temperature and atmospheric pressure, gave rise to the desired ether **11**. This compound was oxygenated photochemically under conditions similar to those described previously for the transformation of **6**→**7** to give the target compound **12.**

Tosylate **17** was also prepared from (-)-α-campholenic aldehyde **9** via a similar synthetic sequence (Scheme 4). Wittig reaction of **9** with the ylid, preformed from (α-methoxyethyl)triphenylphosphonium chloride and *n*-butyllithium, in tetrahydrofuran at room temperature gave enol ether **13**, which was immediately hydrolyzed with a mixture of aqueous 20% perchloric acid and ether (1: 1). Sodium borohydride reduction of ketone **14** thus formed in methanol, followed by tosylation with *p*-toluenesulfonyl chloride in pyridine in the presence of a small amount of 4-dimethylaminopyridine, furnished tosylate **16**. Subsequent photooxidation led to the formation of the α-methylenecyclopentanone **17**.

α-Methylenecyclopentanone derivatives **7**, **12**, and **17** were subjected to anticancer screening and were found to have *in vitro* activity against P-388 cells at the level of $IC_{50}=0.3—1.8\,\mu g/mL$ and against L-1210 cells at the level of $IC_{50}=0.4—2.8\,\mu g/mL$. The results obtained from the *in vivo* screening were, however, disappointing, as no activity was observed against L-1210 cells in mice.

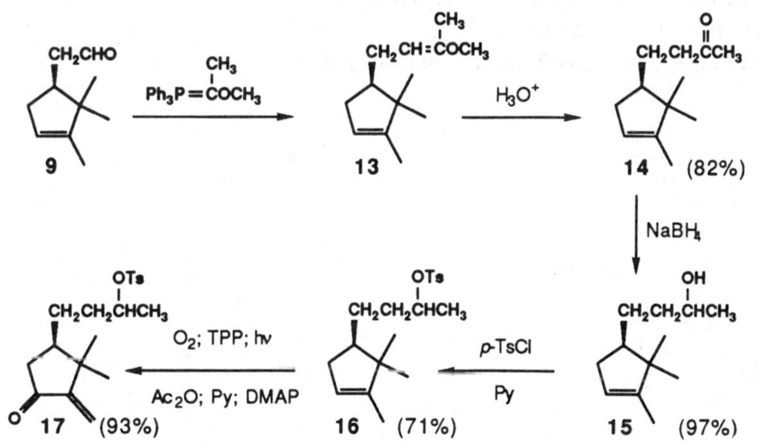

Scheme 4

We are grateful to the Natural Sciences and Engineering Research Council of Canada for financial support, to the Alberta Heritage Foundation for Medical Research for a Studentship to M. R., and to Zenyaku Kogyo Co., Ltd. for anticancer screening.

References

1 Calton, G.J., Ranieri, R.L. and Espenshade, M.A., *J. Antibiot.*, **31**(1978), 38.
2 Ranieri, R.L. and Calton, G.J., *Tetrahedron Lett.*, **499**(1978).
3 Nakagawa, N., Hirota, A., Sakai, H. *et al.*, *J. Antibiot.*, **35**(1982), 778.
4 Hirota, A., Nakagawa, M., Sakai, H. *et al.*, *J. Antibiot.*, **35**(1982), 783.
5 Danishefsky, S., Vaughan, K., Gadwood, R.C., *et al.*, *J. Am. Chem. Soc.*, **102**(1980), 4262; **103**(1981), 4136.
6 Bornock, W.K., Bagwat, S.S., Ponton, J. *et al.*, *J. Am. Chem. Soc.*, **103**(1981), 4647.
7 Burke, S.D., Murtiashaw, C.W., Saunders, J.O. *et al.*, *J. Am. Chem. Soc.*, **104**(1982), 872; Burke, S.D., Murtiashaw, C.W. and Oplinger, J.A., *Tetrahedron Lett.*, **24**(1983), 2949; Burke, S.D., Murtiashaw, C.W., Saunders, J.O. *et al.*, *J. Am. Chem. Soc.*, **106**(1984), 4558.
8 Kende, A.S., Roth, B., Sanfilippo, P.J. *et al.*, *J. Am. Chem. Soc.*, **104**(1982), 5808.
9 Takeda, K., Shimono, Y. and Yoshil, Y., *J. Am. Chem Soc.*, **105**(1983), 563.
10 Schlessinger, R.H., Wood, J.L., Poss, A.J. *et al.*, *J. Org. Chem.*, **48**(1983), 1146.
11 Dewanckele, J.M., Zuttermand, F. and Vandewalle, M., *Tetrahedron*, **39**(1983), 3235.
12 Kon, K., Ito, K. and Isoe, S., *Tetrahedron Lett.*, **25**(1984), 3739.
13 Smith, A.B., III and Konopelski, J.P., *J. Org. Chem.*, **49**(1984), 4094.
14 Piers, E. and Moss, N., *Trtrahedron Lett.*, **26**(1985), 2735.
15 Wender, P.A. and Wolanin, D.J., *J. Org. Chem.*, **50**(1985), 4418.
16 Liu, H.J. and Llinas-Brunet, M., *Can. J. Chem.*, **66**(1988), 528.
17 Sauers, R.S., *J. Am. Chem. Soc.*, **81**(1959), 925.
18 Liu, H.J. and Chan, W.H., *Can. J. Chem.*, **60**(1982), 1081.
19 Mihelich, E.D. and Eickhoff, D.J., *J. Org. Chem.*, **48**(1983), 4135.
20 Arbusow, B. and Mitteil, I., *Ber.*, **68**(1935), 1430.
21 Meinwald, J. and Chapman, R., *J. Am. Chem. Soc.*, **90**(1968), 3218.

Conformational Analysis of the Antineoplastic Pentapeptide Dolastatin 10 and Its Analogue Without Nonstandard Amino Acids

M. Toscano, T. Marino, E. Zasa and N. Russo

(*Dipartimento di Chimica Università della Calabria, I-87030 Arcavacata di Rende* (CS), *Italy.*)

Abstract We present a preliminary report on the conformational analysis of the Dolastatin 10 (Dov-Val-Dil-Dap-Doe) antineoplastic pentapeptide and its analogue (Val-Val-Ile-Pro-Phe) without nonstandard amino acids obtained at nonbonded and Molecular Mechanics levels of theory. Thirteen minima in the range of 10 kcal/mol above the absolute minimum have been found for both systems.

I. Introduction

In the last two decades different new natural peptides with potent cytostatic and antineoplastic activity have been isolated from sea hare *Dolabella Auricularia* and then characterized[1-4]. One of them is the pentapeptide Dolastatin 10 which is the most powerful (i. e. lowest *in vivo* dose) antineoplastic substance known to date[2]. Because of the presence in the Dolastatin 10 backbone of four very unusual amino acid residues, this peptide is very interesting also from a conformational point of view. It is well known that conformational analysis plays a central role in the determination of structure-activity relationships and more in general in the field of molecular biology. Studies in this direction on small peptides containing modified amino acid residues, show that a significant reduction of available conformational space can be expected[5].

In this paper the first results of a conformational study on Dolastatin 10 and its analogue (see Fig. 1) without nonstandard amino acid residues (N-Dolastatin 10) are reported. Conformational analyses of Dolavaline (Dov), Dolaisoleuine (Dil), Dolaproine (Dap) and Dolaphenine (Doe) are also given.

II. Method

Conformational energy calculations have been performed by employing the NB/80[6] package which evaluates the conformational energy as a sum of nonbonded, electrostatic, hydrogen-bond and intrinsic torsional contributions. The net atomic charges as well as the nonbonded parameters have been taken from Ref. [7]. The geometries of the amino acid residues have been optimized using the MODEL package and the MMX

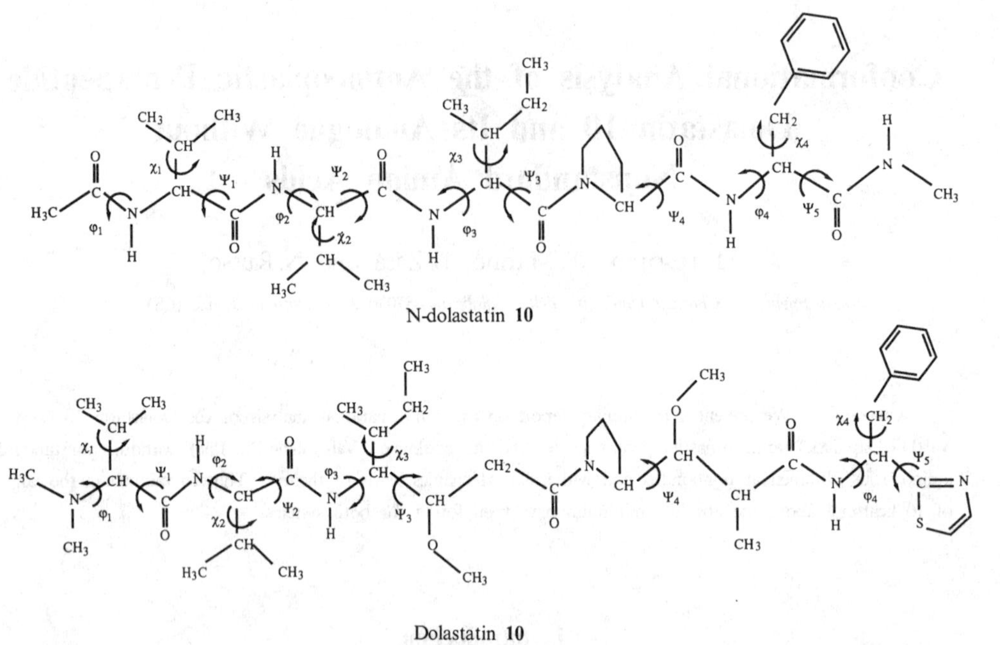

Fig. 1 Schematic drawing of the N-Dolastatin 10 and Dolastatin 10 peptides and labelling of the main dihedral angles.

force field[8].

After an initial search into the whole conformational space (employing a grid mesh of 10°) minimum-energy conformations were obtained in the low energy regions by OPT/80 package using algorithms with analytical evaluation of both the gradient and the Hessian[9]. Conformational energies (in kcal/mol) are expressed as $\Delta E = E - E_0$, where E_0 is the most stable conformation.

III. Results and Discussion

As a first step of the work we have performed the conformational analysis of the amino acid residues present in Dolastatin 10 and N-Dolastatin 10.

The conformational flexibility and structures of valine, isoleucine, proline and phenylalanine are very similar to those previously reported in the literature[10,11]. Concerning the unusual Dov, Dil, and Doe residues our results show a reduction of the conformational space with respect to the correspoding Val, Ile, and Phe residues, while for Dap, two more minima than in Pro are allowed. For dolaisoleuine, only two low conformational minima are possible, while six minima are present in the isoleucine conformational map. The restriction of the conformationally available space with respect to isoleucine is probably due to the presence of the $-OCH_3$ group that increases the steric hindrance.

The two minima of the Dil residue are practically isoenergetic ($\Delta E = 1.1$ kcal/mol). In particular the absolute minimum has a structure similar to that obtained for one of the minima of isoleucine. This also means that the modified amino acid can have Lα helical structures. In the dolavaline residue, the presence of an additional methyl group on the terminal nitrogen atom again reduces the number of low energy conformational minima. In fact, of the six minima of valine only four are present in an energy range of 2 kcal/mol. As mentioned before, for Dap also we found four minima in an energy range of about 12 kcal/mol. The greater number of different minima with respect to the two found for Pro is essentially due to an additional $-CH(OCH_3)CH(CH_3)$ group in the amino acid backbone that increases the conformational degree of freedom (another torsional angle). This effect is only partially compensated by the steric hindrance of the $-OCH_3$ group.

The last residue in the Dolastatin 10 is the thiazole amino acid dolaphenine. For Doe, conformational analysis shows the presence of two minima with a ΔE of only 0.9 kcal/mol. In Phe we found six minima in an energetic range of 5 kcal/mol. The reduction of the available conformational space, in the case of Doe, is due to the thiazole group which increases the repulsive interactions.

Starting from the minima found for the first amino acid (Doe or Val), we have built up the pentapeptides by adding an amino acid each time. Freezing the structure of the first residue, we have explored the conformational space of the dipeptides, scanning the torsional angles of the second residue for each minimum of the first[11].

The minima obtained in the conformational maps of the dipeptides have been optimized but only those in a range of 30 kcal/mol around the absolute minimum have been considered for the tripeptides analysis. Following the same methodology, we have obtained 13 minima for both N-Dolastatin 10 and Dolastatin 10. The search for the absolute conformational minima of the two systems was performed by employing a molecular mechanics method (MMX force field).

Table 1 Optimized Values for the Dihedral Angles of N-Dolastatin 10 (N-D 10) and Dolastatin 10 (D 10) Obtained by NB and MMX Computations

Molecule	φ_1	Ψ_1	χ_1	φ_2	Ψ_2	χ_2	φ_3	Ψ_3	χ_3	φ_4	Ψ_4	χ_4	Ψ_5
						NB							
N-D10	−94.5	82.7	174.0	100.2	−142.0	178.9	−70.0	−20.9	93.7	46.5	123.2	−59.6	33.9
D10	−100.1	3.3	−170.0	−145.4	178.0	177.2	15.4	164.5	142.1	−175.2	177.5	176.3	11.2
						MMX							
N-D10	−141.8	148.5	177.6	171.1	96.8	175.4	60.1	−151.9	−64.9	−70.4	109.9	−170.6	−38.0
D10	61.6	−134.7	−169.9	112.3	−75.7	176.0	−127.8	−79.4	176.5	81.3	63.0	179.9	145.6

The sizes of the main torsional angles are reported in Table 1, while in Fig. 2 the NB absolute minima of Dolastatin 10 and N-Dolastatin 10 are depicted.

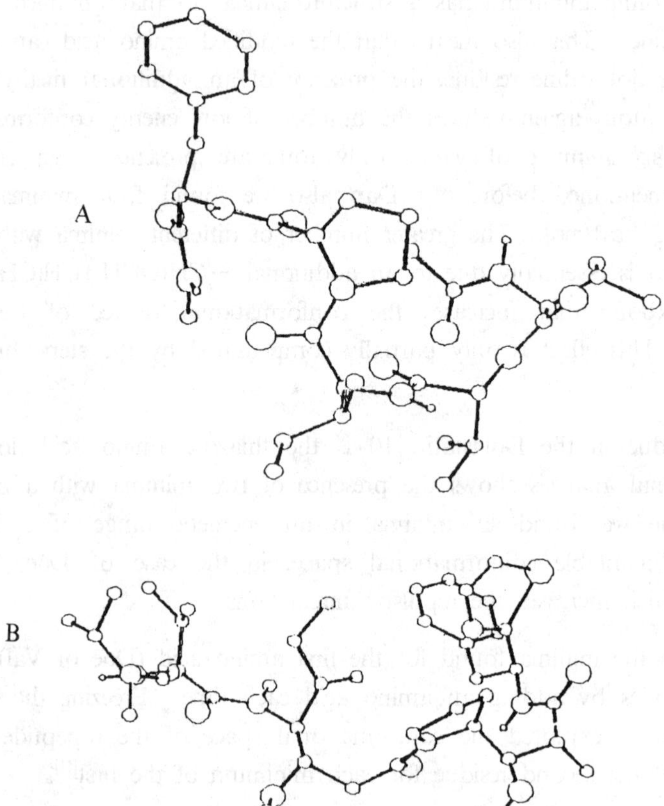

Fig. 2 Structures of the absolute conformational minima of the N-Dolastatin 10 (A) and Dolastatin 10 (B) peptides obtained at an NB level of computation.

Notwithstanding the fact that the conformational flexibility (number of minima) is the same, the relative structures of some minima are quite different in the two pentapeptides. The same structural differences are found for the two absolute minima. Comparison between MMX and NB results shows that the two methods give a different conformation for the absolute minimum for each molecule. Further work is in progress to better characterize the conformational analysis as well as the role of the solvent effect both at the NB level and using a different force field før the MM calculations.

IV. Conclusions

On the basis of our study some preliminary conclusions can be given:

The conformational space of the unusual amino acids dolavaline, dolaisoleuine and dolaphenine is reduced with respect to that of the corresponding nonmodified residues. In the case of dolaproine the low energy minima are in a greater number with respect to those of the phenylalanine.

The conformational flexibility of dolastatine 10 is similar to that of N-Dolastatine 10. This is essentially due to the competition between two effects: the increased degree of freedom and the steric hindrance of additional groups in the peptied backbone.

The structure of the absolute minimum as well as that of some other minima is different in the two molecules.

MMX and NB methods give different conformations for the absolute minima of both the systems.

References

1 Pettit, G. R., Kamano, Y., Herald, C.L. *et al., J. Am. Chem. Soc.,* **109**(1987), 6883.

2 Pettit, G. R., Kamano, Y., Holzapfel, C.W. *et al., J. Am. Chem. Soc.,* **109**(1987), 7581.

3 Pettit, G. R., Kamano, Y., Herald, C. L. *et al., J. Am. Chem. Soc.,* **111**(1989), 5015.

4 Pettit, G. R., Singh, S. B., Hogan, F. *et al., J. Am. Chem. Soc.,* **111**(1989), 5463.

5 Barone, V., Fraternali, F. and Cristinziano, P. L., *Macromolecules,* **23**(1990), 2038 and references therein.

6 Barone, V., Cristinziano, P. L., and Lelj, F., *Programs NB/*80 *and OPT/*80, unpublished.

7 Weiner, S.J., Kollman, P. A., Nguyen, D.T. *et al., J. Comput. Chem.,* **7**(1986) 230 and reference therein.

8 *Program Model, Version* 9.2 *of Steliou K,* Universite de Montreal (Canada).

9 Schlegel, H.B., *Adv. Chem. Phys.,* **67**(1987), 249.

10 Liguori, A.M., *Quant. Rev. Biophys.,* **2**(1969), 65.

11 Roterman, I.K., Lambert, M.H., Gibson, K.D. *et al., J. Biol. Struct. Dynam.,* **7**(1989), 421.

12 Nemethy, G., Pottle, M.S. and Sheraga, M.A., *J. Phys. Chem.,* **117**(1987) 1813 and reference therein.

The Anti-breast Cancer Effect of iRNA

HUANG Huazhang, LI Weilian*, ZHANG Yuqin,
HOU Zizheng and WANG Jinlong

(*Lab. Nucleic Acids and Cancer Research, Tianjin Medical College, Tianjin* 300070, *China*)

Abstract iRNA was prepared from liver, spleen and lymph nodes of breast cancer sensitized mice, rabbit or sheep by the cold phenol method, and showed a typical UV absorption curve, with the ratio of A260/A280 > 2.0, A260/A230 > 2.0 and with an apparent heat hyperchromicity of over 11% after DNase digestion.

On the basis of 6 experiments of iRNA therapy of transplantable mammary carcinoma in mice, we got an average inhibition rate as high as 60.6%, but iRNA therapy had no effect when normal saline, DNA or RNase-treated iRNA was used.

It was observed that in some cases of advanced human breast cancer after treated with iRNA was reduced in size. A follow-up of the 5-year survival rate was carried out on 18 patients treated with iRNA after routine operation, chemotherapy and/or radiotherapy. Another 12 patients having had chemotherapy and radiotherapy after a routine operation were used as a control group. A 83.3% (15/18) survival rate after 5 years was found for the iRNA-treated group and 66.6% for the control group. Thus, the 5-years mortality of control group (33.3%, 4/12) is twice that of the iRNA group (16.7% 3/18). In accordance with these results, we suggest that iRNA has an apparent inhibitory effect on animal and human breast cancer. The inhibitory effect may be due to the following factors. (i) Specific immunity of iRNA. (ii) Nonspecific immunity of iRNA. (iii) The presence of some dsRNA and ds-DNA in the iRNA preparation which can induce IFN production in mice and in human bodies. It is well known that IFN can increase immunity and inhibit viral disease and some kinds of cancer. In our patients, no one caught the common cold during the iRNA injection period, though they were susceptible. Apparently, this is an effect of our iRNA preparation.

Since the discovery of iRNA in 1963 by Fishman and Alder[1], many laboratories have attempted to utilize iRNA in cancer therapy[2-18]. Among them Schlager et al.[16] reported a complete regression of tumors in 10 guinea pigs while Pilch was the first to report the results of clinical trials on human cancers with iRNA. These results were most interesting in this field.

Since 1974 there have been many interesting reports about iRNA including *in vitro* and *in vivo* animal experiments and clinical trials in human patients. It has been used as an anticancer, anti-virus and anti-bacterial agent. Four national iRNA symposia have been held in China, in Hangzhou in 1979, in Shaoxing in 1985, in Hohhot in 1986 and in Changchun in 1988.

---

* Oncology Department, The Second Central Hospital, Tianjin 300120, PRC.

During this period of time some experiments were also done in our laboratory[19–22]. We have found some high inhibition rates on the growth of several tumors in mice. We reported that the iRNA from the liver of immunized animals has the same anti-cancer effect on animals and patients as iRNA from the spleen and lymph nodes of immunized animals.

We used cantharidine skin bleb[21] as an *in vivo* incubation system for the transfer of iRNA information, instead of iRNA incubated with spleen cells *in vitro*. The former is simpler and more effective than the latter. Another study by our graduate students[23,24] was on the comparison of single and combined treatments of iRNA, hyperthermia and X-ray irradiation. It showed that iRNA has the longest survival time in single treatments and iRNA + radiation therapy has a synergistic effect on survival time and tumor inhibition rate.

Then we studied the 5-year survival rate of patients treated with iRNA after a routine operation, irradiation and chemotherapy. In this paper, we report some of the results from our laboratory on the effect of iRNA on breast cancer.

I. Materials and Methods

1. *Immunization of animals and preparation of iRNA*

Routine immunization methods and cold phenol methods for RNA were used as reported previously[22].

2. *Cantharidin skin bleb incubation method*

The skin bleb was prepared by a routine method described by Zhang[25]. The iRNA injection method was as described by Huang[21, 22] (Figs. 1 and 2).

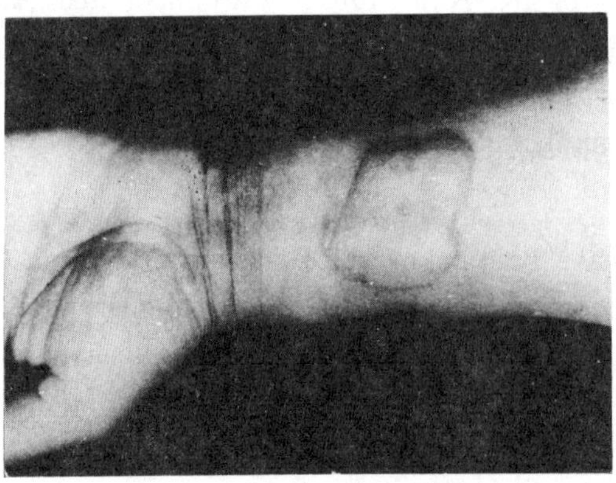

Fig. 1. A 24-h skin bleb on forearm produced by Chinese cantharis tincture.

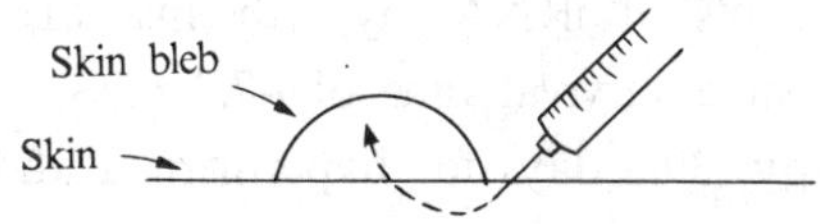

Fig. 2 The injection of RNA solution into the skin bleb.

3. *The selection of patients of breast cancer for observation of 5-year survival rate*

36 patients after routine operations, chemotherapy and radiation therapy were randomly divided into 2 groups equally. The iRNA group was treated with 2 mg of iRNA by the skin bleb incubation method in the first injection, then 2 mg of iRNA was injected sc in the groin or armpit region every 2 days for 1 month (15 × 2 mg iRNA). In the control group, iRNA was substituted with normal saline.

II. Results and Discussion

1. As shown in Table 1 15 of 18 breast cancer patients in the iRNA-treated group survived for longer than 5 years (15/18 or 83.3%). In the control group, contact was lost with 6 patients. The other 12 had a 66.6% or 8/12 survival rate over 5 years.

Table 1 The 5-Year Survival of Breast Cancer Patients

Group	No. of Cases	>5- Year Survival	<5-year Survival
iRNA	18	15/18 or 83.3%	3/18 or 16.7%
Control	12	8/12 or 66.6%	4/12 or 33.2%

The 5-year mortality of the control group was twice that of the iRNA treated group.

In another report by Li Weilian, one of our co-authors[26], the 5-year survival rate of 16 cases of gastric cancer treated with iRNA was 25% or 4/16. This was also better than that of 6.2% or 1/16 for the control group. The results of the 5-year survival rate studies suggest that iRNA may play a role in recovery by increasing the low level immuno-ability of advanced breast cancer patients to a higher level.

2. In our 6 experiments, iRNA from liver or liver+spleen+lymph node of immunized rams, rabbits or mice gave a 60.6% average inhibition of the transplantable mammary cancer in TA-2 mice, while no effect was observed when normal saline or RNase treated with iRNA was used. It shows that iRNA from different sources is effective to the transplantable mammary cancer in mice.

3. In the experiments to study the effects of single or combined treatments of iRNA, hyperthermia or radiotherapy, the results were more significant.

a: The results of single treatments of iRNA, hyperthermia or radiotherapy showed that iRNA gave the longest average survival time of 47.3 days. This was longer than that of 40 days for radiotherapy, 39.3 days for hyperthermia and 23.5 days for the control group (Table 2).

b: In the experiments studying combined treatments, iRNA+radiotherapy gave an excellent result. The survival time was as long as 63 days which was 268.1% that of the control group.

Table 2 Average Survival Days of Mice With the Transplantable Mammary Cancer After Different Treatments

Group	Average Survival Days	Survival Days Longer Than the Control Group
Control	23.5	23.5 (100%)
iRNA	47.3	23.8 (101.3%)
Radiotherapy	40	16.5 (70.2%)
Hyperthermia	39.3	15.8 (67.2%)
iRNA+Hyperthermia	41	17.5 (74.5%)
iRNA+Radiotherapy	63	39.5 (168.1%)

c: The experiments were repeated twice and similar results were obtained. Especially, the results from the iRNA+radiotherapy group showed that a synergistic effect was present, affecting both survival days and tumor inhibition rate. Both were sharply raised (Tables 3 and 4).

Table 3 Average Survival Days of 3 Experiments of the Transplantable Mammary Cancer in Mice Under Different Treatments

Group	Average Survival Days			
	1	2	3	average
Control	23.5	27.2	28.0	26.27
iRNA	47.3	44.3	43.0	44.86
Hyperthermia	39.3	38.4	43.3	40.33
Radiotherapy	40	/	46.5	43.25
iRNA+Hypert.	41	41.5	44	42.17
iRNA+Radiot.	63	60	67.4	63.47

In the past 17 years, many studies related to iRNA have been reported in China with good results; especially in clinical trials in patients of cancers and many other diseases.

Table 4 Average Tumor Inhibition Rate of 3 Experiments of the Transplantable Mammary Cancer in Mice Under Different Treatments

Group	Average Inhibition Rate			
	1	2	3	average
Control	0	0	0	
iRNA	44.7	43.0	50.2	45.97
Hyperthermia	57.5	58.2	59.0	58.23
Radiotherapy	55.6	/	54.0	54.80
iRNA+Hypert.	69.3	54.0	59.8	61.03
iRNA+Radiot.	80.4	73.4	82.0	78.60

The therapeutic effects of iRNA against cancer in our work are also obvious.

The temporary regression of the tumor and the lengthening of the survival time is remarkable. For example, some metastatic lesion of mammary, gastric and kidney cancers regressed sharply in 1 month or less when iRNA was injected and the effect could be observed on X—ray film or by palpation. However, only two lymphosarcoma patients treated with iRNA in 1976 by our collaborator Dr. Zhang Zhepin were cured, got married, have children and are surviving in good health until now. Although some cancer patients treated with iRNA after an operation have survived for over 10 years, many of the patients showed beneficial effects for only a short time (a few months to a year), then suffered a relapse.

Furthermore, the iRNA preparation is a complex mixture of many kinds of RNA; therefore it is difficult to explain the therapeutice effect. It showed both specific immunity[27, 28] and nonspecific immunity and can mediate the production of both antibodies[28] and lymphokines[29, 30]. There is a small portion of dsRNA also present in the RNA-rich preparation of iRNA.

dsRNA can induce the production of a highly effective concentration of interferon (IFN) in human blood[31, 32]. The anti-viral and anti-cancer effects of IFN and its role in immunization arc well known.

An apparent heat hyperchromicity was detected in our DNase-treated preparations and that means some quantity of dsRNA was present. On the other hand, none of our patients caught the common cold during the iRNA injection period, though they were susceptible. Apparently, this is an effect of our iRNA preparation. From our results, we consider that the therapeutic effect of iRNA is complex; it can increase immuno-ability in several ways, but at present the mechanism is not clear.

References

1 Fishman, M. and Alder, F. L., *J. Exp. Med.* **117**(1963), 595.
2 Alexander, P. *et al.*, *Nature*, **213**(1967), 569.
3 Londner, M.V. *et al.*, *Experimentia*, **24**(1968), 598.
4 Rigby, P.G., *Nature*, **221**(1969), 968.
5 Kennedy, C.T.C. *et al.*, *Acta Pathol. Microbiol. Scand*, **77**(1969), 196.
6 Pilch, Y.H. *et al.*, *J. Nalt. Cancer*, **26**(1970), 630.
7 Ramming, K.P. *et al.*, *J. Nalt, Cancer Inst.*, **46**(1971), 735.
8 Deckers P.T. *et al.*, *Nature*, **231**(1971), 181.
9 Pilch, Y.H. *et al.*, *Isr, J, Med, Sci.*, **7** (1971) 1246; CA 75, 33025× (1971).
10 Pilch, Y.H. *et al.*, *Ann. New York Acad. Sci.*, **207**(1973), 409.
11 Deckers, P. T. *et al.*, *Ibid.*, **207**(1973), 442.
12 Ohno, R. *et al.*, *Ibid.*, **207**(1973), 430.
13 Han, T. *et al.*, *Clin Exp Immunol.*, **14**(1973), 213.
14 Fukushima, M. *et al.*, *Exp. Med.*, **112**(1974), 155; *Nucleic Acid Abs.*, **4**, **4n** (1974), 7423.
15 Cohen, E. P. *et al.*, *Immune RNA*, CRC Press, 1976.
16 Schlager, S. I. *et al.*, *Cancer Research*, **35**(1975), 8: 1907.
17 Sinknner, D. G. *et al.*, *J., Urol.*, **115**(1976), 246.
18 Deckers, P. J. *et al.*, *Ann. Ny. Acad. Sci.*, **277**(1976), 575.
19 Dept. of Biochem., Nankai Univ. and Lab. Exp., Cancer Res, Tianjin Med. College, *Scientific Investigation of Tianjin Medical College*, 1975, pp. 1— 7.
20 Tianjin Coperation group for iRNA research *et al.*, *Cancer Communication of Zheijiang*, 1979.
21 Huang H.Z. *et al.*, *Ibid.*, 1979.
22 Huang H.Z. *et al.*, *Proceeding of 2nd International Symposium on the Role of RNA on Development and Reproduction* (edited by Niu M. C. & Chuang H. H.), 1981, pp. 323—342.
23 Hou, Z. Z. *et al.*, *Oncological Supp. of Tumor Clinic*, **10**(1983), 4: 244.
24 Hou, Z. Z. *et al.*, *Tumor Clinic*, **11**(1984), 2: 118.
25 Cancer Research Institute of Chinese Academy of Medical Science., *J. Chinese Med.*, 1976, 4: 229.
26 Li, W. L. and Huang, H. Z., *Immune RNA and Clinic*, Vol. II (edited by Wang, W. Z.), 1989, p. 88.
27 Zheng, C. X., *Qinghua Daxue Xuebao* (in Chinese) (Ziran Kexueban), **27**(1989), 6: 63.
28 Li, S. G. and Yang, M. J., *Chinese Jour., Microbiol. Immunol.*, **8**(1988), 5: 276.
29 Dong, F. M., Yang, M. J. *et al.*, *ibid.*, **5**(1985), 6: 363.
30 Dong, F. M. and Yang, M. J., *ibid.*, **6**(1986), 1: 23.
31 Wang, F.Z., Yang, M. J. *et al.*, *ibid.*, **6**(1986), 2: 92.
32 Lu, Z. Q. *et al.*, *Immune iRNA and Clinc*, Vol. II (edited by Wang, W. Z.), 1989, p. 14.

Presence of a Urokinase Peak in the Urine of Mice Just Before Cancer Metastasis

HUANG Huazhang, LI Guangyu* and ZHANG Yuqin

(*Lab. Nucleic Acids and Cancer Research, Tianjin Medical College, Tianjin 300070, China*)

Abstract Urokinase activity in the urine of several strains of mice during the course of growth of transplanted tumors were studied. Urokinase activity was tested by the fibrin-plate method using 20 μL of urine collected in the morning of the day before transplantation (as control) and every 3 or 4 days after transplantation until the death of each mouse. The tumor and mice strains used were:

(I) Melanoma B16F10 (>90% metastasis on the 18—20th days) in DBF1 mice (repeated 4 times).

(II) B16F10 in TA-2 mice (repeated twice).

(III) Lung adenocarcinoma (100% metastasis on the 8— 10th days).

(IV) Mammary carcinoma MA−74 (no or very low metastasis) in TA-2 mice.

(V) Sarcoma-180 in C57b1/6 mice.

The results are as follows:

1. Urokinase activity increases at the early stage of tumor growth and a sharp peak appears just before metastasis, then decreases to a level lower than the normal value and even to 1/2 of the normal value before death.

2. The higher the metastasis rate, the higher the rise in urokinase activity. For example, it rose to 238% ($P<0.01$) in (III), 170% ($P<0.01$) in (I), 177% ($P<0.01$) in (II) and there was no peak in (IV) and (V).

3. The urokinase peak appeared on the 15— 18 th days just before metastasis (18— 20 th days) in (I); the 18 th day before metastasis (18— 20 th days) in (II); the 5— 8 th days before metastasis (8— 10 th days) in (III) and no peak appeared in non-metastatic cancer.

4. The urokinase level in urine is not proportional to the tumor size especially at the advanced stage of tumor growth.

Urokinase type plasminogen activator or urokinase can transfer plasminogen to plasmin, and plasmin has the ability to degrade many protein components in the extracellular matrix directly. On the other hand urokinase may also degrade some proteins of the extracellular matrix directly. The proteolytic activity of urokinase is related to the invasive growth and metastasis of tumors[1, 2].

A great deal of *in vitro* experimentation indicated that the synthesis and secretion of

* Lab. Immunology, Tianjin Institute of Cancer, Tianjin 300060, P.R.China.

urokinase in cultures of transformed or malignant cells are higher than those in normal cell cultures[3—6]. However, reports of *in vivo* studies are relatively rare.

This work is an attempt to discover if there is any change of urokinase activity in the urine of tumor-bearing animals during the course of tumor growth.

I. Materials and Method

1. *Animals*

(1) DBF1 (C57BL × DBA).
Age: 6— 10 wks, body wt: 18— 26 g, male black mice.
(2) C57BL/6 inbred male black mice.
Age: 10 wks, body wt: 24— 28 g.
(3) TA-2 inbred mice.
Age: 6— 8 wks, body wt: 16— 20 g.
(4) T739 inbred brown-yellowish mice.
Age: 6— 10 wks, body wt: 18— 22 g.

2. *Tumors*

(1) B16F10 melanoma in DBF1 mice[7].
B16F10 melanoma (2.4×10^6 cells in 0.2 ml per mouse) was subdermally transplanted into the right groin of DBF1 mice. Latent period: 4— 6 days, survival period: 19— 25 days. >90% metastasis appeared 18— 20 days after transplantation.

(2) B16F10 melanoma in TA-2 mice (transplanted B16F10 melanoma as in (1)). Latent period: 5— 7 days, survival period: 25— 32 days.

(3) L795 lung adenocarcinoma in T739 mice[8].
2−3 mm graft per mouse was transplanted subdermally into the groin of mice. latent period: 5 — 7 days, survival period: 28 — 33 days, 100% metastasis 8— 10 days after transplantation.

(4) MA75 mammary carcinoma in TA-2 mice.
6×10^6 MA75 cells in 0.2 mL per mouse were transplanted as in (1).
Latent period: 4−6 days, survival period: 28 — 30 days; non-metastasis or very low metastasis.

(5) S180 sarcoma in C57BL/6 mice.
6×10^6 S180 cells in 0.2mL per mouse were transplanted as in (1). Latent period: 4— 5 days, survival period: 14−28 days; non-matastasis.

Table 1 The Changes of Urokinase Activity in Urine of B16F10 Melanoma-Bearing DBFl Mice

Exp. No.	No. of Mice	Urokinase Activity at Days After Tumor Transplantation (iμ / ml urine, $\overline{X}$ ±S. D.)									
		0	2	3	4	5	6	8	9	11	12
1	10	13.74±2.53			17.00±3.65		10.70±2.14		11.80±2.78		22.20±2.62
2	10	13.82±2.22				11.97±3.18		13.8±2.46	14.53±3.55		
3	10	16.20±3.20		8.76±1.33					15.32±1.58		19.50±1.78
4	10	15.19±2.70	16.13=0.85		16.58±2.20				13.36±1.98	16.92±1.68	
			14	15	16	17	19	20	21	22	27
1				23.30±2.07	14.1±3.44		10.70±2.82			11.10±2.32	
				(*P*<0.01)	(*P*<0.01)						
2				16.20±2.80		24.00±2.82	14.60±1.15		12.22±2.36		6.30±0.30
				(*P*<0.01)		(*P*<0.01)					
3			22.0±0.89	27.66±0.42		19.50±3.02	16.00±1.69				
			(*P*<0.01)	(*P*<0.01)		(*P*<0.01)					
4					25.08±1.48		9.45±0.17	9.20±0.23			
					(*P*<0.01)						

3. *Detection of urokinase activity in the urine of mice*

(1) The urine of mice was collected by bladder pressing method in the morning before tumor transplantation (as control sample) and after tumor transplantation (as sample). About 7— 9 samples were collected during the course of survival of the mice at intervals of 2, 3 or 4 days.

(2) The urokinase activity was detected by the fibrin plate method according to Astrupt et al.[9] using 20 μl of fresh urine.

II. Results and Discussion

1. Urokinase activity in the urine of B16F10 melanoma-bearing BDF1 mice during the course of survival: No apparent change of urokinase activity was observed during the latent period, but a sudden rise appeared just before metastasis (the 18th day) as shown in Table 1 and Fig. 1. Then a period of relatively low activity followed. The peak value was 170% of the normal value ($P<0.01$). The experiment was repeated four times.

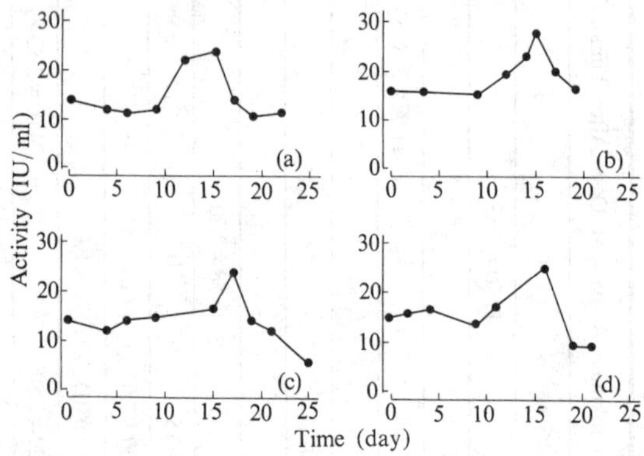

Fig. 1 The changes of urokinase activity in urine of $B_{16}F_{10}$ melanoma-bearing DBF_1 mice.

2. Urokinase activity in the urine of B16F10 melanoma-bearing TA-2 mice during the course of survival: The changes of urokinase activity in the urine of this group were similar to that of B16F10 in BDF1 mice.

The urokinase peak appeared on the 14th – 18th days, as shown in Table 2 and Fig. 2. The peak value was 177% of the normal value ($P<0.01$).

Table 2 The Changes of Urokinase Activity in Urine of $B_{16}F_{10}$ Melanoma-Bearing TA-2 Mice

No. of Mice	Urokinase Activity (iμ/ml urine $\bar{x}\pm$S. D.) at Days After Tumor Transplantation						
	0	4	6	12	15	18	21
10	10.70±2.04	10.70±3.79	13.06±1.11	10.63±2.35	17.50±3.63	19.00±7.63	12.30±4.40
					($P<0.01$)	($P<0.01$)	

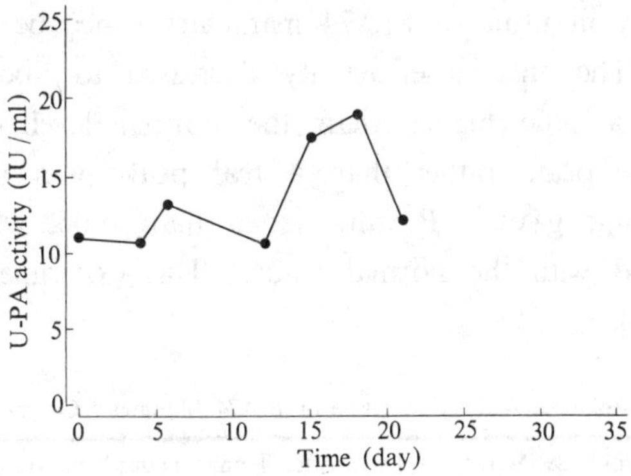

Fig. 2 The changes of urokinase activity in urine of $B_{16}F_{10}$ melanoma-bearing TA-2 mice.

3. Urokinase activity in the urine of L795 lung adenocarcinoma-bearing T739 mice during the course of survival: The urokinase peak appeared in 5— 8 days after tumor transplantation. It is earlier than that of groups I and II. After the peak passed, the urokinase activity reduced to one half of the normal value or less as shown in Table 3 and Fig. 3. The peak value was 238% of the normal value ($P<0.01$).

Table 3 The Changes of Urokinae Activity in Urine of L795 Lung Adenocarcinoma-Bearing T739 Mice

No. of Mice		10		No. of Mice		10	
Urokinase Activity at Days After Tumor Transplantation (iμ/ml, $\overline{X}\pm$S.D.)	0	10.00±1.55		Urokinase Activity at Days After Tumor Transplantation (iμ/ml, $\overline{X}\pm$S.D.)	15	9.63±2.05	
	2	7.00±1.64			18	6.21±1.10	
	4	12.73±2.00			20	5.17±3.48	
	5	23.86±4.30	($P<0.01$)		24	6.67±1.97	
	8	20.88±5.00	($P<0.01$)		30	7.06±3.40	
	12	7.05±2.61			33	3.93±1.00	

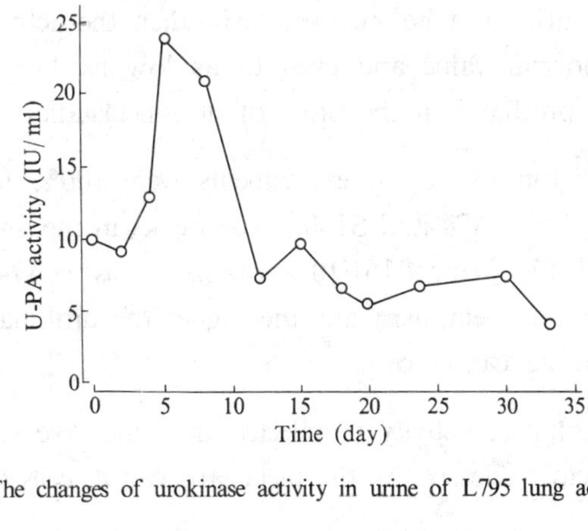

Fig. 3 The changes of urokinase activity in urine of L795 lung adenocarcinoma-bearing T739 mice.

4. Urokinase activity in urine of MA74 mammary cancer-bearing TA-2 mice during the course of survival: The urokinase activity decreased to about 2/3 of the normal level, then increased to a little higher than the normal level. Finally, it decreased again. A false urokinase peak, rather than a real peak, was present since both the lowest and the higher value gave a P value larger than 0.05, which is not statistically significant when compared with the normal value. This experiment was repeated twice. The results are in Table 4.

Table 4 The Changes of Urokinase Activity in Urine of MA74 Mammary Carcinoma-Bearing TA−2 Mice

EXP. No.	No. of Mice	Urokinase Activity at Days After Tumor Transplantation (iμ/ml urine, $\overline{X}\pm$S.D.)								
		0	2	4	6	11	16	20	23	25
1	10	12.20 ±2.40	6.06 ±1.33	12.40 ±5.71	12.42 ±1.99	13.80 ±2.66	16.90 ±6.02 (P>0.05)	7.98 ± 5.72	5.35 ±1.25	7.04 ±3.30
2	10	14.44 ±3.36	9.73 ±2.10	12.20 ±2.12	11.76 ±3.03	15.40 ±1.25	17.67 ±2.08 (P>0.05)	14.72 ±8.09	8.45 ±1.48	11.26 ±3.66

5. Urokinase activity in the urine of S180 sarcoma-bearing C57BL6 mice during the course of survival: The urokinase activity rose slightly during the latent period but it had no statistical significance. It then fell to the normal level or a little lower (see Table 5).

Table 5 The Changes of Urokinase Activity in Urine of S180 Sarcoma-Bearing D57BL/6 Mice

No. of Mice	Urokinase Activity at Days After Tumor Transplantation (iμ/ml urine. $\overline{X}\pm$S.D.)				
	0	5	7	10	20
10	11.90±1.48	17.25±4.31 (P>0.05)	13.81±2.32	11.63±1.25	8.50±1.91

From Tables 1, 2 and 3 and Figs. 1, 2 and 3, it can be seen that a peak in the urokinase activity appears in the urine just before metastasis, then the activity decreases to a level lower than that of the normal value and even to as low as 1/2 of the normal value before death. No peak is produced in the urine of non-metastatic tumor hosts.

The rate of metastasis of the tumors in our experiments were 100% for lung cancer L793>90% for melanoma B16F10>MA74 and S180. The peaks in the urokinase activity were 238% for L793>177% and 170% for B16F10>non-metastasis MA74 and sarcoma 180. So it seems that the higher the metastasis rate, the higher the urokinase peak. This result is similar to that of Yu[6] using cancer cells.

The metastatic increase in urokinase activity is reflected in urine. We suggest that the rise is caused by one or more factors released by the metastatic cancer cells (so called u-PA stimulating factor or USF). It can stimulate the production and release of urokinase in urokinase-producing cells, such as macrophages, granulocytes, epithelial cells of the kidney, tubules and cells of urinary bladder[1]. As Dan[1] reiterated, steroid hormones, polypeptide hormones, CAMP, epidermal growth factor, retinoic acids, phorbol esters and many other factors can influence the urokinase level in cell cultures, intact animals and the human body. The nature of the USF will be further investigated.

A concomitant rise of phagocytic activity in macrophages was observed in this experiment when the urokinase peak rose in B16F10-bearing DBF1 mice.

The B16F10 melanoma cells appeared in the lung tissues of DBF1 mice on the 18th day of transplantation as was confirmed by a lung tissue section which is shown in Fig.4.

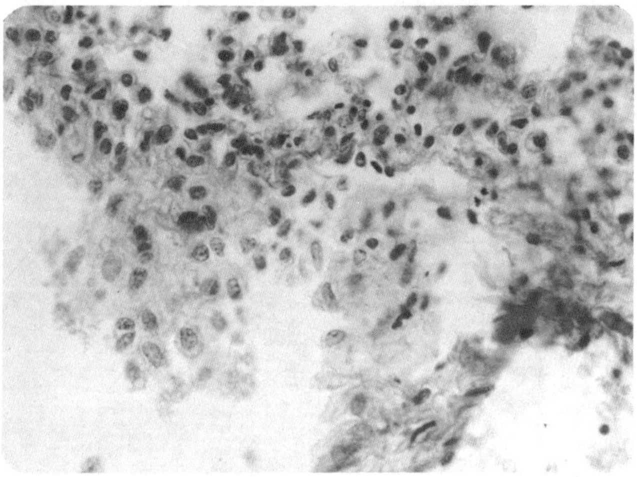

Fig.4 Cancer cells appeared in lung tissues of DBF1 mice 18 days after transplantation. 400X (FIE)

In our experiment the urokinase level in urine was not proportional to the tumor size, especially at the advanced stages of the tumor growth.

Finally, since urokinase is a nonspecific tumor marker, is it possible that it could be an indicator of metastasis and of the prognosis for operation in human cancer patients? This is an interesting problem for further study.

References

1 Dano, K. *et al.*, *Adv. Cancer Res.*, **44**(1985), 139.

2 Goldfarb, R.H. *et al.*, *Thromb. Hemostasis,* **12**(1986), 294.

3 Sappino, A.P. *et al.*, *Cancer Res.* **47**(1987), 4043.

4 Percyra-Alfonso, S. *et al.*, *Int. J. Cancer,* **42**(1988), 59.

5 Duffy, M. J. *et al.*, *Concer* (*Phila*), **62**(1988), 531.

6 Yu, H. *et al.*, *Cancer Res.*, **50**(1990), 7623.
7 Li, X.M., *Chinese Jour. Patho-physiol.*, **2**(1986), 1: 51.
8 Sun, W.Y. *et al.*, *Chinese Tumor Clin.*, **14**(1987), 5: 310.
9 Astrupt, T. *et al.*, *A.B.B.*, **40**(1952), 346.

Supplements

Studies on the Fractal Dimensions for Cancer Growth Paths

ZHAO Huaming and LI Houqiang

(*Department of Chemistry, Sichuan University, Chengdu 610064, China*)

Abstract A brief comment on fractal models of cancer growth so far given in literature has been made. Adopting and combining the merits of the current models, a modified fractal model mainly of diffusion limited aggregate (**DLA**) type for cancer growth has been established and the fractal dimensions have also been assessed by this way.

The growth or the diffusion of cancer cells in a body is a complex process[1, 2]. In general, it is difficult to describe the phenomena by ordinary methods. Since first, the perimeter of the cancer growth is irregular and the unitary pattern is, therefore, not easy to define by classical mathematics. In addition, the growth process of a cancer is influenced by many chaotic factors[3]. To get over the impasse, we have to find a new measure by using the fractal approach to this problem; the cancer growth has, therefore, been studied on the basis of fractal geometry[4]. With this aim in mind, the degree of irregularity or convolution of growth paths is numerically assessed. In particular, we would incline to identify those growth paths that are apparently random and rank among growth paths as the degree of convolution is concerned. We were fortunate to employ the concept of fractals as a logical basis for such a measure, the establishment and development of the fractal conception attributed to Mandelbrot[4].

A fractal is a complex pattern and its natural dimension, or fractal dimension can be used to characterize its shape[4]. Our ultimate goal is to work out a fractal characterization of the irregularity or straightness of cancer growth paths. The measure of a straight growth path should be completely one-dimensional ($D=1$) and that of a random growth path approaches a fractal of two-dimensionality ($D \to 2$). The fractal dimension (D) for the cancer growth paths may be computed by making use of the equation[5]:

$$D=\ln(n) \ / \ \ln(nd/L),$$

where d is the diameter of the growth path (the greatest distance between two points), L is the total length of the growth path, and n is the number of time intervals. For cancer chemistry, one of the premise for the immediate applications of this fractal characterization is the classification of diffusion paths of cancer cells. The movement of a cell is the result of complex processes—it is usually the product of a number of underlying mechanisms and, in addition, stochasticism often plays a significant role. For complicated interplay of the parameters, the patterns described by diffusion paths tend to become both complex and variable. To categorize such variable complex patterns, one needs a natural quantitative measure for the complexity that can be applied to sporadic cases. To compare such patterns, it is of necessity to use standard statistics. Our assessment of the fractal dimension fulfills both of these requirements. Moreover, fractal characterization is generally applicable to curve in a plane, and it may alse prove useful in other non-biological disciplines.

Here, we are concerned with probabilistic growth models which, in turn, can lead to complex structures that mimic certain types of cancer pattern formation. These models display structures in which the fractal dimensionality (D) is distinctly smaller than the Euclidean dimensionality (d) of the space or lattice in which the growth process is in the making[6]. For fractal objects, the D is the exponent which describes how the mass M of the object can be scaled with some characteristic length L which describes the overall size, $M \propto L^D$. This mass-length scaling relationship is the basis for all methods to measure the fractal dimensionality of real objects or objects generated in computer simulation.

One of the earliest examples of probabilistic growth models is the "Eden" (Eden, 1961) model[7] in which each vacant surface site has the same probability of becoming occupied at all stages of growth. A closely related model which includes competing growth and decay process was developed by Williams & Bjerknes (1972)[8] as a model for the growth of skin cancer. They found that for their model the "surface" perimeter size S depended on the total mass or number of occupied sites in the cluster N according to the power law relationship

$$S = N^{0.55}.$$

This result suggests that the surface of cancers may have a fractal geometry. However, more recent work with this model suggests that the surface is simply rough rather than fractal-like.

In recent years a variety of cancer growth models have been studied. To our knowledge, however, none of these leads to structures with well-defined fractal dimensionality. For example, the network formation model of Meinhardt (1982)[9] generates a uniform (non-fractal) network of occupied lattice sites leading to a type of structure which results from a combination of non-linear chemical reaction processes and diffusion. Models of this type may lead to fractal structures under some conditions which, however, have not been found yet.

Recently interest in the non-equilibrium growth processes of cancers has been stimulated by the demonstration by Witten & Sander (1981)[10] that structures with a well-defined fractal geometry are generated by a simple diffusion-limited aggregation (DLA) process in which cancer cells are added one at a time to a growing cancer cluster via random walk trajectories. This model has generated considerable theoretical interest and has led to the development of a number of more or less closely related models that also generate fractal structures. It has also stimulated interest in experimental investigations resulting in a typical two-dimensional Witten-Sander cancer cluster. The growth of cancer systems may be limited by the diffusion of nutrients in the systems or the diffusion of toxic metabolites away from the system. Looking like ordinary DLA model Witten-Sander may provide new insight into the morphology of certain cancer systems.

For computer simulations of cancer nonequilibrium growth processes three mass-length scaling relationships are commonly used to measure the fractal dimensionality. These are $R_8 \propto N^{1/D_\epsilon}$ (1), $M(L) \propto L^{D_r}$ (2) and $C(r) \propto r^{(D_\alpha - d)}$ (3), where R_8 is the radius of gyration and N is the mass (number of cancer cell) of the growing object $M(I)$ is the mass contained within the distance L measured from some occupied site (generally L is measured from the initial growth site or "seed") and $C(r)$ is the two-point density-density correlation function at a distance r. For all real cancer systems and systems generated by finite size simulations these mass-length scaling relationships are applicable only to a finite range of length scales bounded by upper and lower cutoffs. Consequently, the exponents D_α, D_β and D_γ are effective fractal dimensionalities. Such systems also display the property of self-similarity (or statistical self-similarity in the case of a random fractal). In other words, they are scale invariant and look the same under different magnifications. As in the case of the mass-length scaling relationships, this property of self-similarity does not extend over an infinite range of length scales for real cancer systems[11].

The model we are going to discuss below is similar to Eden model in that growth takes place by the random occupation of vacant surface sites. Yet here we assume that the rate of growth (growth probability) depends on the local concentration of some substance which diffuses from a surrounding exterior source and is consumed by the growing system. If the process is diffusion-limited, with the rate of growth directly proportional to the local nutrient concentration, the model becomes very similar to the Witten-Sander model. Under such a case, a structure with a fractal dimensionality of about 1.7 established in $2d$ simulations or in three dimensions a structure with a fractal dimensionality of about 2.5 is obtained. If the growth probability (P) is proportional to some power (ε) of the local concentration (C), $P \propto C^\varepsilon$, then the model becomes equivalent to the dielectric breakdown model which was developed by Niemeyer et al. (1984)[12]. Such being the case the fractal dimensionality generated by the model depends on the exponent ε and may vary from 1.0 to d, the Euclidean dimensionality of the space in which the growth process is embedded.

The simulations of a two-dimensional square lattice were made by Meakin[13]. He started with a single occupied lattice site surrounded by an exterior source of nutrient of low concentration. The nutrient is supplied by the boundary conditions which maintain a fixed concentration ($C=1.0$) of nutrient on a circle of lattice sites surrounding the growing cluster. Initially this circle has a radius of 15 lattice units, but it grows with the cluster so that its radius is always significantly larger than the maximum radius of the cluster R_{max}. In most of simulations the nutrient is supplied at a distance of 2.0 R_{max} or 2.5 R_{max} from the origin of the growth. The early stage of one of the simulations resembles something like the so called Koch island in fractal morphology.

In the most simple version of the model we assume that a nutrient concentration of zero is maintained on the lattice sites occupied by the cluster at all times and that the diffusion process is fast as compared with growth process. Under these conditions, the concentration field will reach a steady state determined by the boundary conditions before each growth event, i. e. $\frac{dc}{dt}=D_d\nabla^2C=0$, where D_d is the diffusion coefficient. In order to approximate the conditions $\nabla^2C=0$ before each growth step, the concentration field is "relaxed" by replacing the concentration on each lattice site by the average of the concentrations on the four nearest neighbor lattice sites. In most simulations, this process is repeated 10 or 20 times before each growth step.

The fractal dimensionalities of the cancer clusters generated using growth exponents ε of respectively 0.5, 1.0 and 2.0 were estimated from both the dependence of the radius of gyration on cluster size (D_β) and from the density-density correlation function (D_α). An effective fractal dimensionality D_α can be obtained using the expression

$$D_\alpha=d+d\ln[C(r)]/d\ln(r),$$

where $C(r)$ is the density-density correlation function at a distance r. This equation is applicable to cases with intermediate length scales where $\ln C(r)$ depends linearly on r. The results for both D^α and D^β are summarized in Table 1.

Table 1 Values of D_α and D_β by DLA Growth Model

Growth Exponent	D_α $(2\leqslant r\leqslant 20)$	D_β $(0.1N_{max}\leqslant N\leqslant N_{max})$	D_β $(0.5N_{max}\leqslant N\leqslant N_{max})$
0.5	1.86	1.92	1.94
1.0	1.71	1.72	1.70
2.0	1.44	1.39	1.36

Note: The effective dimensionality D_α was obtained from the density-density correlation function, and D_β, from the dependence of the radius of gyration on the mass of the growth.

We do not expect that a change in boundary condition will be sufficient to change the fractal dimensionality of structures generated by the diffusion-limited growth model discussed above. However, a change in the boundary conditions from those associated with the model used to generate the results in Table 1 may lead to interesting and potentially important new effects in the same way by which diffusion-limited deposition on fibers and surfaces has led to new quantities which are not found in DLA on single growth sites.

To sum up, the fractal dimensions are good parameters characterizing degrees of irregularity of cancer growth and cancer cell diffusions. The larger fractal dimension is, the more irregular and complex the cancer growth will be. It has been shown that cancer growth is a recurrent process[11], which is associated with the multiplicity of the structure, self-organization and catastrophe theory. The multifractal theory[14] may be used to describe the heterogeneous distribution of cancer in the body. We believe that the unity fractal model of cancer growth will be established in the near future and any research achievements in this regard are helpful to obtain a better understanding of the morphology and mechanisms existing in cancer systems.

References

1 Harris, R. *et al.*, *Nature*, **233**(1971), 556.

2 Schmahl, D. *et al.*, *Cancer Treat Rev.*, **5**(1978), 175; *Int. J. Cancer*, **23**(1979), 706.

3 Li, H. Q. and Cheng, G. Y., *Fractals and Fractal Dimensions*, Sichuan Education Press, 1990.

4 Mandelbrot, B.B., *Fractal Geometry of Nature*, W. H. Freemen Sanfransisco, 1984.

5 Katz, M. J. and Geogre, E. B., *Bull. Math. Bio.*, **47**(1985), 2 : 273.

6 Vicsek, T., *Fractal Growth Phenomena*, Word Scientific, Singapore, 1989.

7 Eden, M., *Proc. Fourth Berkeley Symposium on Mathematics Statistics and Probability* (Ed. Neeyman, J.), 1961. Vol Ⅳ, 223, Berkeley University of California Press.

8 Williams, T. and Bjerknes, R., *Nature*, **236**(1972), 19.

9 Meinhardt, H., *Models of Biological Pattern Formation*, New York, Academic Press, 1982.

10 Witten, T. A. and Sander, L. M., *Phys. Rev. Lett.*, **47**(1981), 1400.

11 Li, H. Q., *J. Biomed. Eng.*, **2**(1988), 82.

12 Niemeyer, L. *et al.*, *Phys. Rev. Lett.*, **52**(1984), 1033.

13 Meakin, P., *Adv. Colloid Interface Sci.*, **28**(1988), 249.

14 Feder, J., *Fractals*, Plenum Press, 1988.

Effect of a Chinese Traditional Prescription "White Tiger Soup" to the Patient With High Fever After Chemotherapy

HAO Qinling
(*Jiaozuo Tumor Institute*)

and ZHANG Jinghua
(*Qinyang City People's Hospital*)

Abstract 6 cancer patients were administered with "Baihutang"(white tiger soup), a traditional Chinese prescription, along with the routine treatment, their high fever symptoms were controlled, but the two among seven control cases died of high fever.

Chemotherapy as one of the three main treatment methods has been playing an important role in treatment of tumors, but it brings the patients serious side effects, such as immunodepression and depressed bone marrow function; its mechanism is that chemotherapeutic agents can kill the immunocytes and reduce their phagocytosis and bactericidal activities[1]. The patients may have infection and high fever after chemotherapy (cxcept cancer fever and medicamentous fever). It is difficult to control the high fever symptoms[2]. It is dangerous to the patients if the high fever cannot be controlled in time. It is reported in the paper that thirteen cases of patients with high fever after chemotherapy were researched and divided into two groups randomly. A satisfactory effect was obtained got in the group receiving "Baihutang" (i.e. "white tiger soup" a direct translation from Chinese, a Chinese traditional medicine prescription).

I. Patients and Methods

Thirteen patients were selected, 9 men, 4 women, aged betwccn 24 and 80 (averaging 40). They were all suffering from high fever after chemotherapy, with an average of 40°C (39.5°C – 41°C). The patients were divided into two groups randomly. Six in research group were administered with " white tiger soup" which consisted of Dangshen 30 g, Astragalus Membranaceous 30 g, Gypsum 30 – 60 g, Anemarrhena 9 g, Lonicera 30 g, dry fruit of Forsythia 15g, dry leaf of Polygonum Tinctori Lour 30 g, dry root of lsatin Tinctori 30 g, polished round-grained Nonglutinous rice 30 g, Glycyrrhiza 6 g, one dose daily, taken in decoction for three days. 7 in control group were treated with conventional treatment, such as an antibiotic antipyretic.

II. Results

After treatment, the high fever in research group was controlled the day after drinking "white tiger soup", while in the control group it could be controlled temporarily with conventional treatment, but they still had high fever after stopping medicine. Two of the seven patients died of high fever.

III. Discussion

Chemotherapeutic agents have a strong depressive effect on the body's immunity, so the patients can easily catch infection after chemotherapy. From the Chinese medical viewpoint, the patients' vital energy becomes weak after chemotherapy; the unhealthy environment can easily affect the patients; the patients can catch feverish diseases which can dehydrate the patient; losing liquid may exhaust the patients' vital energy. Treatment principle: strengthen patients' vital energy, provide liquid, lower temperature[3]. In the prescription of "white tiger soup", Gypsum can lower temperature in combination with Anemarrhena, the Nonglutinous rice and Glycyrrhiza can strengthen vital energy, and the above four Chinese medicines have an antipyretic action. Dangshen and Astragalus Membranuceous can also strengthen vital energy, protect the body from harmful agents and increase the body's immunity. Lonicera, dry leaf of *Polygonum tinctoria* Lour and its root can reduce temperature; they also have antibiotic action[4]. In the control group, antibiotic and anti-pyretic can merely reduce temperatures temporarily. They could not strengthen the patients' resistance, so the patients' high fever in the control group continued.

References

1 Nobuyuki *et al.*, *Cancer.*, **66**(1990), 4: 684.
2 Zhang Zi-yi *et al.*, *Chemotherapy of Malignance*, Shanghai Scientific and Technical Publishing House, 1984, p. 126.
3 Hebel New Medical University, *Chinese Medicine*, Hebei New Medical University, 1974, p. 96.
4 *Dictionary of Chinese Herbal Medicine*, 1972.

The Action of Chemotherapy in the Combined Therapy for Carcinoma of the Nasopharynx

—— A Report of 49 Cases

SHENG Hongzheng

(Department of Otolaryngology, Futian Hospital, Shenzhen 518033, China)

and ZHENG Guangwen

(Otolaryngological Department, First Teaching Hospital of Henan Medical University, Zhengzhou 450002, China)

From Apr., 1986 to Jun., 1989, 49 patients (29 male, 20 female) aged between 20 and 70 who developed carcinoma of the nasopharynx (including 15 with relapses) were treated with neoadjuvant regional chemotherapy, followed by radiotherapy or cryosurgery and radiotherapy.

Thirty-three of the patients had squamous cell carcinoma of poor differentiation, 4 had squamous cell carcinoma of well differentiation, 11 have undifferentiated, and one has cystadeno carcinoma. Tumors were treated in three ways: (1) inductive regional chemotherapy with temporal artery incubation as well as superselective intra-arterial chemotherapy of the femoral artery (chemotherapeutants-P. D. V. M and P. D. M programs); (2) liquid nitrogen cryosurgery in 25 cases; (3) radiotherapy for 2 weeks after cryosurgery or immediately applied to those without cryosurgery after chemotherapy.

The data showed that C R and P R were 40 cases (81.6%) and M R were 9cases (10.3%) in regional chemotherapy. All of the patients were followed up more than one year, and 48 of them survived(97.9%). 35 cases were followed up over 2 years and 28 of them survived (80.0%). 20 cases were followed up over 3 years, and 12 of them survived (60.0%).

Treatment by of regional chemotherapy and cryosurgery in combination for carcinoma of nasopharynx were discussed in this paper.

I. Introduction

Carcinoma of nasopharynx is a common malignant tumor in China and southeast Asia. Traditionally, radiotherapy was the chief treatment, and it has cured many patients. Attached Tumor Hospital of Zhongshan Univ. reported in 1974 that the survival rate of patients with cancer of various stages reached 46.3—49.5% after 5 years' radiotherapy. But the 5-year survival rate should still be investigated. From Apr., 1986 to Jun., 1989, 49 cases of carcinoma of nasopharynx (including 15 patients with relapses) were tr ated with neoadjuvant regional chemotherapy, followed by radiotherapy cryotherapy and radiotherapy. 45 cases of them were at the third or fourth stage of cancer (91.8% of the total number). Of the 20 followed up for more than three years, 12 survived (the 3-year survival rate was 60.0%). There is hope for the combination treatment to raise it, although the 5-year survival rate remains to be observed further.

II. Materials and Methods

1. *Sex and age*

The 49 patients (29 male, 20 female) were aged between 20 and 70 (Table 1) and more than half of them were aged 41 – 60 (55.1%).

Table 1 Distribution of Carcinoma of Nasopharynx by Age

Age	Number
<30	5
31 – 40	10
41 – 50	13
51 – 60	14
>60	7

2. *Pathology*

Pathological findings with regard to the carcinoma of nasopharynx appear in Table 2.

3. *Symptoms and signs*

(1) The metastasis to lymph nodes in the neck. 34 cases were seen to have metastasis in lymph nodes in the neck in this group (69.3%), among whom 18 cases were bilateral, and the majority were superior group of lymphatic nodi of cervicales profundi, with only 5 cases of lympha nodes around accessory nerve who had relapses after radiotherapy.

(2) Symptoms of the ears and noses. The most common symptoms of nasopharyngeal carcinoma was mild nasal or postnasal bleeding (16 cases), and 12 cases showed severe otitis media.

(3) Symptoms of the cranial nerves. 18 patients had severe headaches and invasions of cranial nerves, and the fifth and sixth cranial nerves of 12 cases were invaded. The base of the skull bone was obviously destroyed in 4 cases, the seventh and

eighth cranial nerves were damaged in 2 cases and the hoarseness and palsy of the twelfth nerve occurred from the ninth, the tenth and the twelfth cranial nerves invaded by lymphonodi cervicales profundae.

(4) Distant metastases. Two cases were found to have distant metastases. X-ray film showed that one of the patients had metastases in the lung and another to the liver.

Table 2 Distribution of Carcinoma of the Nasopharynx by Pathology

Pathological Findings	Number
Pathological types	
Squamous cell carcinoma with poor differentiation	33
Squamous cell carcinoma with well differentiation	4
Undifferentiated carcinoma	11
Cystadeno carcinoma	1
Originated site of neoplasms	
Lateral wall (including Rosenmuller fossa)	31
Postero-superior wall	14
Anterior wall	4
Appearance of neoplasm	
Nodules form	20
Cauliflower form	12
Infiltrative growth	16
Infiltration of the submucosa	1
Direction of expansion	
Cranial nerves form	15
Cervical metastases of lymph nodes	21
Mixed form	13
Staging	
T_1	0
T_2	2
T_3	19
T_4	26

4. *Regional chemotherapy*

(1) Artery intubation and point for attention A. The temporal artery was first selected, and a facial artery was selected in cases where the temporal artery was obstructed. The depth of intubation was about 10 – 11cm so that it was beyond the opening of arteriae pharyngea ascendens; B. intra-arterial chemotherapy were given to each patient 15 times, and 7 or 8 times of bilaterial intubations were needed if the patient had bilaterial metastases of cervicales lymphonodi or wideranging damage of the nasopharynx; C. supenselective intra-arterial chemotherapy of femoral artery — the intubations lead directly to arteriae pharyngea ascendens and maxillaris internal after angiography, and 3 cases had femoral artery intubations in the group.

(2) The drugs of chemotherapy. Programmes applied are as follows.

A. P D V M therapy— First, cell cycle non-specific agents, such as P M (20 mg/m^2 each time, D D P (30—50 mg/m^2 each time) were administered (to a total dose of 100 mg and 150 mg); second, cell cycle specific agents such as V C R (2 mg each time), H D-MTX (500—1000 mg each time) were given, and two hours later C F was intramuscularly injected for three days for detoxication at a dose of 12 mg of over 6 h. 11 cases in this group were treated in this way.

B. P D At therapy— this therapy was applied in 10 cases at an earlier stage in this group, P M (20 mg/m^2 each time), D D P (30—50 mg/m^2 each time) and At-1258 (40—60 mg/m^2 each time) were administered twice a week for a total of 15 times.

C. P D M therapy— This therapy was essential when C F was deficient, P M (20 mg/m^2 each time), D D P(30—50 mg/m^2 each time) and M T X (30 mg/m^2 each time) were given to 25 cases in this group twice a week to a total of 15 times.

D. P D Adm therapy— This therapy was used with superselective femoral artery intubation. The drugs were given once at a dose of P M 30 mg, D D P100 mg and Adm 60 mg, 60 min after starting a 2 h i.v. hydration program with 2000 ml of fluid. Sodium hyposulfite 12 g, Maxolon 40 mg and Benadryl 150 mg were once given i. v. for detoxication. 3 cases were treated this way in this group.

5. *Liquid nitrogen cryosurgery*

(1) The patients who valunteered for cryosurgery were givenliquid nitrogen cryosurgery of the nasopharynx under endotracheal anesthesia in the trendelenhurg's position.

(2) Two catheters were separately inserted into the nares taken out from the soft palate and bound tightly with the soft palata so as to lift it up and expose the nasopharynx before cryosurgery.

(3) The head of the cryosurgical apparatus was inserted from the oropharynx to the nasopharynx and its direction was adjusted acoording to the preoperative examination, so that it could touch the cancerous focus as close as possible.

(4) The spraying or touching cryosurgery to the cancerous focus was carried out 3 or 4 times 3—5 min each time. The frozen and thawed area was so large that the whole cancerous focus was involved. The direction of the head of the cryosurgical apparatus was adjusted for separate cryosurgery if the cancerous focus was large.

(5) In order to avoid frostbite of the soft palate or the respiratory tract, the hypopharynx cavity was obstructed with dry gauze and the head of the cryosurgical apparatus was wrapped in oil-gauze. Twenty-five patients in this group received

cryosurgery.

6. *Radiotherapy*

(1) The radiotherapy was normally applied half month after cryotherapy but the patients who had not had cryosurgery were directly treated with radiotherapy after regional chemotherapy.

(2) The source of irradiation was Cobalt-60, and the field of irradiation was routinely designed. 60—70 GY was given to primary focus and 40—50 GY to metastasis focus of cervical lymphonodus.

III. Results

Among all the cases with carcinoma of the nasopharynx, 25 were treated with regional alchemotherapy and radiotherapy (i. e. two-combination), and 25 with regional chemotherapy, cryotherapy and radiotherapy (i. e. three-combination). The results are as follows.

1. *The curative effect of regional chemotherapy*

(1) The standard of effectiveness. The curative effect was divided into three levels according to the proposal put forward by the Research Association of Head and Neck Surgery. A. Obvious effects: complete of less than 2/3 and more than half of the tumor have been reduced by treatment; B. Minor response: The tumor removed by treatment was less than 1/2, but more than 30%; C. Non response: The tumor reduction was less than 30% or indefinite.

(2) The results (see Table 3). It was effective that all of the patients with this therapy (including 15 cases with relapse).

The obvious response was 81.6%(40/49), much higher than that of the treatment for cancers of the nasal cavity and sinuses in our department (14/35)[2].

Table 3 Treatment and Effectiveness

Treatment	No. of Cases	CR + PR	MR	NR
P D V M	11	10	1	0
P D M	25	21	4	0
P D A t	10	7	3	0
P D Adm	3	2	1	0
Total	49	40 (81.6%)	9 (18.3)	

2. *Follow-up*

All the patients were followed up for 1—4 years, and the results are given in Table 4.

Table 4 Results of Follow-up

Time	Patients	Survivals	Survival Rate (%)
Over 1 year	49	48	97.9
Over 2 years	35	28	80.0
Over 3 years	20	12	60.0

Table 4 shows that death occurred mostly within two years.

One patient died of destruction of the base of the skull bone and massive haemorrhage one year after this treatment. Of the 35, followed up for 2 years, 6 died, of whom 4 died of relapse after radiotherapy, one died of obvious destruction of the base of the skull bone and another was a 70-year old patient. Of the 20 followed up for more than 3 years, 12 survived but 8 died, and one died after 1 year of treatment; 5 died after 2 years and 2 died after 3 years. Local relapse was responsible for the death.

IV. Discussion

1. *The action of regional chemotherapy in the combinative treatment for carcinoma of the nasopharynx*

(1) Regional chemotherapy had obvious recent-term effects. The obvious response was seen in 81.6% in this group. The faith of the patients in the treatment was greatly increased when the tumour disappeared or was obviously reduced in 2 weeks after treatment. It has been reported that regional chemotherapy is applicable to some cranial nerves, but our study shows that it is satisfactory in all types. Regional chemotherapy is likely to come into play although the carcinoma of nasopharynx is quite infiltrative. It was possible that clinical metastasis is decreased; therefore the survival period was prolonged because regional chemotherapy can reduce clinical focus as well as any metastatic focus.

(2) The action of radiotherapy can be sensitized by regional chemotherapy. As a preparation before radiotherapy, the cells deficient in oxygen can be oxygenated and sensitized by regional chemotherapy, so better efficacy can be gained. 15 with relapse (30.6% of the total number) are also benefited from regional chemotherapy in this group. It has been evidently confirmed that regional chemotherapy is an important way to treat carcinoma of nasopharynx. Radiotherapy would be all the more effective because it can be sensitized by regional chemotherapy.

(3) Regional chemotherapy can help radiotherapy to function smoothly. Many patients with carcinoma of nasopharynx have such large cervical tumors that, without chemotherapy, the radiotherapeutic area has to be enlarged, which brings about not only stronger reaction to radiotherapy but also poor effects. In this group there was one

patient with undifferentiated carcinoma of the nasopharynx, whose tumor of bilateral cervicalmetastases of lymph nodes looked like a"cow's neck" with two extensive ulcerations. Radiotherapy in other hospital did not produce any effect on him. But after two applications of superselective intra-arterial chemotherapy of the femoral artery, his cervical tumor disappeared and the ulcerations were cured, then radiotherapy was successful applied and good efficacy was achieved. This suggests that chemotherapy can, on the one hand, made radiotherapy easy to carry out in those who are not suitable for radiotherapy at first, and, on the other hand, reduce the dosage and reaction of radiotherapy.

(4) Regional chemotherapy should be applied before radiotherapy Untreated patients have a better blood supply to local tumors. That is quite benefical to the absorption and distribution of anticancer drugs. As a result, local concentrations of medicine, compared with general chemotherapy, are greatly increased and the general toxic reaction is reduced. The obvious effects in this group were 81.6%, which is much higher than that of general chemotherapy. The good results seem relative to the fact that most of the patients were untreated before. In fact, whether regional chemotherapy can prolong the survival time of those with cancer of head and neck at a late stage is still in dispute, but there is in sufficient evidence against chemotherapy for carcinoma of the nasopharynx. In cases where regional chemotherapy was used, good results and an increase in the survival rate of later carcinoma of nasopharynx are possible.

2. *The action of cryosurgery in combinative treatment for carcinoma of the nasopharynx*[3,4]

(1) Cryosurgery can increase the effectiveness of radiotherapy. The healing period of cryosurgery usually lasts 3 weeks. If radiotherapy is carried out 2 weeks after the operation before the recrudescence of the remnant tumor, the curative effect will be reinforced and the possibility of recrudescence greatly decreased. At the same time, the dosage of radiotherapy can be reduced so as to lessen the reaction to radiotherapy.

(2) The immune response brought about by cryosurgery can help the prevention of the recrudescence and distant metastasis of the tumor.

References

1 Guan Zhong-Zheng, *Recent advances in cancer chemotherapy*, lst ed., Jinan, Shandong Scientific & Technical Publishers, 1987, pp. 320—325.

2 Sheng Hong-zheng, Neoadjuvancet regional chemotherapy for head and nech cancer—a report of 80 cases, *Chinese Journal of Cancer*, **8**(1989), 6: 431.

3 Ablin, R. J., *Handbook of Cryosurgery*, lst ed., New Your and basd Marcel Dekker, INC. 1980, pp. 3—12; 69—79.

4 Sheng Hong-zheng, in *Chinese Association of Refrigeration etc. Advances in Cryosurgery*, lst ed., Oxford, New York, Beijing etc. International Academic Publishers, 1989, pp. 562— 566.

On Essentials of Acupuncture Channel

JIN Chengzhe

(*Yanbian Agriculture Insitute, Yanji 133400, China*)

The acupuncture is an important and special measure to cure diseases in the traditional Chinese medicine. Two thousand years ago, the acupuncture was described in the earliest Chinese medicinal book "Nei Jing" (Scripture of Internal Medicine). It has been reported in ancient classic medicine books, that there are over 300 yuxues (acupuncture points) on a human body, and through the acqupuncture to these yuxues some diseases can be cured. The acupuncture points discovered by more recent doctors are named strange xues.

It is well known that the acupuncture effect can be transferred remotely from the point to the focus of the disease, so it is considered that there must have the acupuncture channels called jingluo in Chinese language in the traditional Chinese medicine. This paper reviews the proposed theories of the essentials of the acupuncture channel, considering that the acupuncture channel might be constituted from some sorts of protein with α-helix or β-structure. The quantum chemical calculation of protein molecule will be reviewed in this paper, too.

Discussion from Dai Qianhuan

Based upon the reports from the doctors of the traditional Chinese medicine, it seems that the acupuncture can play a certain limited role on the provention of the patients from a certain cancer disease, which might be related to the strenthening of the immunity system excited by the acupuncture. According to a recent interesting report, it is said that if a solid malignant tumor appears in an internal organ, an anomalous temperature increase will be observed at the related acupuncture point exposed on the surface of the skin. It might not only be an evidence of the effect of the acupuncture channel, but also become a diagnose method of the cancer in an early phase through a physical marker other than the well investigated chemical markers.

The one hundred most important acupuncture points can be divided into two sorts. Some points are neighbouring with the focus of the illed organ or position, while the most of them are in a remote distance to the focus. Almost all the acupuncture points of the latter case are distributed over the four limbs with the most musclar muscle or around the central axis of the body. It is a pity that there is still a gap between the modern molecular biology and the traditional acupuncture theories. It would be possible that the mysterious acupuncture channel, evidenced certainly by the practice in the traditional Chinese medicine, might be just an ordered network formed through a more dense fibrous muscle cell line, the recognition of the fine structure of the myofibril can be traced back to the 1950s in Huxley's works, and the pulse of the acupuncture might be transferred by the myosins, a protein with α-helix form in a remarkably long slender structure, through the known myosin-ATP-actin interaction along the network formed from the bound muscle cell lines. Based upon the modern knowledge on muscle cell, the different positions on ears representing different internal organs asserted in the traditional ear acupuncture medicine might be a possible fact through a certain network of the muscle cell lines.

A Regression Analysis of Influence of Atmospheric Pollution on Cancer Incidence

HAN Zhinong, BAI Yunfeng

(Jilin Institute of Chemical Technology, Jilin, China)

and HUANG Zhuhan

(JCIC Worker Hospital, Jilin, China)

Jilin, the second biggest city of Jilin Province, has a population of 5 million. The population in every one of the six districts of the city is over 600 thousands. The quantitative indices of the main atmospheric pollutions in annual average, i. e. the concentrations of CO_2, CO, NO_x, SO_2, CH_x (total hydrocarbons) and the amount of total suspended particulate (TSP), have been recorded by the environmental monitoring stations in every district, and the total incidences of the cancer disease have been recorded by the epidemic prevention stations in every district. Through the statistic method of multiple regression, the concentration of SO_2 and the amount of TSP show a remarkable positive correlation with the total incidence of cancer disease.

Discussion from Dai Qianhuan

In China, the comprehensive treatment, by combining the epidemiological materials and the data of environmental chemical analysis, might be of special significance for the epidemiology of cancer disease. The large population of this country, even a small town with a population of 100 thousand, would provide a more convinced conclusion based upon the statistics.

The pollutions caused by SO_2 and TSP might imply the major contribution of the coal combustion, the main energy resource in this country, to the higher cancer incidence. Therefore, the TSP is directly correlative with the pollution of carcinogenic polycyclic aromatic hydrocarbons (PAH), both the amount of TSP and the concentration of SO_2 would run parallel to the quantity of coal combustion, which exhausts much more PAH to air environment than other combustion sources. However, the regression analysis by using the data of different cities might give a more reliable result than the analysis within a single city, because the transference of the pollutant would disturb the investigation in a certain degree.

